A Textbook of Clinical
Embryology

A Textbook of Clinical Embryology

Eliezer Girsh
Barzilai Medical Center, Ashkelon

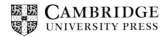

CAMBRIDGE
UNIVERSITY PRESS

CAMBRIDGE
UNIVERSITY PRESS

University Printing House, Cambridge CB2 8BS, United Kingdom

One Liberty Plaza, 20th Floor, New York, NY 10006, USA

477 Williamstown Road, Port Melbourne, VIC 3207, Australia

314–321, 3rd Floor, Plot 3, Splendor Forum, Jasola District Centre, New Delhi – 110025, India

79 Anson Road, #06–04/06, Singapore 079906

Cambridge University Press is part of the University of Cambridge.

It furthers the University's mission by disseminating knowledge in the pursuit of education, learning, and research at the highest international levels of excellence.

www.cambridge.org
Information on this title: www.cambridge.org/9781108744386
DOI: 10.1017/9781108881760

© Cambridge University Press 2021

First published 2021

Printed in Singapore by Markono Print Media Pte Ltd

A catalogue record for this publication is available from the British Library.

ISBN 978-1-108-74438-6 Paperback

Contents

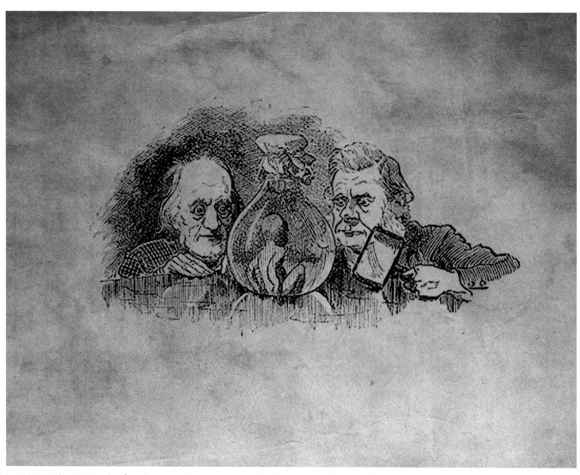

In 1674, Nicolaas Hartsoeker found sperm cells in the seminal fluid under magnification. Observing human sperm through a microscope, Hartsoeker believed that he saw tiny men inside the sperm, which he called Homunculus. The theory of Homunculus (1694) claimed that a tiny, formed child exists in the head of a sperm cell, which becomes engulfed in the uterus, where it grows as in an incubator. The same idea underlies the base of IVF, i.e. to grow a child in a laboratory flask instead of in the mother's womb.

Chapter Co-authors

Irina Ayzikovich
Assistant Professor, Department of Obstetrics and
Gynecology, Novosibirsk State Medical University,
Novosibirsk, Russia

Mira Malcov
Director of PGT Lab at IVF Unit and Genetic
Institute, Tel Aviv Sourasky Medical Center, affiliated
to Tel Aviv University, Tel Aviv, Israel

Raoul Orvieto
Professor of Obstetrics and Gynecology, Sackler
Faculty of Medicine, Tel Aviv University, Tel Aviv,
Israel; Director of Infertility and IVF Unit,
Department of Obstetrics and Gynecology, Sheba
Medical Center, Ramat Gan, Israel

Acknowledgments

I want to express my deep gratitude to the co-authors of my textbook for their participation and help in writing some chapters:

Professor Raoul Orvieto (M.D.) for contribution in Chapter 6 and Chapter 7.

Dr. Irina Ayzikovich (M.D.) for contribution in Chapter 11.

Dr. Mira Malcov (Ph.D.) for contribution in Chapter 17.

Mrs. Polina Ryabko for preparation of illustrations.

Dr. Yorgos Nikas (M.D.), Athens Innovative Microscopy, Greece, for his kind and generous provision of original electron-scans in Chapter 5.

I gratefully acknowledge the following individuals who have provided me with helpful suggestions to this text:

Dr. N. Koudinova (M.D., Ph.D.) – The Weizmann Institute of Science, Rehovot, Israel.

Dr. G. Liberty (M.D.) – The Barzilai Medical Center, Ashkelon, Israel.

Dr. J. Rabinson (M.D.) – The Barzilai Medical Center, Ashkelon, Israel.

Dr. A. Harlev (M.D.) – The Barzilai Medical Center, Ashkelon, Israel.

Physiology of Reproduction

Introduction

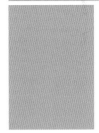

Evidence of infertility complications dates back to biblical times, when the foremother, Sarah, failed to conceive. Many centuries later, in 1667 the Danish scientist Anton van Leeuwenhoek, a glazier by profession, serendipitously invented a magnifying glass and in 1674 Nicolaas Hartsoeker, a Dutch scientist, assisted by Leeuwenhoek, found sperm cells in the seminal fluid under magnification (Figure 0.1). Observing human sperm through a microscope, Hartsoeker believed that he saw tiny men inside the sperm, which he called Homunculus. The theory of Homunculus (1694) claimed that a tiny, formed child exists in the head of the sperm cell, which becomes engulfed in the uterus, where it grows as if in an incubator until the moment of birth (Figure 0.2). It

was then that the idea of in vitro fertilization (IVF) was born, i.e., to grow a child in a laboratory flask instead of in the mother's womb. The understanding that the embryo is formed by fertilization of the oocyte by the sperm cell came only later. Almost 100 years had passed when an Italian Catholic priest and scientist, Lazzaro Spallanzani, investigated functions of sperm cells. Spallanzani created perhaps the first frog contraception, crafting little taffeta pants for his male subjects to test whether semen was essential for fertilization of ova. He was also the first to artificially inseminate a dog, again demonstrating that semen is critical for reproduction.

One of the first pioneers of IVF was Gregory Pincus, a Harvard scientist who, in 1934, experimented

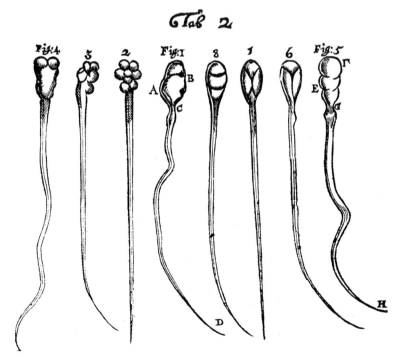

Figure 0.1 Animal sperm cells in the seminal fluid under magnification (Nicolaas Hartsoeker, 1674).

1

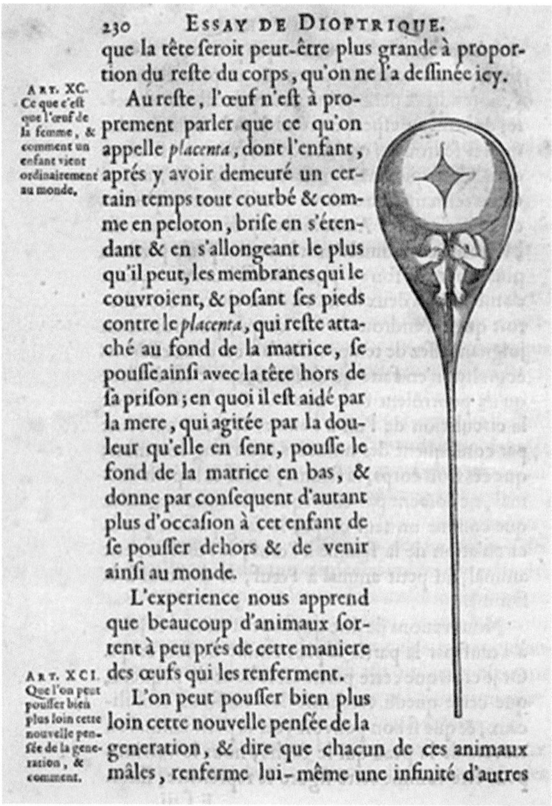

230 ESSAY DE DIOPTRIQUE.

que la tête feroit peut-être plus grande à proportion du refte du corps, qu'on ne l'a deffinée icy.

ART. XC. Ce que c'eft que l'œuf de la femme, & comment un enfant vient ordinairement au monde.

Au refte, l'œuf n'eft à proprement parler que ce qu'on appelle *placenta*, dont l'enfant, aprés y avoir demeuré un certain temps tout courbé & comme en peloton, brife en s'étendant & en s'allongeant le plus qu'il peut, les membranes qui le couvroient, & pofant fes pieds contre le *placenta*, qui refte attaché au fond de la matrice, fe pouffe ainfi avec la tête hors de fa prifon; en quoi il eft aidé par la mere, qui agitée par la douleur qu'elle en fent, pouffe le fond de la matrice en bas, & donne par confequent d'autant plus d'occafion à cet enfant de fe pouffer dehors & de venir ainfi au monde.

L'experience nous apprend que beaucoup d'animaux fortent à peu prés de cette maniere des œufs qui les renferment.

ART. XCI. Que l'on peut pouffer bien plus loin cette nouvelle penfée de la generation, & comment.

L'on peut pouffer bien plus loin cette nouvelle penfée de la generation, & dire que chacun de ces animaux mâles, renferme lui-même une infinité d'autres

Figure 0.2 The theory of Homunculus claimed that a tiny, formed child exists in the head of sperm cell (Nicolaas Hartsoeker, 1694).

with artificial insemination of rabbits and openly stated that this technique is applicable to humans, which led to his expulsion from the university and suspension of his scientific work. In 1937, John Rock hired Miriam Menkin, Pincus' former technician, as a research assistant and, in 1944, they succeeded in artificially fertilizing ova. This marked the first successful IVF of a human oocyte. In 1969, Robert Edwards and Patrick Steptoe published the results of their successful IVF experiments in the journal *Nature.* They succeeded in fertilizing an oocyte and accepting of early embryo, but they had not yet attempted implantation of the embryo back into a woman. After their 103 unsuccessful trials to get a normal pregnancy, Louise Joy Brown, the world's first "test tube baby" was born in Oldham (UK) on July 25, 1978. This date was adopted as the date of birth of IVF and the date of emergence of clinical embryology, an entirely new profession in medicine.

Embryology is a story of biological marvels, describing the means by which a new human life begins and the steps by which a single microscopic cell is transformed into a complex human being.

The objective of this book is to provide an introduction to "everything that a clinical embryologist should know," and is intended mainly for students and trainees.

Development of Reproductive Systems at the Embryo Stage

The Fetal Gonads

The female and male reproductive tracts originate from the same embryonic/fetal tissue. The gonads and internal and external genitalia begin as bipotential tissues. The indifferent gonad consists of a medulla and cortex. Human female and male embryos develop in the same way for the first 6 weeks, regardless of genetic sex (46,XX or 46,XY karyotype) (Figure 1.1). The one way to tell the difference between 46,XX and 46,XY embryos during this time period is by looking for a Barr body ("inactive" one X chromosome) or a Y chromosome. The medulla of the XY embryo will develop into the testes and the cortex will regress. In the XX embryo, the ovary will originate from the cortex and the medulla will decline. A complete 46,XX chromosomal complement is necessary for normal ovarian development. The second X chromosome contains elements essential for ovarian development.

The Fetal Ovary

The development of the human ovary during fetal life can be divided into five stages:

1. Indifferent gonad stage
2. Stage of differentiation
3. Period of oogonia formation (mitosis and migration)
4. Period of oocyte formation (meiosis and differentiation)
5. Stage of follicle formation (follicle assembly)

The gonads begin with development from the mesothelial layer of the peritoneum. The ovary differentiates into a central part – the medulla, which is covered by a surface layer, called the germinal epithelium. At approximately 4–5 weeks of gestation, the paired gonads structurally form the gonadal ridges [1]. The immature ova originate from 50 to 80 germ cells of the dorsal endoderm of the yolk sac (Figure 1.2). These progenital or primordial germ cells (PGCs) mul-

tiply by mitosis, to yield approximately 30 000 at migration. By the time they reach the gonadal ridge (between 5 and 6 weeks of gestation), they are called oogonia (diploid stem cells of the ovary with underdeveloped endoplasmic reticulum and differentiated nucleus) [2–3]. The factors that initiate and direct the migration of the germ cells are not known. Migrating PGCs still express core pluripotency genes such as *SOX2*, *OCT4*, and *NANOG* that are characteristic for early embryonic stem cells [4]. After migration, PGCs begin to express *Mvh* [5], which marks the end of their migration and the beginning of sexual dimorphic development in the undifferentiated gonadal ridge and thus their development into primary oogonia. *DAX1* is a gene typically expressed in both testicular and ovarian tissues (a short arm of the X chromosome). *DAX1* downregulates the effectiveness of the male sex reversal Y gene (*SRY*) or its downstream elements, resulting in an ovary.

At approximately week 6–7 of development, in the absence of anti-Müllerian hormone (AMH) (from Sertoli cells), the Müllerian ducts develop into the female internal genitalia. The development of female internal and external structures is gonad independent.

The source of the gonadal somatic cells is still uncertain. Besides germ cells, the earliest recognizable gonad contains somatic cells derived from at least three different tissues: coelomic epithelium, mesenchyme, and mesonephric tissue. Ultrastructural studies have even suggested that both the coelomic epithelial and underlying mesonephric cells offer the somatic cells that are intended to become follicular cells. The germ cells are first identifiable at the end of the third week after fertilization and can be found in the primitive endoderm at the caudal end in the dorsal wall of the adjacent yolk sac. At 6–8 weeks, the first signs of ovarian differentiation are reflected by the rapid mitotic multiplication of germ cells, reaching 6–7 million oogonia by weeks 16–20 (Figure 1.3). Oogonia go into prophase of the first

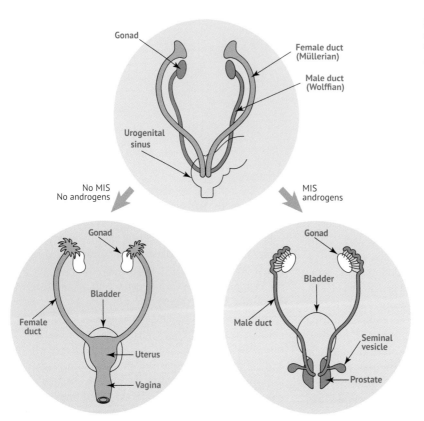

Figure 1.1 Human male and female embryos develop similarly for the first 6 weeks, regardless of genetic sex. MIS, Müllerian-inhibiting substance.

meiotic division and form clusters (oogonia surrounded by a single layer of flattened follicular cells) called primordial follicles.

Around gestation week 10, the primary oocytes, which are arrested at the diplotene stage in prophase of the first meiotic division, cluster together in germ cell nests, in a structure known as ovarian cords, which can be found either in the developing ovary medulla or in the cortex. Around gestation week 20, the germ cell nests of the medulla of the ovary break down. While the exact mechanisms involved in germ cell nest breakdown are unknown, it is associated with a wave of oocyte apoptosis, ultimately resulting in the establishment of primordial follicles. Oogonia become fully surrounded by a layer of coelomic epithelial cells (pregranulosa cells, derived from both the peritoneum and mesonephros), and form the rudiments of the ovarian follicles. Interstitial theca cells originate from two sources: coelomic epithelium and mesonephros.

A pituitary follicle-stimulating hormone peak can be observed at 20–23 weeks, and circulating levels peak at 28 weeks. The ovary begins to express gonadotropin receptors in the second half of pregnancy. The loss of oocytes during fetal life cannot be solely explained by the decline in gonadotropins. During meiosis progression and follicle formation, approximately 70% of germ cells are eliminated [6]. The reason underlying constitutive germ cell death remains poorly understood, but has been suggested to ensure the elimination of germ cells exhibiting defective nuclear or mitochondrial genomes. The constitutive elimination of germ cells during ovarian differentiation may, thus, be a critical process, which could, intriguingly, favor reproductive success. Tight control of the balance between germ cell survival and death is, however, critical in preventing excessive germ cell death leading to premature ovarian failure.

The Fetal Testicle

Human embryos, as mentioned, develop similarly for the first 6 weeks, regardless of genetic sex. The testes-determining factor, a product of a single gene located

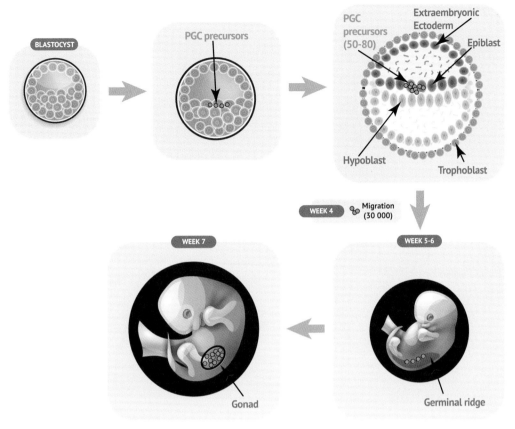

Figure 1.2 Human embryonic primordial germ cell (PGC) migration.

on the Y chromosome, within a region of *SRY*, is the factor that determines whether the indifferent gonad will become a testis. This gene is expressed in the Sertoli cells [7] and its expression results in a cascade of events leading to the development of the seminiferous tubules. As the seminiferous tubules form, the PGCs enter the gonad and associate with the tubules. Through the rete testis, the seminiferous tubules become connected with outgrowths from the mesonephros, which form the efferent ducts of the testis. In contrast to the female, male PGCs do not start meiotic division and do not differentiate to spermatozoa before puberty.

At approximately the seventh week of development, the embryo Sertoli cells (following up *SRY* expression) secrete AMH, also named Müllerian-inhibiting substance, to suppress the development of the Müllerian ducts, leading to their degeneration and stimulating the differentiation of Leydig cells (secreting testosterone a week later, at week 8) from

mesenchymal cells. The prostate, seminal vesicles, and bulbourethral glands develop at 10–13 weeks. Although AMH suppresses the development of the Müllerian ducts, mutations in the AMH receptor gene results in the presence of the uterus, Fallopian tubes, and the upper vagina in 46,XY men with normal external virilization.

Androgen secretion increases in conjunction with increasing Leydig cell numbers and Leydig cell hypertrophy, elicited by human chorionic gonadotropin, until a peak is reached at 15–18 weeks of embryo development. At this time, Leydig cell regression begins, and, at birth, only a few Leydig cells are present.

In the presence of testosterone, secreted by the Leydig cells, and functional androgen receptors, encoded by a gene located on the long proximal arm of the X chromosome (locus Xq11-Xq12), the Wolffian ducts develop into the epididymides, vasa deferentia, and seminal vesicles [8]. In the process of masculine

5

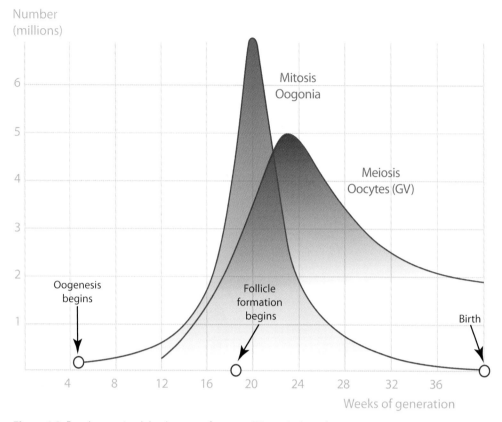

Figure 1.3 Female gestational development of oocytes. GV, germinal vesicle.

differentiation, the development of these Wolffian duct structures is dependent on testosterone as the intracellular mediator, whereas development of the urogenital sinus (scrotum) and urogenital tubercle (penis) into the male external genitalia, urethra, and prostate requires the conversion of testosterone to dihydrotestosterone (DHT). In this manner, the development of the internal and external genitalia in the male is dependent on both testicular testosterone and DHT.

Although the initial testosterone production and sexual differentiation are in response to the fetal levels of adrenocorticotropic hormone (ACTH) and human chorionic gonadotropin (hCG), further testosterone production and masculine differentiation are maintained by the fetal pituitary gonadotropins. If the testes fail to secrete testosterone, or the androgen receptors do not function properly, the Wolffian ducts degenerate.

Rare cases of phenotypic, infertile males with a 46,XX karyotype have been reported; the male differentiation is due to a translocation (meiotic recombination) of a Y chromosome fragment containing *SRY* to an autosome or an X chromosome in 75% to 90% of sporadic cases. In XY gonads, *SRY* induces autosomal *Sox9*, a gene closely related to *SRY* structurally, and involved in testes differentiation, and tips differentiation toward testis development. Duplication of SOX9 transcription factor may be responsible for some familial cases of XX sex reversal. In XX gonads lacking *SRY*, *DAX1* represses *Sox9* and promotes ovary development. Most male genes (*Dhh*, *Sox9*, *Cbln1*) are activated in XY gonads. Many female genes (*Irx3*, *Wnt4*, *Msx1*) are repressed in XY gonads.

References

1. Eddy EM, Clark JM, Gong D, Fenderson BA. Origin and migration of primordial germ cells in mammals. *Gamete Res.* 1981; 4:333–362.

2. Konishi I, Fujii S, Okamura H, Parmley T, Mori T. Development of interstitial cells and ovigerous cords in the human fetal ovary: an ultrastructural study. *J. Anat.* 1986; 148:121–135.

3. Francavilla S, Cordeschi G, Properzi G, et al. Ultrastructure of fetal human gonad before sexual

differentiation and during early testicular and ovarian development. *J. Submicrosc. Cytol. Pathol.* 1990; **22**:389–400.

4. Ulloa-Montoya F, Kidder BL, Pauwelyn KA, et al. Comparative transcriptome analysis of embryonic and adult stem cells with extended and limited differentiation capacity. *Genome Biol.* 2007; **8**:R163.

5. Eguizabal C, Shovlin TC, Durcova-Hills G, Surani A, McLaren A. Generation of primordial germ cells from pluripotent stem cells. *Differentiation* 2009; **78**:116–123.

6. Baker TG. A quantitative and cytological study of germ cells in human ovaries. *Proc. R. Soc. Lond. B. Biol Sci.* 1963; **158**:417–433.

7. Li Y, Zheng M, Lau YF. The sex-determining factors SRY and SOX9 regulate similar target genes and promote testis cord formation during testicular differentiation. *Cell Rep.* 2014; **8**:723–733.

8. Hannema SE, Hughes IA. Regulation of Wolffian duct development. *Horm. Res.* 2007; **67**:142–151.

Chapter 2

Reproductive Puberty

Puberty is a process in which a child's body matures into an adult body capable of sexual reproduction and involves physiologic, somatic, and constitutional changes associated with further development of the internal and external genitalia and secondary sex characteristics. On average, girls begin the process at the age of 10–11 and end puberty at around 15–17, while boys begin at around the ages of 11–12 and end at around 16–17. Puberty which starts earlier than average is known as precocious puberty and puberty which starts later than usual is known as delayed puberty. The onset of puberty is the consequence of a complex sequence of maturation in the central nervous system (CNS) that is not fully understood. A critical body mass is required before the CNS begins to activate puberty [1]. Two autonomous but associated processes, controlled by different mechanisms, but strictly linked temporally, are involved in the amplified secretion of sex steroids in the peripubertal and pubertal period. One process has been designated "adrenarche," and involves an increase in adrenal androgen secretion [2], and the second event, "gonadarche," involves the pubertal activation of the hypothalamic–pituitary gonadotropin–gonadal apparatus [3]. These two events and their role in puberty shall be measured separately.

Adrenal System ("Adrenarche")

Social behavior (childhood experience) is related to the adrenal axis, which produces cortisol and dehydroepiandrosterone (DHEA) and its sulfate (DHES). Increases in the production of DHEA/DHES by the adrenal gland begin around the age of 8 and continue until the mid-20s [4], thereby roughly bracketing the progression of pubertal development from ages 10 to 18. The increase in DHEA/DHES production in males appears to extend some 5 years beyond that in females [4], suggesting important sex differences in the onset of reproduction potential.

DHEA/DHES is the most shared hormone in the human body and is well known for its key role as a precursor for estrogen production during fetal development [5] and for its rise during maturation [6]. DHEA/DHES is a neurosteroid, and is produced in the brain as well as in the adrenal gland [7]. DHEA/DHES binds to neurotransmitter gamma-aminobutyric acid type (GABA$_A$) receptors, acting as an antagonist [8], and presumably impacting neural mechanisms. In peripheral tissues, DHEA/DHES is converted to estrogen and testosterone [9], and may thereby also elicit effects, such as bone and muscle growth, through testosterone and estrogen receptors in systems other than the brain [10]. Premature adrenarche has been revealed to have effects on both cognition and psychosocial development [11–12].

Hypothalamic–Pituitary System ("Gonadarche")

Reproductive maturation involves maturation of the hypothalamic–pituitary–gonadal axis (Figure 2.1). The hypothalamic neurons mature in accordance with a genetic (familial) pattern. In mammals, activation of gonadotropin-releasing hormone (GnRH) neurons is the key event gating the onset of puberty. However, the mechanisms that trigger GnRH secretion at puberty remain one of the enigmas of modern science.

Kisspeptin stimulates GnRH secretion by a direct effect on GnRH neurons, which express the kisspeptin receptor, GPR54. Kisspeptin expression is upregulated in the anteroventral periventricular nuclei (AVPV) and downregulated in the arcuate nuclei (ARC) of the hypothalamus by sex steroids. Compared with male, the female AVPV contains a much higher number of kisspeptin neurons, which are critical for the luteinizing hormone (LH) surge under estradiol regulation. Expression of *Kiss1* in the ARC appears to be involved in the negative feedback regulation of GnRH/LH by

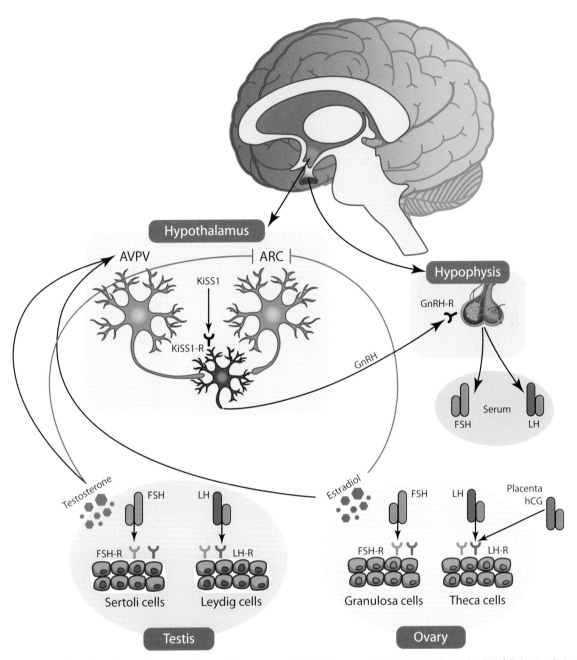

Figure 2.1 Hypothalamic–pituitary–gonadal axis. ARC, arcuate nuclei; AVPV, anteroventral periventricular nuclei; FSH, follicle-stimulating hormone; GnRH, gonadotropin-releasing hormone; hCG, human chorionic gonadotropin; LH, luteinizing hormone.

sex steroids and induces slow pulses of GnRH, which activate follicle-stimulating hormone (FSH) pulses. The expression of *Kiss1* mRNA in the ARC is inhibited by estradiol, progesterone, and testosterone. These same hormones induce *Kiss1* mRNA expression in the AVPV, where kisspeptin neurons are thought to

be involved in the positive feedback regulation of GnRH/LH [13]. GnRH neurons also integrate information from the body through hormones such as neuropeptide Y and adiponectin.

Migration of GnRH-secreting neurons from the nasal olfactory epithelium to the basal hypothalamus occurs during embryogenesis. *KAL1* (on X chromosome) is involved in the migration of the GnRH neurons, with mutations of *KAL1* responsible for 30–70% of Kallmann syndrome cases [14]. Kallmann syndrome, a familial disorder characterized in 1944, is manifested by failure of the hypothalamus to produce and release GnRH, which results in a complete lack of FSH and LH (hypogonadotropic hypogonadism). Other developmental anomalies, i.e., craniofacial distortion, harelip, cleft palate, and cryptorchidism, are also frequently associated with it. Inheritance of the disorder appears to be autosomal recessive, dominant with incomplete expressivity, or X-linked associated with partial deletion of the short arm of the X chromosome.

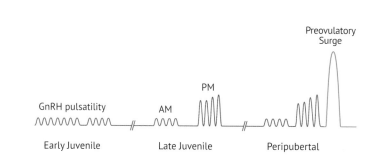

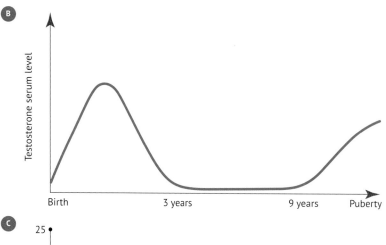

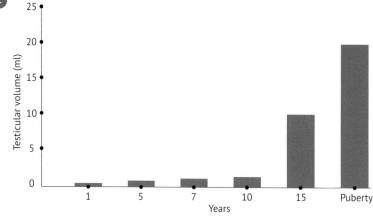

Figure 2.2 (A) GnRH pulsatility from juvenile to pubertal ages. (B) Male serum testosterone levels and (C) testicular volume.

GnRH is released from the medial basal hypothalamus in a pulsatile pattern, approximately every 70–90 minutes [15], and its half-life is 2–5 minutes. GnRH contributes to the release of both LH and FSH from the anterior part of the pituitary. GnRH binds to its receptor on pituitary cells within 1 minute of release and activates the G protein (phospholipase C and ERK pathways); the GnRH receptor then undergoes desensitization in 5 minutes and becomes active again within 30 minutes [16]. FSH is the first gonadotropin to rise at puberty, in response to low-frequency GnRH pulses in the ARC; small changes in LH levels are seen in parallel. FSH levels begin to increase at the age of ~7–8 years in females and 9–11 years in males; however, LH does not begin to rise until the age of 9–12 years [17]. With the acceleration of GnRH pulse frequency, FSH and LH reach adult levels (Figure 2.2). GnRH release is regulated by feedback signals from testosterone, inhibin, activin, estrogen, progesterone, and others. Low levels of estrogen have little effect on LH secretion, but inhibit FSH secretion. High levels of estrogen induce the LH surge at female midcycle, and high steady levels of estrogen lead to sustained elevated LH secretion [18]. Low levels of progesterone, acting at the level of the pituitary gland, enhance the LH response to GnRH and are responsible for the FSH surge at midcycle. High levels of progesterone inhibit the pituitary secretion of gonadotropins by inhibiting GnRH pulses at the level of the hypothalamus [18]. Corticotropin-releasing hormone (CRH), secreted during stress, as well as opiates, downregulate GnRH secretion [19].

Both FSH and LH are secreted from the anterior hypophysis (pituitary). Both hormones have the same α-subunit; however, β-subunits are different [20]. FSH has a plasma half-life of ~149 minutes (95–250 minutes), which is about five times longer than the ~30 minutes half-life of LH. The LH pulses are more frequent (interval between LH pulses is ~120 minutes) and of greater amplitude than those of FSH. The amplitude of LH pulses is highly variable, both within and between individuals.

FSH release is controlled by the feedback of inhibin from the gonads. The disturbed pulse frequency of GnRH is followed by increased FSH levels. LH release is controlled by the feedback of steroids from the gonads. Androgen plays central negative feedback roles in both the hypothalamus and hypophysis. Gonadal hormones act at different sites along the hypothalamic–pituitary axis to modulate the frequency and amplitude of gonadotropin release. LH and FSH also control their own release by feeding back to the hypothalamus.

References

1. Frisch RE, Revelle R. Height and weight at menarche and hypothesis of menarche. *Arch. Dis. Child.* 1971; **46**:695–701.

2. Grumbach MM, Richards GE, Conte FA, Kaplan SL. Clinical disorders of adrenal function and puberty: an assessment of the role of the adrenal cortex in normal and abnormal puberty in man and evidence for an ACTH-like pituitary adrenal androgen stimulating hormone. In: Serio M, ed., *The Endocrine Function of the Human Adrenal Cortex.* New York: Academic Press. 1978; 583–612.

3. Grumbach MM, Roth JC, Kaplan SL, Kelch RP. Hypothalamic-pituitary regulation of puberty in man: evidence and concepts derived from clinical research. In: Grumbach MM, Grave GD, Mayer FE, eds., *Control of the Onset of Puberty.* New York: John Wiley & Sons. 1974; 115–166.

4. Worthman CM. The epidemiology of human development. In: Worthman CM, Panter-Brick C, eds., *Hormones, Health and Behavior.* Cambridge: Cambridge University Press. 1999; 47–104.

5. Parker CR Jr. Dehydroepiandrosterone and dehydroepiandrosterone sulfate production in the human adrenal during development and aging. *Steroids* 1999; **64**:640–647.

6. Orentreich N, Brind JL, Vogelman JH, Andres R, Baldwin H. Long-term longitudinal measures of plasma dehydroepiandrosterone sulfate in normal men. *J. Clin. Endocrinol. Metab.* 1992; **75**:1002–1014.

7. Baulieu EE. Neurosteroids: a novel function of the brain. *Psychoneuroendocrinology* 1998; **23**:963–987.

8. Majewska MD. Neuronal actions of dehydroepiandrosterone. Possible role in brain development, aging, memory and affect. *Ann. N. Y. Acad. Sci.* 1995; **774**:111–120.

9. Labrie F, Belanger A, Simard J, Luu-The Van, Labrie C. DHEA and peripheral androgen and estrogen formation: intracinology. *Ann. N. Y. Acad. Sci.* 1995; **774**:16–28.

10. Argquitt AB, Stoecker BJ, Hermann JS, Winterfeldt EA. Dehydroepiandrosterone sulfate, cholesterol, hemoglobin, and anthropometric measures related to growth in male adolescents. *J. Am. Diet. Assoc.* 1991; **91**:575–579.

11. Dorn LD, Hitt SF, Rotenstein D. Biopsychological and cognitive differences in children with premature vs. on-time adrenarche. *Arch. Pediat. Adolesc. Med.* 1999; **153**:137–146.

12. Nass R, Baker S, Sadler AE, Sidtis JJ. The effects of precocious adrenarche on cognition and hemispheric specialization. *Brain Cogn.* 1990; **14**:59–69.

13. Gottsch ML, Cunningham MJ, Smith JT, et al. A role for kisspeptins in the regulation of gonadotropin secretion in the mouse. *Endocrinology* 2004; **145**:4073–4077.

14. Cariboni A, Pimpinelli F, Colamarino S, et al. The product of X-linked Kallmann's syndrome gene (KAL1) affects the migratory activity of gonadotropin-releasing hormone (GnRH)-producing neurons. *Hum. Mol. Genet.* 2004; **13**:2781–2791.

15. Ferris HA, Shupnik MA. Mechanisms for pulsatile regulation of the gonadotropin subunit genes by GNRH1. *Biol. Reprod.* 2006; **74**:993–998.

16. Liu F, Austin DA, Mellon PL, Olefsky JM, Webster NJ. GnRH activates ERK1/2 leading to the induction of c-fos and LHbeta protein expression in LbetaT2 cells. *Mol. Endocrinol.* 2002; **16**:419–434.

17. Scherf KS, Behrman M, Dahl RE. Facing changes and changing faces in adolescence: a new model for investigating adolescent-specific interactions between pubertal, brain and behavioral development. *Dev. Cogn. Neurosci.* 2012; **2**:199–299.

18. Bouchard P, Wolf JP, Hajri S. Inhibition of ovulation: comparison between the mechanism of action of steroids and GnRH analogues. *Hum. Reprod.* 1988; **3**:503–506.

19. Bethea CL, Centeno ML, Cameron JL. Neurobiology of stress-induced reproductive dysfunction in female macaques. *Mol. Neurobiol.* 2008; **38**:199–230.

20. Booth RA Jr, Weltman JY, Yankov VI, et al. Mode of pulsatile follicle-stimulating hormone secretion in gonadal hormone-sufficient and -deficient women – a clinical research center study. *J. Clin. Endocrinol. Metab.* 1996; **81**:3208–3214.

Chapter 3

Physiology of the Male Reproductive System

The male reproductive system consists of organs that function to produce, transfer, and introduce mature sperm cells into the female reproductive tract, where fertilization can occur (Figure 3.1). The initial development of the male reproductive organs begins before birth when the reproductive tract differentiates into the male form. Several months before birth, the immature testes descend behind the parietal peritoneum into the scrotum, guided by the fibrous gubernaculum. The testes and other reproductive organs remain in an immature form. They remain incapable of providing reproductive function until puberty when levels of reproductive hormones stimulate the final stages of their development (Figure 3.2). Prepubertal boys have no spermatogenesis; however, spermatogonia preserve in their testicles. Sexual maturity and ability to reproduce are reached at puberty. A gradual decline in hormone production and testicular cell count during adulthood may decrease sexual desire and fertility.

Testes

The testes measure about 4 × 2.5 cm, with a volume of ~25 ml and a weight of 30–45 g each. The left testis is generally located approximately 1 cm lower in the scrotal sac than the right testis. A dense, white, fibrous capsule called the tunica albuginea encases each testis and then enters the gland, sending out septa that radiate through its interior, dividing it into ~200–350 cone-shaped lobules (pyramids). Each lobule of the testis contains interstitial cells (Leydig cells, fibroblasts, and macrophages), lymphatic and blood vessels, and one to three tiny, coiled seminiferous tubules, which contain Sertoli cells and germ cells. The tubules from each lobule assemble to form a plexus called the rete testis. Efferent ductules then drain the rete testis and enter the genital duct, the head of the epididymis (Figure 3.3).

Leydig cells. In 1850, histologist Franz von Leydig (1821–1908), a professor at the University of Bonn, was the first to describe Leydig cells, which he observed surrounding connective tissue septa. Only at 1935 testosterone was isolated from these cells.

The Leydig cell numbers decrease markedly from 3 to 6 months of age to the end of the first year of life, and from 6 years onwards the number of Leydig cells progressively increase. The Leydig cells are presented in clusters, contain an amount of smooth endoplasmic reticulum, and are responsible, under stimulation by luteinizing hormone (LH), for testosterone secretion. LH binds to a G protein-coupled receptor on the Leydig cells and induces increases in cAMP levels, which subsequently leads to activation of the side-chain cleavage of cholesterol, as well as other events which culminate in increased steroidogenesis and the production of testosterone and other androgens from cholesterol. The pathway begins with the conversion of cholesterol to pregnenolone, which takes place in the mitochondria. Pregnenolone is then converted to testosterone by microsomal enzymes, and the testosterone is released into the circulation (Figure 3.4) and regulates its own production by negative feedback on the hypothalamus and pituitary to modulate or suppress LH secretion.

In the plasma, 54% of the testosterone binds to sex hormone-binding globulin (SHBG, which is synthesized in the liver), 45% binds to human serum albumin (HSA), and only 1% circulates as free testosterone. **Testosterone bioavailability** is represented by the free androgen index. In many tissues, testosterone is reduced to two other potent androgens, dihydrotestosterone (DHT) and 5α-androstenediol.

Leydig cells also produce oxytocin [1] and small amounts of estrogens [2]. Follicle-stimulating hormone (FSH) and prolactin receptors have been identified on the Leydig cells. Prolactin has been shown to enhance LH-stimulated testosterone secretion, while FSH regulates LH receptors, rendering prolactin and FSH stimulators of the Leydig cell response to LH [3]. FSH induces rapid hypertrophy and hyperplasia of interstitial cells that transform into mature Leydig cells.

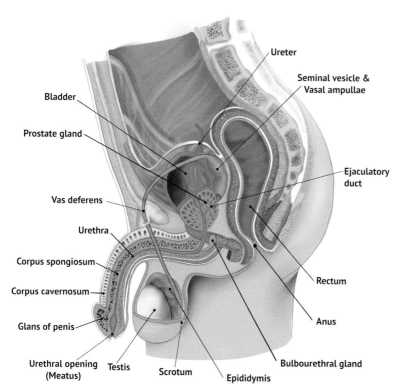

Figure 3.1 Male reproductive system.

In both testes of a 20-year-old male the number of Leydig cells is up to 700 million and diminishes by one-half by the age of 60 [4], and consequently, plasma testosterone levels decline [5]. No division of Leydig cells has been observed in the testes of adult men.

Peripheral production of estrogen increases (adipose tissue is capable of aromatizing testosterone to estradiol) with male age, resulting in a decreased androgen/estrogen ratio and increased estrogenic (female) effect. This is believed to underlie the development of benign prostatic hypertrophy and gynecomastia in elderly men. Aromatase inhibitors, e.g., letrozole and anastrozole, can decrease estradiol levels. Tamoxifen, an estrogen receptor antagonist, can disrupt the interaction between estrogen and its receptor, thereby decreasing the estrogenic effect.

Sertoli cells. A regular testicle contains 600–1200 seminiferous tubules with a total length of approximately 250 m. Seminiferous tubules are made up of layers of Sertoli cells, germ cells, and myoid cells. The adult seminiferous tubule contains an epithelium of five to eight layers of Sertoli cells. On their basal side, each Sertoli cell has tight junctions (TJs) and basal adherens junctions (AJs), with all Sertoli cells side by side, creating the blood–testis barrier (BTB) [6]. The TJs integrate membrane proteins, such as occludin, claudin, and junctional adhesion molecules, which are stimulated by testosterone. The AJs include complexes of membrane proteins, such as cadherin–catenin, nectin–afadin–ponsin, integrin–laminin–actinin. Loss of one of these junction proteins could lead to loss of cell–cell adhesion. Cadmium chloride and other smoking products have been known for decades to induce infertility in males [7], and this effect may be mediated by BTB damage in the testis. The BTB must open periodically to permit germ cell transport, to ensure the successful and continual production of sperm cells, and also plays a vital role in spermatogenesis [6, 8].

FSH binds to its receptor on the Sertoli cells of the seminiferous tubules, increases cAMP levels, protein synthesis, and androgen binding in the tubules. The Sertoli cells produce the androgen-binding protein (ABP), which displays a high affinity to testosterone. ABP is secreted into the lumen of the seminiferous tubule and then transported to the epididymis, where it is taken up, and 80% is degraded. The remaining 20% is released into the blood, likely from the base of Sertoli cells. Sertoli cells also produce inhibin (α- and β-subunits), which serves as a negative feedback in the

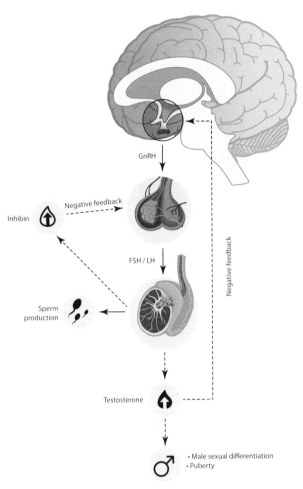

Blood test

HORMONE	RANGE
FSH	1-10 mIU/ml
LH	1-10 mIU/ml
Prolactin	50-400 mIU/L
Testosterone	2.65-9.15 ng/ml

Figure 3.2 Male reproductive hormonal axis. FSH, follicle-stimulating hormone; GnRH, gonadotropin-releasing hormone; LH, luteinizing hormone.

pituitary to regulate FSH, but not LH. Increased inhibin B levels may be initiated by ductal obstruction or anomalies within the seminiferous tubules.

During aging, there is a reduction in Sertoli cell numbers (from 600 million/testis at 20–48 years to 300 million/testis at 50–85 years), which can affect the integrity of the BTB [9], reducing the sperm production rate, motility, and morphology [10]. Loss of BTB function during aging is apparently irreversible.

Spermatogenesis

Primordial germ cells give rise to germ type A cells. Type A stem cells form additional type A spermatogonia and differentiate into type B spermatogonia cells all through early puberty. Type B cells differentiate during late puberty and in the adult form primary spermatocytes, secondary spermatocytes, and spermatids. These events initially occur through mitosis, after which, chromosome numbers are halved through meiosis. The spermatogonium (diploid, 2 n) is a most immature male germinal cell, and is located at the basal membrane of seminiferous tubules and undergoes mitotic division (six cycles) before migration through the TJ. The number of spermatogonia in prepubertal testes is influenced by the rate of proliferation, apoptosis, and differentiation into more advanced germ cells. The number of spermatogonia per tubular cross-section tends to decrease from 2.5 to 1.2 (from $30 \times 10^6/cm^3$ to $19 \times 10^6/cm^3$, respectively) over the first 3 years of life, followed by a two-fold increase until it peaks at 2.6 at the age of 6–7 years, then plateaus ($48 \times 10^6/cm^3$) until the age of 11 years,

15

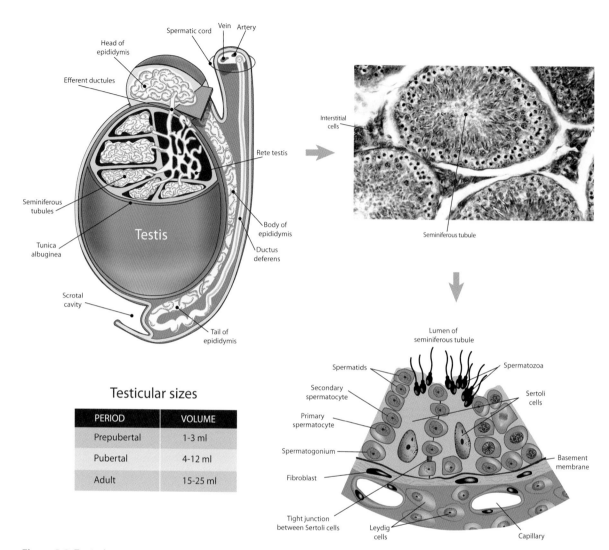

Testicular sizes

PERIOD	VOLUME
Prepubertal	1-3 ml
Pubertal	4-12 ml
Adult	15-25 ml

Figure 3.3 Testicular structure.

after which it rises to values of 7 ($100 \times 10^6/cm^3$), marking the onset of puberty [11]. Proliferation and differentiation of spermatogonia are induced by elevated FSH and LH, as well as increased inhibin B and testosterone secretion. FSH fuels the proliferation of immature Sertoli cells, causing the dispersion of spermatogonia across the elongating seminiferous tubules. Rapid spermatogonia proliferation is associated with increased levels of gonadotropins [12], the last wave of Sertoli cell proliferation followed by maturation [13–14], and enhanced germ cell differentiation, resulting in complete spermatogenesis [12].

In the human testis, three types of spermatogonium are usually considered: dark type A spermatogonia (Ad), characterized by densely staining chromatin and which

serve as reserve stem cells; these cells divide (mitotically) into daughter, active stem cells and pale type A spermatogonia (Ap), which are characterized by palely staining granular chromatin and which mature (mitotically divide) into type B or differentiating spermatogonia (Figure 3.5). The classification is based on the nuclear features, the presence of mitochondria aggregations, and the presence or absence of glycogen granules. The proliferation of Ap spermatogonia occurs constitutively, independent of gonadotropin stimulation, whereas the differentiation of these cells into B spermatogonia is gonadotropin dependent and driven by either LH or FSH [15].

Type B spermatogonia are the precursors (mitotically divide) of primary spermatocytes, which are

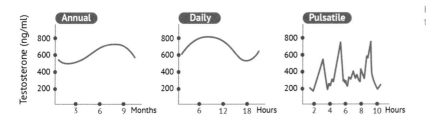

Figure 3.4 Secretion pattern of testosterone.

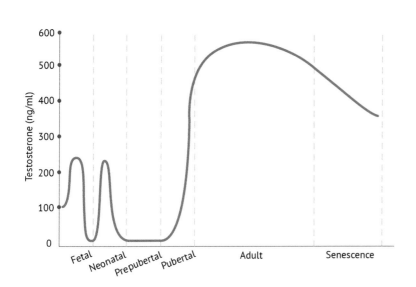

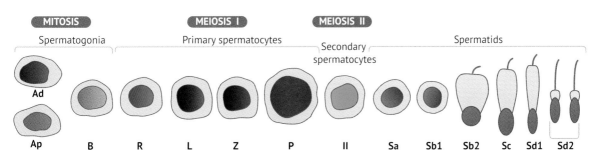

Figure 3.5 Spermatogenesis. Ad, dark spermatogonia; Ap, pale spermatogonia; B, type B primary spermatocyte; R, resting primary spermatocyte; L, leptotene stage spermatocyte; Z, zygotene stage spermatocyte; P, pachytene stage spermatocyte; II, secondary spermatocyte; Sa–Sd, spermatids at various stages of differentiation.

recognized by their large nuclei (chromosome set: 44 +XY), into which they transform before doubling internal DNA and before entering the first meiotic division (stages of preleptotene [R], leptotene [L], zygotene [Z], and pachytene [P]) to produce secondary spermatocytes. Primary spermatocytes differentiate from type

B spermatogonia behind the BTB at the basal compartment of the seminiferous epithelium and must traverse the BTB at preleptotene and leptotene stages (transitional stage from primary to secondary spermatocytes) and move into the adluminal compartment for further development. The new TJs are formed under the migrating preleptotene and leptotene spermatocytes. Every 16 days, preleptotene and leptotene spermatocytes enter the TJ of the BTB and give 256 mature spermatozoa into the ejaculate. Secondary spermatocytes go directly through the second meiotic division to produce haploid spermatids. Since neither DNA reduplication nor recombination of the genetic material occurs, the second meiosis can occur quickly (lasting around 5 hours). From this stage, no further divisions take place, and each spermatid begins its transformation into a spermatozoon [16]. This spermatogenic cycle takes ~62–65 days (Figure 3.5).

Spermiogenesis. Next, the spermatids undergo spermiogenesis, which involves the Sa (formation of acrosome), Sb_1 and Sb_2 (nuclear changes), Sc (development of flagellum), and Sd_1 and Sd_2 (reorganization of the cytoplasm and organelles) stages. Residual cytoplasm, including mitochondria, undergoes phagocytosis by Sertoli cells and spermatozoa are released from the seminiferous epithelium into the tubule lumen, in a process termed spermiation (Figure 3.6). A small residual cytoplasmic droplet may remain attached to the spermatozoa. As the cell undergoes further maturation during transit across the epididymis, this cytoplasmic droplet migrates along the tail and is finally lost.

During the elongating spermatid stage of spermiogenesis, sperm chromatin undergoes a complex transition in which histones are extensively replaced first by transition proteins and then by protamines (a process called protamination). At the nuclear level, histones, which are associated with DNA and preserve the DNA chain in a coiled configuration, are replaced by protamines leading to a highly compact condensed chromatin structure (Figure 3.7). Protamines (protamine 1 [P1] and protamine 2 [P2]) are 27–65 amino acid-long proteins, rich in arginine and cysteine, amino acids that are highly positively charged. The replacement of most histones by P1 and P2 facilitates the high order of chromatin compaction and packaging, due to their stronger binding than histones to negatively charged DNA. This compaction is necessary for normal sperm function and may also be necessary for DNA silencing and imprinting changes within the sperm cell [17]. P1 and P2 are usually expressed in nearly equal quantities (1:1), but abnormal P1/P2 ratios are observed in some infertile men and are often associated with severe spermatogenesis defects, DNA fragmentation, lower fertilization rates, poor embryo quality, and reduced pregnancy rates [18]. Elevated P1/P2 ratios have been taken as evidence of nuclear immaturity. In contrast to most mammals, whose spermatozoa contain only one P1 type of protamine, humans contain a second type of protamine (P2), which is deficient in cysteine residues. Therefore, human sperm chromatin has a potentially less stable structure than that of species that contain P1 only [19]. Transition protein is important for DNA condensation. Approximately 20% of the DNA in spermatozoon remains decorated by histones. It remains unclear which genes are compacted by histones and which by protamines, and what the

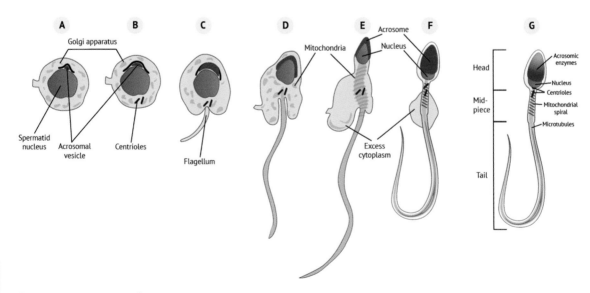

Figure 3.6 Spermiogenesis (from spermatid to spermatozoa).

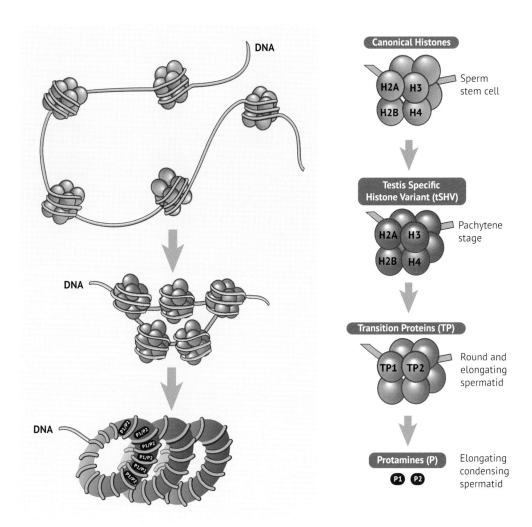

Figure 3.7 Sperm cell DNA compaction process. Substitution of canonical histones (spermatogonia) to protamines (spermatids).

physiological significance of the different compaction may be. This histones/protamines rate cannot be altered by exogenous hormonal treatment. It has already been shown that some infertile patients have anomalies in protamine content [20–21].

Mature spermatozoa bear a centrosome, which contains a pair of centrioles. The oocyte has none. Sperm centrioles are absolutely essential for the formation of the centrosome, which will form a spindle, enabling the mitotic division of the zygote.

At the end of spermiation, the seminiferous tubule contracts by myoid cells, in a hormone-dependent manner. Tubular fluid builds up pressure, and spermatozoa are released from the tubule and pass to the epididymis.

Epididymis

The epididymis is a 3–4 cm-long structure with a tubular length of 4–5 m, whose primary functions include post-testicular maturation (enabled by the unique microenvironment within the lumen of the duct that helps transform immotile, immature testicular spermatozoa into fully mature spermatozoa) and storage of fertile spermatozoa in a viable state within the cauda with their passage from the testis to the vas deferens. Testosterone and DHT are the major androgens controlling epididymal function. Other participant in this process include prolactin, which increases the number of LH receptors [22] and uptake of testosterone by the caput epididymis. The microenvironment and lower temperature of 30–32°C are thought to be major contributors to sperm cell survival.

The epididymis is divided into three functionally distinct regions: head, body, and tail or cauda. Different proteins exist in the functionally distinct regions of the epididymis, and during sperm cell maturation, membrane lipids undergo distinct physical and chemical alterations [23]. Two major functions of the epididymis have been described: adsorption and secretion. Much of the testicular fluid that transports sperm cells from the seminiferous tubules to the epididymis is resorbed in the caput, resulting in the concentration of the spermatozoa increasing by 10- to 100-fold. The epididymal plasma, in which the spermatozoa are suspended within the epididymis, is secreted by the epididymal epithelium. The epididymal fluid is rich in glycosyltransferases and glycosidases. Variations in the lipid composition of the plasma membrane of sperm cells during maturation are thought to underlie the sensitivity of ejaculated spermatozoa to cold shock, when compared with testicular sperm.

One of the most important changes in the spermatozoa during epididymal maturation is the tail axonemal complex "maturity" and the development of sperm cell motility. The motility of mature spermatozoa is dependent on the intracellular cAMP generated by adenylate cyclase and on subsequent successive phosphorylation of proteins, including protein kinase A, A-kinase anchor proteins, and many others [24].

As many as half of the spermatozoa released from the testis die within the epididymis and are routinely resorbed by the epididymal epithelium (principal cells) after spermiophagy by macrophages.

Sperm take roughly 2 weeks to get through the epididymis (from caput to cauda). Sperm cells are put in storage near the tail portion and in the vas deferens until they are ejaculated. After prolonged sexual inactivity, caudal spermatozoa first lose their fertilizing ability, followed by their motility and then their vitality. This process is one of the reasons for the maximal 3-day sexual abstinence limitation prior to the collection of ejaculates for semen analysis.

Inflammation of the epididymis, epididymitis, is often caused by infection or by sexually transmitted diseases such as chlamydia. Gonorrhea frequently destroys the distal section of the epididymis and spares the caput. The vas deferens may be affected (sclerosis), in addition to the epididymis. Patients with epididymal obstruction present with semen containing no sperm cells (azoospermia) or semen with low sperm cell counts (severe oligozoospermia), and elevated serum FSH levels.

Hormonal control. The male reproductive system is under tight hormonal control. Negative feedback mechanisms operate between the hypothalamus, the anterior pituitary gland, and the hormone-producing cells of the testes, i.e., Leydig cells producing testosterone and Sertoli cells producing inhibin.

Inhibin secretion by the Sertoli cell is stimulated by FSH and inhibited by LH, the latter presumably acting via Leydig cell-derived testosterone. Inhibin acts in negative feedback control of FSH release at the pituitary level, whereas testosterone acts in a negative feedback loop inhibiting LH secretion at the hypothalamic and pituitary levels. Like gonadotropins, prolactin also plays an important role in male reproduction. Low prolactin levels (hypoprolactinemia) have been associated with reduced ejaculate (seminal vesicles) volume in infertile subjects [25], erectile dysfunction, and premature ejaculation. Men with abnormally elevated prolactin levels present with gynecomastia, diminished libido, and erectile dysfunction. Prolactin inhibits the production of gonadotropin-releasing hormone, LH, and FSH. Elevated titers of plasma prolactin were shown to induce spermatogonia apoptosis [26]. Blockade of the portal veins by adenoma may prevent the hypothalamic prolactin-inhibiting factor from reaching the hypophysis and induce elevation of plasma prolactin levels.

Vascular System

The testicular arteries have their origin from three different blood vessels: (1) the abdominal aorta, which elongates to form the testicular artery as the testes migrate, (2) the inferior epigastric artery, and (3) the internal iliac artery, which supplies blood to the vas deferens.

The veins leaving the testis divide near the dorsal pole to form a venous plexus called the pampiniform plexus. The venous blood then drains into the spermatic vein. The right spermatic vein collects blood from the right testis to the inferior vena cava, while the left spermatic vein drains blood from the left testis into the left renal vein. This anatomical difference is important for the detection of varicocele, with those on the left side easily detectable. The pressure in the right spermatic vein is around 10 mm Hg. The pressure in the inferior vena cava is on average 0 mm Hg. The patient cannot raise hydrostatic pressure in the inferior vena cava above the pressure in the right spermatic vein and right spermatic vein backflow cannot be evoked on the right side, so right varicocele cannot be detected by palpation; however, it can be clearly seen on venography.

Arterial blood is cooled from body temperature to scrotal temperature by the venous blood, which leaves the testis at a temperature similar to that prevailing under the scrotal skin (scrotal skin has a very thin epidermis and is well supplied by blood vessels resulting in scrotal blood cooling). In the healthy male, the temperature of the scrotal skin is symmetrically distributed and does not exceed 32.5°C. This temperature has importance in normal spermatogenesis. Impaired testicular thermoregulation is commonly implicated in abnormal spermatogenesis and impaired sperm function with outcomes ranging from subclinical infertility to sterility.

Structure of Spermatozoa

Spermatozoa in the seminal fluid were observed for the first time under the magnifying glass and drawn by Anton van Leeuwenhoek (1632–1723) in 1667. Overall, sperm cell length is ~50–60 μm, including the head, mid-piece, and elongated tail. The mature spermatozoon has an oval flat-shaped, 4.0–5.5 μm-long, and 2.5–3.5 μm-wide head, with a pale anterior part (acrosome, 40–70% of the head area) and darker posterior region. The head has a highly compact package of genetic chromatin material. The cylindrical midpiece is ~7–8 μm long and characterized by a helical arrangement of its mitochondria, which provide energy for sperm locomotion. Spermatozoa can be motile under anaerobic conditions without mitochondrial activity due to the utilization of fatty acids. The tail is ~10 times the length of the head (~45 μm), and is divided into a principal piece, about 40 μm long, and a short end piece (5–10 μm in length).

The central portion of the sectioned sperm tail is a cylinder composed of nine dense doublet microtubules (periaxoneme), arranged around two single microtubules in the center (axoneme). The 9 + 2 arrangement of microtubules is also associated with dynein, which is an ATPase motor protein that hydrolyzes ATP and then undergoes conformational changes, forcing the microtubules to move past each other. The dense fibers dictate the structure that limits the flexibility of the flagella and allows the progressive movement (ahead) of a spermatozoon.

Ejaculate

During sexual arousal before ejaculation, the Cowper's glands (bulbourethral exocrine glands located posterior and lateral to the urethra at the base of the penis) secrete a clear mucoid alkaline pre-ejaculatory fluid that may appear at the tip of the penis [27]. This fluid aids in urethral lubrication and neutralizes the acidity of the urethra in preparation for the passage of sperm cells. During intercourse, a short burst of activity in sympathetic adrenergic nerves liberates norepinephrine that stimulates α_1 adrenergic receptors on smooth muscle cells in the cauda epididymides and vasa deferentia. This results in the peristaltic transfer of the contents of the distal cauda to the prostatic part of the urethra. The same mechanism is responsible for the emission of prostatic fluid in which the emitted spermatozoa are suspended. It also causes the normally delayed emission of seminal vesicular fluid. The sympathetic autonomic nerves also stimulate contraction of the smooth muscle tissue of the bladder neck, hindering the reflux of urethral contents into the bladder. Dilation of the urethra evokes a reflex (ejaculation) caused by the somatic nervous system, leading to rhythmical contractions of the striated bulbo- and ischio-cavernous muscles. These contractions increase the pressure in the urethra, and with the bladder neck closed, the contents are ejected out of the penis. The expulsion is divided into several fractions: generally, ejaculate is composed of the first fraction of prostatic fluids (~25%), and a second fraction containing both vesicular fluids (~65%) (seminal vesicles and vasal ampullae) and fluids from bulbourethral glands (~10%). Others divided ejaculate into six fractions [28]. A typical ejaculate contains 300×10^6 spermatozoa in 3 ml (Figure 3.8). The daily production is estimated at $80–100 \times 10^6$ spermatozoa. The alkaline pH of semen protects spermatozoa from the acidic environment of the vagina.

After ejaculation, human semen spontaneously coagulates within approximately 1 minute of coitus and then liquefies enzymatically [29] within 5–30 minutes under normal physiological conditions [30]. Semen proteins are involved in coagulation and liquefaction processes. Protein concentration in human seminal plasma has been estimated at 45 mg/ml [31]. Semenogelin-I (50 kDa) and -II (63 kDa) are secreted from the seminal vesicle and represent the most

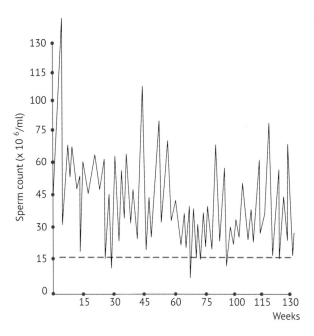

Figure 3.8 Variability in sperm cell count from a man with normozoospermia.

abundant components (about 20–40%) of the human semen coagulum [32]. Prostate-specific antigen (PSA, or human kallikrein 3) is a serine protease that is synthesized in prostate tissue and involved in semenogelin breakdown, causing liquefaction of the semen coagulum [33]. Free spermatozoa from liquefied sperm rush in advance and were found in the endocervix 1.5–3 minutes after ejaculation [34]. Sperm cells that enter the cervical mucus appear to do the cervical way within 15–20 minutes [35].

Spermatozoa cannot penetrate the zona pellucida (ZP) of the oocyte immediately after ejaculation. Capacitation is defined as the process by which spermatozoa acquire the capacity to undergo the acrosome reaction and then penetrate ZP to fertilize eggs.

Capacitation of spermatozoa. The mechanism of capacitation is poorly understood. Capacitation begins with the separation of spermatozoa from the seminal plasma. The time required for human sperm capacitation in vitro appears to vary considerably (minimum time 1 hours) and is unknown in vivo (some report estimate about 6 hours).

During ejaculation, seminal plasma proteins prime sperm cells to undergo capacitation. Capacitation likely involves the removal of cholesterol from the sperm cell plasma membrane, performed by sterol acceptors present in the female tract secretions. Contact between the spermatozoon membrane and the female tract activates Ca^{2+} influxes to the sperm cell, through the Ca^{2+}-permeable channel CatSper. Female cumulus cells secrete progesterone in the range of 10–100 μM. Progesterone, via its receptor ABHD2, activates the calcium channel CatSper in the sperm cell membrane and allows Ca^{2+} to enter [36]. A marked activation in sperm cell motility (hyperactivation) is associated with a Ca^{2+} influx [37]. Calcium-binding protein (CABYR) is proposed to play a role in this sperm cell hyperactivation. A defective sperm cell response is associated with reduced fertilization rate and subfertility [38].

Capacitation is related to activation of a signal transduction cascade leading to an increase in protein tyrosine phosphorylation. In brief, capacitation starts with Ca^{2+} binding to CABYR, followed by activation of protein kinase C. Heat shock protein-90 becomes tyrosine phosphorylated during capacitation. This is an important step in the activation of nitric oxide synthase at the midpiece, which is associated with capacitation [39]. The flagellum acquires hyperactivated movement, a key attribute of the capacitated state. Hyperactive spermatozoa exhibit high amplitude of flagellum, asymmetric flagellar movement, increased side-to-side head displacement, and nonlinear motility [40]. Capacitation leads to an acrosome reaction.

Acrosome reaction.

The acrosome is a membrane-bound, Golgi-derived organelle that covers the anterior one-half to two-thirds of the sperm cell head. The acrosome develops at the stage of spermiation, and primarily contains the hyaluronidase (splits the hyaluronic acid of the extracellular matrix between cumulus cells), proacrosin (a serin protease), acrosin (a trypsin-like enzyme) and β-galactosidase. Upon completion of capacitation, spermatozoa are ready to undergo the acrosome reaction, which is induced by binding of the spermatozoon to glycoprotein ZP3 in the ZP. Sperm surface β1,4-galactosyltransferase-I satisfies all the criteria expected of a ZP3 receptor. During the acrosome reaction, specific components of the acrosomal matrix may stabilize sperm adhesion to the zona matrix. Candidates include sp56, zonadhesin, and fusion protein – Izumo. Fertilin (α- and β-subunits), disintegrin, metalloproteinase (ADAM) family, and cyritestin are sperm cell surface proteins, which were found to be required for spermatozoon–oocyte fusion. Fusion between the outer acrosomal and sperm cell plasma membranes leads to the massive influx of Ca^{2+}. Sperm cell intracellular Ca^{2+} inactivates plasma membrane Na^+/K^+-ATPase and rapidly leads to an increase in intracellular Na^+. This action causes an H^+ efflux, producing a rise in the intracellular pH. High intra-acrosomal pH activates acrosomal enzymes, such as phospholipase A_2, which have been implicated in the final destabilization of the outer acrosomal and plasma membranes, which completes membrane fusion.

A fusion between the sperm cell and oocyte leads to the introduction of oocyte activation factor phospholipase C zeta (PLCζ) from the spermatozoa to the oocyte [41]. In fertile men, PLCζ is located along the inner acrosomal membrane [42]. Studies have demonstrated genetic links between PLCζ defects and infertility [43–44].

Seminal Vesicles

The paired seminal vesicles (5–6 cm long and 1–2 cm wide), arising from the vas deferens, are lateral to the ampulla of the vas deferens, posterior to the urinary bladder, and superior to the prostate. The gland is divided into stroma and parenchyma with two types of epithelial cells: glandular and basal. The vesicular fluid is yellowish, viscous, and alkaline, and comprises two-thirds of the ejaculate volume. Fructose is a marker specific for the vesicular fluid and is under androgenic regulation. The fructose of seminal fluid is formed from blood glucose (which undergoes isomerization and dephosphorylation) and appears to provide a source of energy for the spermatozoa. Prolactin may play a key role in the availability of seminal fructose [45]. The seminal fluid also includes ascorbic acid, inorganic phosphorus and potassium, and prostaglandins (predominantly group PGE). The major clotting protein, semenogelin (isoform I and isoform II) is the specific marker for seminal fluid and characterized by a high zinc-binding capacity.

The seminal vesicles and vas deferens share an embryonic origin. This fact can be used in determining the etiology of azoospermia, as only in cases of azoospermia due to congenital absence of the vas deferens, obstruction of ejaculatory ducts, or retrograde ejaculation is there an absence of seminal fructose. In cases of azoospermia due to blockage at the epididymal level, seminal fructose is in the normal range.

Prostate

The prostate completely surrounds the urethra below the neck of the bladder. It is an aggregate structure formed from 30 to 50 acinar glands of different sizes and shapes and is divided into an anterior lobe and two lateral and posterior lobes. Its 16–32 excretory ducts open into the urethra. Prostatic fluid is homogeneous and slightly milky, with a pH in the range of 6.6–7.2. The prostatic fluid does not coagulate spontaneously and contains the fibrinolytic enzymes responsible for liquefaction of coagulated vesicular secretion. More specifically, it contains citrate, prostatic acid phosphatase, PSA, zinc, magnesium, glycerylphosphorylcholine (that converts to choline), sodium, albumin, aliphatic polyamines (spermine, spermidine, and putrescine). Polyamines and zinc were found to enhance sperm motility. Spermine and zinc also prevent microbial growth, which may explain the difficulties in culturing semen for bacteriology testing. PSA is an androgen-regulated serine protease that cleaves semenogelin (I and II) in the seminal coagulum. PSA in the serum was demonstrated to be a clinically important measure for monitoring of prostate cancer. The secretory activity of the epithelial cells of the male accessory sex glands is primarily under the control of testicular androgens. Testosterone in the prostate (and seminal vesicles) is converted to DHT by 5α-reductase. The DHT/testosterone ratio is increased in patients with prostatic hypertrophy due to the activity of 5α-reductase [46].

Bulbourethral Glands

The bulbourethral (Cowper's) glands are paired bodies (3–5 mm in diameter) which are homologous to the Bartholin's glands in the female. These glands exhibit the typical arrangement of stroma and parenchyma seen in all male accessory sex glands. Cowper's glands secrete clear and mucoid, sialoprotein-rich fluid during erection, which presumably aids in urethral lubrication [27].

Other Accessory Glands

Additional small glands are scattered throughout the male reproductive tract and include the urethral (Littre's) and preputial (Tyson's) glands. Their secretions are discharged close to their location, where they function as urethral lubricants. Preputial glands are modified sebaceous glands, and as such, produce a fatty secretion that seems to be primarily associated with pheromone functions.

Male Reproductive Aging

All physiological functions of organisms decrease with age. Diminishing male gonadal hormonal activity arouses "male menopause" as "andropause," which primarily occurs in middle-aged and elderly men when testosterone production and its plasma levels are reduced. This phenomenon can be associated with impaired spermatogenesis. Reduced levels of testosterone affect most male systems and tissues, including the central nervous system, endocrine and cardiovascular systems, muscles and bones, as well as sexual and fertility functions. In contrast to menopause, andropause progresses gradually over the years and is therefore now termed "late-onset hypogonadism"; however, it can also be determined as permanent periandropause.

Late-onset hypogonadism stems from the gradual and slow aging of testicular tissue. The tissue structure can be functionally separated into two major compartments, i.e., seminiferous tubules housing a Sertoli cell section, and spermatogenic cells and interstitial tissue containing a Leydig cell section and a source of testosterone production. Both compartments are inalienable elements in the spermatogenic process, and both are affected by the aging process. Sertoli cell functionality and spermatogenesis are directly dependent upon androgen and the function of Leydig cells; therefore, one testicular compartment is closely influenced by the other. Pituitary FSH acts on the Sertoli cells, mainly to increase spermatogenesis, while pituitary LH acts on the Leydig cells, mainly to increase steroidogenesis. As such, the control of male fertility requires accurate endocrine, paracrine, and autocrine communications along the hypothalamic–pituitary–gonadal axis [47].

Seminal volume, spermatozoa concentration and total count, and overall motility and progressive motility of spermatozoa gradually decline between 22 and 80 years of age [10; 48]. The risk of spontaneous miscarriage is higher for fathers older than 35 years, compared with those younger than 35 [49–50]. Semen samples show an increasing level of sperm cells with highly damaged DNA in men aged 36–57 years, compared with those aged 20–35 years [51]. Sperm cell DNA damage is linked with a significantly increased risk of pregnancy loss [52]. Increasing paternal age is also significantly associated with delayed conception and diminished pregnancy in a population of fertile couples, which is a mark of declining fecundity in older men [53–54]. Moreover, advanced paternal age is associated with increased risks of birth defects, including heart defects, tracheo-oesophageal atresia, musculoskeletal/integumental anomalies, achondroplasia, autism, Down syndrome, and other chromosomal anomalies [55–58].

Testosterone levels begin to decline in early middle age and then progressively decline in a linear manner [59]. While low testosterone levels are critical for male sexual function, there is a variation between individuals [60]. An abnormally low concentration of testosterone (hypotestosteronemia) may be the consequence of a testicular (primary hypogonadism) or a hypothalamic–pituitary (secondary hypogonadism) dysfunction. These types of hypogonadism can be either congenital or acquired. By the age of 80 years, serum total testosterone concentrations fall by about 75% and serum free testosterone concentrations to about 50% of what they are at the age of 20 [59].

Clinical manifestations of androgen deficiency can be classified as physical, behavioral, and sexual. Physical manifestations of androgen deficiency include loss of bone mineral density, muscle wasting and weakness, loss of male body hair, gynecomastia, and small or shrinking testes. Behavioral manifestations of androgen deficiency include decreased cognitive functions and memory, depressed mood, irritability, low energy, poor motivation, sleep disturbance, increased sleepiness, and reduced libido. Sexual manifestations of androgen deficiency include erectile dysfunction and infertility.

Male aging is associated with an increase in body fat and reduced muscle mass and strength. This could be explained by an age-associated decline in growth hormone concentrations, which, itself, is associated with an increase in SHBG and, therefore, a reduction in bioavailable testosterone [61]. In overweight men, adipose tissue is capable of aromatizing testosterone to estradiol, and it is speculated that reduced total testosterone production in obese men affects the function of the seminiferous epithelium, as well as the synchrony of spermatogenesis. Estrogens have a marked impact on proliferative and apoptotic events in the testis, and, as such, serve as key local modulators of the production, transport, and maturation of spermatozoa [62].

A decline in sexual interest and potency is usually related to aging [62]. Such changes in sexual behavior are androgen dependent but are not verified in all cases. Emotional symptoms have long been associated with low levels of testosterone, whereas depressed mood significantly correlates with low levels of bioavailable testosterone in older men [63]. Although the percentage of men complaining of erectile dysfunction rises dramatically with age, only 50% of men between the ages of 50 and 70 years report on potency loss [64].

Androgens also have an important role in the development of cognitive functioning and strong correlations exist between testosterone concentrations and visuospatial abilities in certain domains [65]. Administration of pharmacological doses of testosterone to aging men has been shown to be associated with improved visuospatial skills [66], bone metabolism [67], muscle mass [68], and reduced cardiovascular risk factors [69].

References

1. Nicholson HD, Hardy MP. Luteinizing hormone differentially regulates the secretion of testicular oxytocin and testosterone by purified adult rat Leydig cells in vitro. *Endocrinology* 1992; **130**:671–677.

2. Carreau S, Bilinska B, Levallet J. Male germ cells. A new source of estrogens in mammalian testis. *Ann. Endocrinol.* 1998; **59**:79–92.

3. Waeber C, Reymond O, Reymond M, Lemarchand-Beraud T. Effects of hyper- and hypoprolactinemia on gonadotropin secretion, rat testicular luteinizing hormone/human chorionic gonadotropin receptors and testosterone production by isolated Leydig cells. *Biol. Reprod.* 1983; **28**:167–177.

4. Neaves WB, Johnson L, Petty CS. Age-related change in numbers of other interstitial cells in testes of adult men: evidence bearing on the fate of Leydig cells lost with advanced age. *Biol. Reprod.* 1985; **33**:259–269.

5. Gray A, Berlin JA, McKinley JB, Longcope C. An examination of research design effects on the association of testosterone and male ageing: results of a metaanalysis. *J. Clin. Epidemiol.* 1991; **44**:671–684.

6. Cheng CY, Mruk DD. The blood-testis barrier and its implications for male contraception. *Pharmacol. Rev.* 2012; **64**:16–64.

7. Ragheb AM, Sabanegh Jr ES. Smoking and male fertility: a contemporary review. *Arch. Med. Sci.* 2009; **5**:S13–S19.

8. Lee NPY, Cheng CY. Nitric oxide/nitric oxide synthase, spermatogenesis, and tight junction dynamics. *Biol. Reprod.* 2004; **70**:267–276.

9. Johnson L, Zane RS, Petty CS, Neaves WB. Quantification of the human Sertoli cell population: Its distribution, relation to germ cell numbers, and age related decline. *Biol. Reprod.* 1984; **31**:785–795.

10. Girsh E, Katz N, Genkin L, et al. Male age influences oocyte-donor program results. *J. Assist. Reprod. Genet.* 2008; **25**:137–143.

11. Masliukaite I, Hagen JM, Jahnukainen K, et al. Establishing reference values for age related spermatogonial quantity in prepubertal human testes: a systematic review and meta-analysis. *Fertil. Steril.* 2016; **106**:1652–1657.

12. Paniagua R, Nistal M. Morphological and histometric study of human spermatogonia from birth to the onset of puberty. *J. Anat.* 1984; **139**:535–552.

13. Trainer TD. Histology of the normal testis. *Am. J. Surg. Pathol.* 1987; **11**:787–809.

14. Sharpe RM, McKinnell C, Kivlin C, Fisher JS. Proliferation and functional maturation of Sertoli cells, and their relevance to disorders of testis function in adulthood. *Reproduction* 2003; **125**:769–784.

15. Hecht NB. Molecular mechanisms of male germ cell differentiation. *Bioassays* 1998; **20**:555–561.

16. Hecht NB. The making of a spermatozoon: a molecular perspective. *Dev. Genet.* 1995; **16**:95–103.

17. Gill-Sharma MK, Choudhuri JD, Souza S. Sperm chromatin protamination: an endocrine perspective. *Protein Pept. Lett.* 2011; **18**:786–801.

18. Carrell DT, Emery BR, Hammoud S. Altered protamine expression and diminished spermatogenesis: what is the link? *Hum. Reprod. Update* 2007; **13**:313–327.

19. Jager S. Sperm nuclear stability and male infertility. *Arch. Androl.* 1990; **25**:253–259.

20. Oliva R. Protamines and male infertility. *Hum. Reprod. Update* 2006; **12**:417–435.

21. Carrell DT, Emery BR, Hammoud S. The aetiology of sperm protamine abnormalities and their potential

impact on the sperm epigenome. *Int. J. Androl.* 2008; **31**:537–545.

22. Brumlow WB, Adams CS. Immunocytochemical detection of prolactin or prolactin-like immunoreactivity in epididymis of mature male mouse. *Histochemistry* 1990; **93**:299–304.

23. Dacheux JL, Dacheux F. New insights into epididymal function in relation to sperm maturation. *Reproduction* 2014; **147**:R27–R42.

24. Turner RM. Moving to the beat: a review of mammalian sperm motility regulation. *Reprod. Fert. Dev.* 2006; **18**:25–38.

25. Lotti F, Corona G, Maseroli E, et al. Clinical implications of measuring prolactin levels in males of infertile couples. *Andrology* 2013; **1**:764–771.

26. Rastrelli G, Corona G, Maggi M. The role of prolactin in andrology: what is new? *Rev. Endocr. Metab. Disord.* 2015; **16**:233–248.

27. Zukerman Z, Weiss DB, Orvieto R. Does preejaculatory penile secretion originating from Cowper's gland contain sperm? *J. Assist. Reprod. Gen.* 2003; **20**:157–159.

28. Björndahl L, Kvist U. Sequence of ejaculation affects the spermatozoon as a carrier and its message. *RBM Online* 2003; **7**:440–448.

29. Lilja H, Lundwall A. Molecular cloning of epididymal and seminal vesicular transcripts encoding a semenogelin-related protein. *Proc. Natl. Acad. Sci. U. S. A.* 1992; **89**:4559–4563.

30. Zaneveld LG, Tauber PF. Contribution of prostatic fluid components to the ejaculate. *Prog. Clin. Biol. Res.* 1981; **75A**:265–277.

31. Tomar AK, Sooch BS, Singh S, Yadav S. Differential proteomics of human seminal plasma: a potential target for searching male infertility marker proteins. *Proteomics Clin. Appl.* 2012; **6**:147–151.

32. Peter A, Lilja H, Lundwall A, Malm J. Semenogelin I and semenogelin II, the major gel-forming proteins in human semen, are substrates for transglutaminase. *Eur. J. Biochem.* 1998; **252**:216–221.

33. Suzuki K, Kise H, Nishioka J, Hayashi T. The interaction among protein C inhibitor, prostate-specific antigen, and the semenogelin system. *Semin. Thromb. Hemost.* 2007; **33**:46–52.

34. Sobrero AJ, Macleod J. The immediate postcoital test. *Fertil. Steril.* 1962; **13**:184–189.

35. Perloff WH, Steinberger E. In-vitro penetration of cervical mucus by spermatozoa. *Fertil. Steril.* 1963; **14**:231–236.

36. Publicover S, Harper CV, Barratt C. [Ca2+]i signaling in sperm—making the most of what you've got. *Nat. Cell Biol.* 2007; **9**:235–242.

37. Rode B, Dirami T, Bakouh N, et al. The testis anion transporter TAT1 (SLC26A8) physically and functionally interacts with the cystic fibrosis transmembrane conductance regulator channel: a potential role during sperm capacitation. *Hum. Mol. Genet.* 2012; **21**:1287–1298.

38. Krausz C, Bonaccorsi L, Luconi M, et al. Intracellular calcium increase and acrosome reaction in response to progesterone in human spermatozoa are correlated with in-vitro fertilization. *Hum. Reprod.* 1995; **10**:120–124.

39. Ankri R, Friedman H, Savion N, et al. Visible light induces nitric oxide (NO) formation in sperm and endothelial cells. *Lasers Surg. Med.* 2010; **42**:348–352.

40. Suarez SS. Control of hyperactivation in sperm. *Hum. Reprod. Update* 2008; **14**:647–657.

41. Nomikos M, Kashir J, Swann K, Lai FA. Sperm PLCζ: from structure to Ca2+ oscillations, egg activation and therapeutic potential. *FEBS Lett.* 2013; **587**:3609–3616.

42. Escoffier J, Yassine S, Lee HC, et al. Subcellular localization of phospholipase Cζ in human sperm and its absence in DPY19L2-deficient sperm are consistent with its role in oocyte activation. *Mol. Hum. Reprod.* 2015; **21**:157–168.

43. Heytens E, Parrington J, Coward K, et al. Reduced amounts and abnormal forms of phospholipase C zeta (PLCzeta) in spermatozoa from infertile men. *Hum. Reprod.* 2009; **24**:2417–2428.

44. Kashir J, Konstantinidis M, Jones C, et al. A maternally inherited autosomal point mutation in human phospholipase C zeta (PLCzeta) leads to male infertility. *Hum. Reprod.* 2012; **27**:222–231.

45. Küċükkömürcü S, Delogne-Desnoeck J, Robyn C. Prolactin and fructose in human seminal fluid. *Int. J. Fertil.* 1980; **25**:117–121.

46. Meikle AW, Stephenson RA, Lewis CM, Wiebke GA, Middleton RG. Age, genetic, and nongenetic factors influencing variation in serum sex steroids and zonal volumes of the prostate and benign prostatic hyperplasia in twins. *Prostate* 1997; **33**:105–111.

47. Chianese R, Cobellis G, Chioccarelli T, et al. Kisspeptins, estrogens and male fertility. *Curr. Med. Chem.* 2016; **23**:4070–4091.

48. Eskenazi B, Wyrobek AJ, Sloter E, et al. The association of age and semen quality in healthy men. *Hum. Reprod.* 2003; **18**:447–454.

49. Slama R, Bouyer J, Windham G, et al. Influence of paternal age on the risk of spontaneous abortion. *Am. J. Epidemiol.* 2005; **161**:816–823.

50. Sartorius GA, Nieschlag E. Paternal age and reproduction. *Hum. Reprod. Update* 2010; **16**:65–79.

51. Singh NP, Muller CH, Berger RE. Effects of age on DNA double-strand breaks and apoptosis in human sperm. *Fertil. Steril.* 2003; **80**:1420–1430.

52. Robinson L, Gallos ID, Conner SJ, et al. The effect of sperm DNA fragmentation on miscarriage rates: a systematic review and meta-analysis. *Hum. Reprod.* 2012; **27**:2908–2917.

53. Ford WCL, North K, Taylor H, et al. Increasing paternal age is associated with delayed conception in a large population of fertile couples: evidence for declining fecundity in older men. The ALSPAC Study Team (Avon Longitudinal Study of Pregnancy and Childhood). *Hum. Reprod.* 2000; **15**:1703–1708.

54. Hassan MA, Killick SR. Effect of male age on fertility: evidence for the decline in male fertility with increasing age. *Fertil. Steril.* 2003; **79**:1520–1527.

55. Yang Q, Wen SW, Leader A, et al. Paternal age and birth defects: how strong is the association? *Hum. Reprod.* 2007; **22**:696–701.

56. Orioli IM, Castilla EE, Scarano G, Mastroiacovo P. Effect of paternal age in achondroplasia, thanatophoric dysplasia, and osteogenesis imperfecta. *Am. J. Med. Genet.* 1995; **59**:209–217.

57. Lauritsen MB, Pedersen CB, Mortensen PB. Effects of familial risk factors and place of birth on the risk of autism: a nationwide register-based study. *J. Child. Psychol. Psychiatry* 2005; **46**:963–971.

58. Lawson G, Fletcher R. Delayed fatherhood. *J. Fam. Plann. Reprod. Health Care* 2014; **40**:283–288.

59. Gray A, Berlin JA, McKinlay JB, Longcope C. An examination of research design effects on the association of testosterone and male aging: results of a meta-analysis. *J. Clin. Epidemiol.* 1991; **44**:671–684.

60. Nieschlag E. The endocrine function of the human testis in regard to sexuality. *Ciba Found. Symp.* 1978; **14**:183–208.

61. Diver MJ, Imtiaz KE, Ahmad AM, Vora JP, Fraser WD. Diurnal rhythms of serum total, free and bioavailable testosterone and of SHBG in middle-aged men compared with those in young men. *Clin. Endocrinol. (Oxf.)* 2003; **58**:710–717.

62. Davidson JM, Chen JJ, Crapo L, et al. Hormonal changes and sexual function in aging men. *J. Clin. Endocrinol. Metab.* 1983; **57**:71–77.

63. Johnson JM, Nachtigall LB, Stern TA. The effect of testosterone levels on mood in men: a review. *Psychosomatics* 2013; **54**:509–514.

64. Hawton KE. Sexual problems associated with physical illness. In: Weatherall DJ, Ledingham JG, Warrell DA, eds., *Oxford Textbook of Medicine.* Oxford: Oxford University Press. 1997; 4243–4247.

65. Lašaitė L, Čeponis J, Preikša RT, Žilaitienė B. Effects of two-year testosterone replacement therapy on cognition, emotions and quality of life in young and middle-aged hypogonadal men. *Andrologia* 2017; **49**(3):10.1111/and.12633.

66. Janowsky JS, Oviatt SK, Orwoll ES. Testosterone influences spatial cognition in older men. *Behav. Neurosci.* 1994; **108**:325–332.

67. Finkelstein JS. Androgens and bone metabolism. In: Nieschlag E, Behre HM, eds., *Testosterone: Action, Deficiency, Substitution.* Berlin: Springer Verlag. 1998; 187–207.

68. Bhasin S, Storer TW, Berman N, et al. Testosterone replacement increases fat-free mass and muscle size in hypogonadal men. *J. Clin. Endocrinol. Metab.* 1997; **82**:407–413.

69. Haider A, Yassin A, Haider KS, et al. Men with testosterone deficiency and a history of cardiovascular diseases benefit from long-term testosterone therapy: observational, real-life data from a registry study. *Vasc. Health Risk Manag.* 2016; **14**:251–261.

Physiology of the Female Reproductive System

The physiological importance of the female reproductive system is the production of offspring. The female produces gametes that can be fertilized by the male gamete to form the first cell of the offspring. The sequence of events is tightly dependent on the proper functionality of the endocrine system.

Much of the endocrine system is governed by rhythms, some of which are intrinsic, while others are influenced by the environment. Rhythms that are longer than 24 hours, the infradian rhythms, include the seasonal breeding patterns in some animals and the female menstrual cycle. Circadian or 24-hour rhythms include the sleep–wake cycle and the increase in gonadotropin secretion seen at night in adolescents. Finally, cycles of less than 24 hour, the ultradian cycles, include the pulsatile release of luteinizing hormone (LH), follicle-stimulating hormone (FSH), growth hormone, and prolactin.

The reproductive axis is a finely controlled system consisting of three endocrine organs: the hypothalamus, pituitary (hypophysis), and gonads (Figure 4.1). Each of these organs secretes hormones critical for normal reproduction. The hormones feedback, at multiple levels of the reproductive axis, to control their synthesis and secretion, resulting in a tightly regulated system.

Hormonal Regulation of Reproduction

Puberty is the event that switches the reproductive system on and is restrained by higher levels of central nervous system control. The earlier endocrine event of puberty is an increase in the sensitization in kisspeptin pulses at night and an increase in the pulsatile release of the hypothalamic decapeptide gonadotropin-releasing hormone (GnRH) in an episodic pattern of pulses into the hypothalamic–pituitary portal system [1]. GnRH travels through the hypophysial portal blood system to the anterior pituitary, where it binds to the GnRH receptors on the cell surface of the gonadotropes. This is reflected by an increase in

FSH and LH secretion. The secretion of FSH and LH at the appropriate frequency and amplitude is critical for normal fertility in the female. Gonadal steroids are produced due to positive feedback of gonadotropin stimulation. The pubertal growth start results from an increase in growth hormone production induced by sex steroids, as well as by local production of growth factors. Positive feedback leads to the onset of ovulation and menses in girls by mid-puberty or later.

Low levels of estradiol (E_2) have little effect on LH secretion and inhibit FSH secretion. High levels of E_2 induce the LH surge at midcycle, and high steady levels of E_2 lead to sustained elevated LH secretion. Low levels of progesterone (P_4), acting at the level of the pituitary gland, enhance the LH response to GnRH and are responsible for the FSH surge at midcycle. High levels of P_4 inhibit the pituitary secretion of gonadotropins by inhibiting GnRH pulses at the level of the hypothalamus. The hypothalamic–pituitary axis is described in detail in Chapter 2.

The Vagina

The vagina is a tubular muscular organ, about 7–8 cm long, and is capable of great distention (Figure 4.2). The organ extends from its external orifice in the vestibule between the labia minora of the vulva to the cervix. It is composed mainly of smooth muscle and is lined with a mucous membrane. The vaginal mucosa contains tiny exocrine glands (Bartholin's glands) that secrete lubricating fluid during sexual response. During sexual intercourse, the vagina triggers the ejaculation of semen and serves as a receptacle for semen. The vagina also serves as the lower portion of the birth canal.

The "normal" microbiome of the vagina in nonpregnant, healthy women predominantly includes a variety of *Lactobacillus* species, which provide a healthy, supportive environment [2]. In healthy individuals, *Lactobacillus* species dominate this ecosystem at a concentration of 10^7–10^8 colony forming

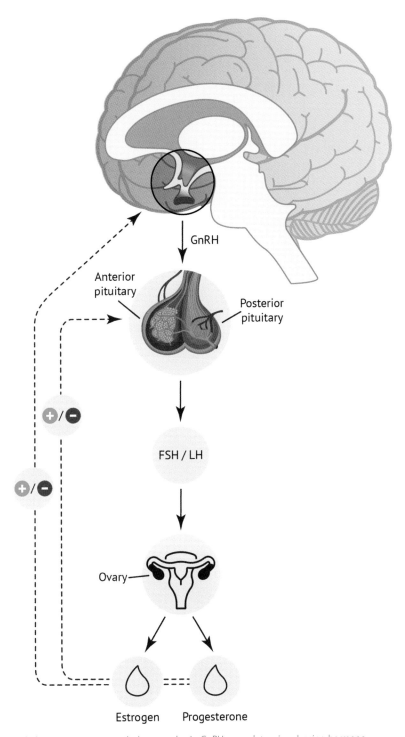

Figure 4.1 Female hypothalamic–pituitary–gonads–hormonal axis. GnRH, gonadotropin-releasing hormone.

units per gram of vaginal fluid. Broadly, the vaginal microbiota (VMB) can be classified into different community groups or grades. In an analysis of VMB samples collected from healthy, nonpregnant women, Grade I, characterized by a dominance of *Lactobacillus crispatus*, was found in 26.2% of the sampled

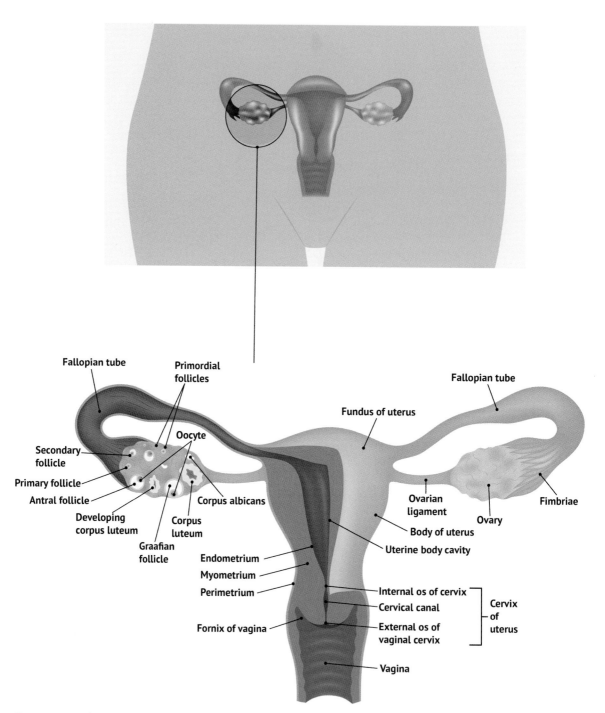

Figure 4.2 Female reproductive anatomy.

population, while Grades II (6.3%), III (34.1%), and V (5.3%) were characterized by a dominance of *Lactobacillus gasseri*, *Lactobacillus iners*, and *Lactobacillus jensenii*, respectively. These four main groups were isolated primarily from White and Asian women. Grade IV, found mainly in Black and Hispanic women, was classified by the dominance of non-*Lactobacillus* species, and included *Gardnerella*,

Prevotella, Corynebacterium, Atopobium, Megasphaera, and *Sneathia* [3]. Lactobacilli and other bacteria metabolize glycogen to glucose and maltose and further to lactic acid, resulting in a vaginal pH of 3.8–4.4, which is defined as normal.

The Uterus

The uterus serves as the site of embryo implantation and development. In a woman who has never been pregnant, the uterus is pear-shaped and measures approximately 7.5 cm in length, 5 cm in width at its widest part, and 3 cm in thickness. The uterus has two main parts: the body at the top, and the cervix, a lower, narrow "neck" (Figure 4.2).

The uterine wall comprises three layers: an inner endometrium, middle myometrium, and an incomplete outer layer of the parietal peritoneum. The endometrium lines the mucous membrane, and is composed of three layers: a compact surface layer of partially ciliated, simple columnar epithelial cells called the stratum compactum, a spongy middle layer of loose connective tissue called the stratum spongiosum and a dense inner layer termed the stratum basale that attaches the endometrium to the underlying myometrium. Throughout menstruation and after delivery of a baby, the compact and spongy layers slough off. The endometrium varies in thickness from 0.5 mm just after menstruation, to about 5 mm near the end of the endometrial cycle (before menstrual flow). The endometrium has a rich supply of capillaries, as well as numerous exocrine glands that produce mucus and other substances onto the endometrial surface.

The myometrium consists of three layers of smooth muscle fibers that extend in all directions, and give the uterus great strength.

The peritoneum is the serous membrane covering the abdominal cavity. This peritoneal lining of the cavity supports many of the abdominal organs and serves as a conduit for their blood vessels, lymphatic vessels, and nerves.

The cavity of the uterine body is directed downward and constitutes the internal os, which opens into the cervical canal. The cervical canal forms the external os, which opens into the vagina. The mucous glands in the lining of the cervix produce mucus that changes in consistency during the female reproductive cycle. Most of the time, cervical mucus acts as a barrier to sperm. Cervical mucus becomes more slippery and facilitates the movement of sperm through the cervix around the time of ovulation.

The uterus obtains a generous supply of blood from uterine arteries, which branch off from the internal iliac arteries. Also, the ovarian and vaginal arteries anastomose with the uterine vessels, thereby serving as an additional blood source. Arterial vessels penetrate the layers of the uterine wall as arterioles and then break up into capillaries between the endometrial glands. Uterine, ovarian, and vaginal veins return venous blood from the uterus to the internal iliac veins.

As in the vagina, the "normal" microbiome of the uterus in nonpregnant, healthy women predominantly includes a variety of *Lactobacillus* species. The low abundance of *Lactobacillus* in the endometrium is associated with poor reproductive and IVF outcomes [2].

Mayer–Rokitansky–Küster–Hauser (MRKH) syndrome, a well-established uterine anomaly, involves an uncommon variation in the prenatal development of the female genital tract. Its incidence is approximately 1 in 4000–5000 female births, and its underlying cause is unknown. The syndrome features include an absent or very short vagina and a uterus that can be absent or immaturely formed. Females with MRKH syndrome have functioning ovaries, normal external genitalia, and the genetic appearance of 46,XX female chromosome pattern. Breast development and growth of pubic hair are also typical. Associated renal and/or skeletal abnormalities are shared. MRKH syndrome is also known as Müllerian (female internal sex organs) agenesis (no growth) syndrome. The usual external appearance of MRKH females makes it difficult to diagnose until puberty – often when a girl visits a physician because she has not started to menstruate. In some cases, a young woman may have attempted unsuccessfully to have intercourse. The average age of diagnosis usually is between 15 and 18 years, although occasionally, a girl may be diagnosed at birth or during childhood because of other health problems. A pelvic ultrasound may be used to determine the presence or absence of the uterus and its condition.

The Uterine Tubes

The uterine tubes are also called Fallopian tubes or oviducts. The first correct anatomical description of uterine tubes was in 1561 by Gabrielis Fallopius. In 1566, Fallopius described the extension of these tubes from the uterus to the ovaries. Reinier de Graaf defined the function of the Fallopian tubes in 1672.

The Fallopian tubes are approximately 10 cm long and are attached to the uterus at its upper outer angles. The same three layers (mucous, smooth muscle, and serous) of the uterus compose the tubes. Inflammation of the uterine tubes may lead to scarring and partial or complete closure. The pH in the female reproductive tract is graduated, with the lowest pH in the vagina (~pH 4.4) increasing toward the Fallopian tubes (~pH 7.9), reflecting variation in the site-specific microbiome and acid–base buffering at the tissue/cellular level.

The Ovary

The female gonads, or ovaries, are homologous (in origin) to the testis in the male. The adult ovaries weigh about 4–8 g each. They are paired and located on each side of the uterus (Figure 4.2). The ovary consists of three main parts: the outer cortex (the major bulk of follicles), the inner medulla, and the hilum. The hilum is the part of the ovary which attaches along its anterior margin by a double fold of peritoneum, the mesovarian ligament (mesovarium), and broad ligament. The ovarian ligament anchors it to the uterus. It includes blood support and nerves. The rete ovarii, the ovarian analog of the rete testis, is present in the hilus of all ovaries. After menopause, the ovaries typically shrink to a size approximately one-half that has been seen in the reproductive period.

The ovary is not quiescent during childhood. Follicles begin to grow at all times and frequently reach the antral stage. The lack of gonadotropin support prevents full follicular development and function. There is no evidence that ovarian function is necessary until puberty. However, before puberty, the oocytes are active and synthesize mRNAs and protein. Ovariectomy in prepubertal monkeys has indicated that the prepubertal suppression of GnRH and gonadotropins is partially dependent on the presence of ovaries, suggesting some functional activity of the ovary in childhood.

Female fertility depends on the supply and maturation of the ovarian germ cells, i.e., the oocytes, and the differentiation and proliferation of the ovarian somatic cells, i.e., granulosa cells (GCs) and theca cells (TCs). Assembly of oocytes and somatic cells into follicular structures, a process also called initial folliculogenesis, marks the last step of ovarian differentiation. During folliculogenesis, oocytes grow in size, and are surrounded by an increasing number of GC layers; from the preantral stage onward, TCs differentiate outside the follicle. GCs are delimited by a thin basement membrane and bordered outside by mesenchymal cells.

When a primordial follicle enters the growth phase, its surrounding flat GCs become cuboidal and proliferative. Follicles reach the primary (one layer of flattened GCs), preantral (number of GCs), and antral (antral cavity) stages [4]. As maturation advances, the number of granulosa layers increases, and the cells begin secreting increasing amounts of an estrogen-rich fluid that pools around the oocyte in a space called an antrum. From puberty onward, the follicle can pass into the preovulatory follicle stage in which the oocyte resumes meiosis and becomes arrested again in metaphase II. The oocyte is then ovulated in the oviduct, rendering it ready for fertilization. Subsequently, TCs and GCs differentiate into luteal cells and form the corpus luteum (CL), which produces P_4 (Figure 4.3).

Follicular growth and atresia are not interrupted by pregnancy, ovulation, or periods of anovulation. This dynamic process continues at all ages, including infancy, and around menopause. At puberty, ovaries contain approximately 300 000–400 000 follicles; however, from this large reservoir, about 400–500 follicles will ovulate during a woman's reproductive years. The antral follicle count (AFC) positively correlates with age and declines at a rate of 3.8% per year [5]. Follicular decline (atresia/apoptosis) causes the elimination of more than 99% of germ cells from a cohort of the ovary.

Folliculogenesis

During the reproductive era, primordial follicles are found in clusters in the superficial cortex. They contain a primary oocyte, measuring 40–70 μm in diameter, surrounded by a single layer of flattened, mitotically inactive GCs, resting on a thin basal lamina. When follicles enter the growth phase, they increase, both by a proliferation of GCs and by an increase in the size of the oocyte. The first morphological evidence of follicular growth is the assumption of a cuboidal to columnar shape among GCs. Although primary and preantral follicles can grow in the absence of gonadotropins, optimal development may require these hormones. In contrast, beyond the antral follicle stage, follicular growth, maturation, and survival are dependent on gonadotropins [4]. When early-growing follicles become vascularized, they are

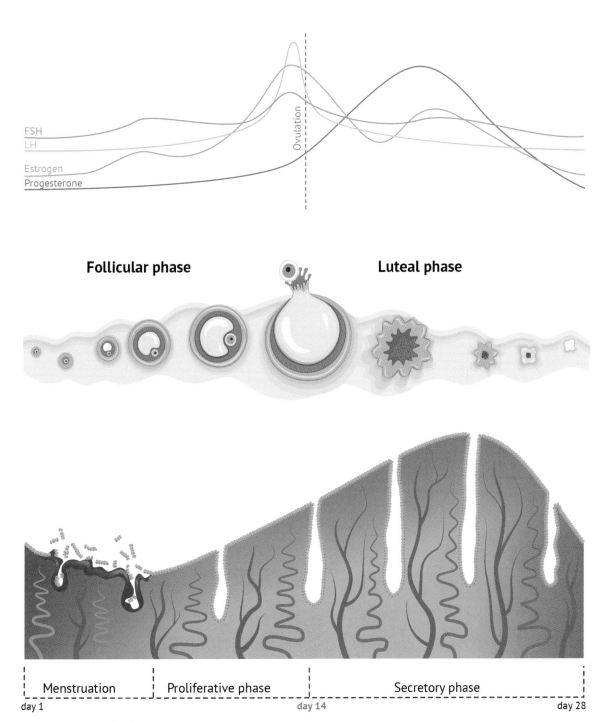

Figure 4.3 Menstrual cycle.

directly exposed to factors circulating in the blood. Circulating FSH is the earlier regulator of ovarian folliculogenesis. However, despite the presence of FSH receptors on GCs [6], the role of FSH in

sustaining early follicular growth remains unclear, as follicles at this stage seem to be unresponsive to gonadotropins [7–9]. Indeed, follicles smaller than 2 mm do not display any change in GC proliferation upon cyclic changes in FSH levels [4]. Under conditions of FSH deprivation, the development of early-growing follicles can be continued by local factors. However, it appears possible that these factors are less efficient at sustaining growth than they are when they act in synergy with FSH.

At this stage of growth, a system of gap junctions, i.e., intercellular channels that allow nutrients, inorganic ions, second messengers, and small metabolites to pass from cell to cell, appear in the GC layer. These channels are composed of connexins (Cx), with connexin 43 (Cx43) being the most abundant Cx in the ovary and expressed in the GCs from the start of folliculogenesis.

Paracrine factors and intercellular gap junctions ensure complex bidirectional communication between the oocyte and its surrounding somatic cells during folliculogenesis, for the coordinated development of both somatic cell and germ cell compartments [10–11]. In this dialog, the oocyte plays a vital role in the early stages of follicular growth on somatic cells [12]. Among the oocyte-specific factors potentially involved in GC proliferation are three members of the transforming growth factor-beta (TGF-β) superfamily, i.e., growth differentiation factor 9 (GDF-9), bone morphogenetic protein 15 (BMP-15) and BMP-6 [13]. Oocyte factors potentially involved in the initiation of follicular growth include KIT, a receptor activated by GC-derived KIT ligand (KL), as well as fibroblast growth factor 2 (FGF2) [14–15]. Other molecules have been reported capable of stimulating the initiation of follicular growth, with a body of evidence demonstrating a role for neurotrophic factors, including nerve growth factor (NGF), brain-derived neurotrophic factor (BDNF), and neutrophins [16–18]. Oocytectomy of rabbit preovulatory follicles led to the early luteinization of follicles and increased P_4 production [19]. Similarly, GCs from rat antral follicles transform into luteal cells after oocytectomy [20]. Gradually, follicles become secondary follicles, i.e., follicles with three or more complete layers of GCs surrounding the oocyte that are served by one or two arterioles, terminating in an anastomotic network just outside the basal lamina. The importance of this event is highlighted by the fact that the follicle becomes directly exposed to factors circulating in the blood. At this stage, an acellular layer, the zona pellucida (ZP), arises and encases the oocyte. Its formation is usually attributed to the GC, but the oocyte may also play a role.

Simultaneously, the surrounding ovarian stroma cells near the basal lamina become aligned parallel to each other and constitute the theca layer. As the follicle enlarges, the TCs differentiate into two parts. The outer part, named theca externa, is composed of cells that do not differ from undifferentiated TCs. In the inner part, named theca interna, some fibroblast-like precursor cells assume the appearance of typical steroid-secreting cells, also referred to as epithelioid cells. From the time of appearance of epithelioid cells, the secondary follicle is defined as a preantral follicle and constitutes the first class of growing follicles, with classification based on morphological aspects and the total number of GCs in each follicle [4]. GCs of preantral, small antral, and mid-antral follicles (5–8 mm) exclusively produce anti-Müllerian hormone (AMH) [21] and make the greatest contribution (~60%) to serum AMH. In more developed follicles, follicles >10 mm in diameter, the GCs fail to produce AMH. AMH was first discovered in follicular fluid (FF) in 1993. AMH inhibits follicular development and recruitment and suppresses primordial follicle activation. Both AMH gene expression and concentrations in FF negatively correlate with the E_2 concentration [22]. Absolute serum levels of AMH do not necessarily reflect the number of ovarian follicles; although detection of serum AMH indicates the presence of secondary or early antral follicles, one cannot rule out the presence of non-AMH-secreting primordial follicles. Patients with undetectable AMH levels have responded to hormonal treatment due to the presence of residual primordial follicles. Thus, the detection of serum AMH ensures the presence of secondary follicles but does not accurately reflect ovarian reserve.

The first evidence of antrum formation occurs in follicles measuring 200–400 μm in diameter. When small fluid-filled cavities merge to form the antrum, the follicle enters the early antral phase and possesses FF with a composition similar to that of the blood serum. From this time, the GCs surrounding the oocyte proliferate and differentiate to form the "cumulus oophorus," which contains the oocyte in its center and protrudes into the antrum. Since there is great importance of wide interactions between the oocyte and follicular tissues, the GC–oocyte gap junctions play a critical role during folliculogenesis. Also, within the large antral follicle, the oocyte plays a role in the establishment of the various functions of the two GC subpopulations, i.e., mural GC and granulosa-derived cumulus cells (CCs). After gonadotropin stimulation, mural GCs express LH receptors [23–24], while CCs do not express LH receptors, P450, or P_4 receptors, but do synthesize hyaluronic acid, an extracellular matrix component enabling the expansion of the cumulus within the follicular cavity [25]. LH receptor concentrations are highest in the cells closest to the basement membrane and are lowest in those that surround the oocyte [26]. Growing oocytes accelerate follicular development, suggesting that the oocyte may act as a "folliculogenesis clock."

With the accumulation of fluid in the antral cavity and proliferation of GCs and TCs, the follicle progresses at an increasing rate through following stages of development, until it reaches a size of 2–3 mm, and becomes a selectable follicle. The early-growing follicle reaches the preantral stage within 2–3 months, and 70 additional days are necessary for the preantral follicle to become early antral reaching a size of approximately 2 mm [27].

Healthy selectable follicles are detected at all stages of the menstrual cycle. During the late luteal phase, their number rises in response to elevating peripheral FSH levels [28]. At this point, there are between 3 and 11 selectable follicles per ovary in women between the ages of 24 and 33 years [29], but counts significantly decline with age. The follicle intended to ovulate during the subsequent cycle will be selected from this bank of follicles [28; 30]. Whereas early-growing follicles are unresponsive to cyclic hormonal changes, selectable follicles are more receptive to these alterations, owing to the increased expression of LH receptors [31], which

heightens sensitivity to an elevating LH pulse frequency (every 90 minutes) during the early follicular phase [32], and later stages of the follicular phase (every 60 minutes) [33], as well as to the positive effect of GDF-9 on androgen production (via activity of enzymes involved in androgen production) by TCs [34]. When follicles reach the selectable phase, their GCs are characterized by increasing concentrations of FSH receptors, which are responsive to the proliferation-related FSH effects, but not to its impact on estrogen production.

The ovarian cycle can be readily assessed via serial ovarian ultrasound scans and serum hormone measurements throughout the menstrual cycle (Figure 4.4). During the menstruation, there are numerous antral follicles in the ovaries measuring 4–8 mm in diameter. These follicles develop from primordial follicles through both gonadotropin-independent and gonadotropin-sensitive phases of growth [35]. It is not very easy to determine how long this process takes, but evidence from tissue transplantation studies proposes that it is longer than 3 months [36]. These antral follicles are gonadotropin dependent and will not continue to grow without gonadotropin stimulation.

The rate of follicle growth can vary from cycle to cycle and from woman to woman (Figure 4.5). Differences in the length of a menstrual cycle depend on the variations in the length of early- to mid-follicular phases. However, when the leading follicle reaches 12 mm in diameter, generally on day 9 or 10 of the menstrual cycle, it continues to grow at an

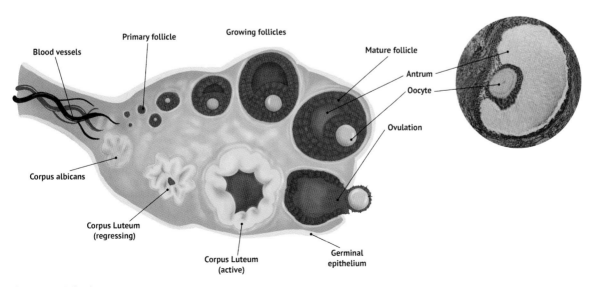

Figure 4.4 Folliculogenesis.

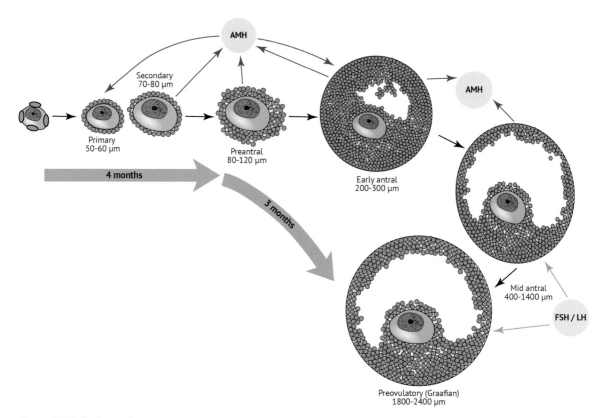

Figure 4.5 Folliculogenesis.

average of 2 mm in diameter each day. This growth is associated with rapidly increasing E_2 concentrations that exert negative feedback on the pituitary to reduce FSH secretion. Follicles larger than 12 mm in diameter will already be expressing LH receptors on their GCs, and LH will maintain follicle growth and function in the presence of declining FSH concentrations. This machinery is responsible for the follicular selection and uni-follicular ovulation; however, it means that follicles reaching 12 mm or more may also ovulate in response to an LH surge. Increasing E_2 secretion from the dominant follicle promotes a switch to positive feedback at the hypothalamus and pituitary that results in a gonadotropin surge. The dominant follicle will generally measure between 17 and 23 mm in diameter at the time of the LH surge, which usually occurs on days 14–15 of a regular menstrual cycle. Generally, the length of the menstrual cycle is 28 days (22–44 days), time to ovulation is close to 14.8 days (9–33 days), and the postovulatory phase is close to 13.2 days (7–17 days).

At the late follicular phase, LH secretion frequency accelerates to occur every 65 minutes. The major effect of LH binding is the activation of G protein, which, in turn, activates adenylate cyclase and increases the production of cAMP [37]. The cAMP-dependent protein kinase A (PKA) pathway is significant; however, LH receptor binding also activates Phospholiase C/inositol phosphate signaling independent of the cAMP/PKA pathway. Other cellular pathways involving ERK and AKT are associated with LH receptor signaling and may have a part in non-steroidogenic processes, such as cell proliferation, differentiation, and cell survival in the follicle [38]. At least 20–30 isoforms of both FSH and LH circulate in the blood during the menstrual cycle [39], each of which may bear different bioactivity.

The dominant healthy follicle appears to be the selected follicle. It grows at a quicker rate than do other subordinate follicles [27], contains a detectable level of FSH [40], and differs substantially from selectable follicles by a concomitant increase in E_2 receptors within the GC and the E_2 levels within the FF.

In addition to E_2, FF contains a broad profile of active compounds such as classical hormones (FSH, LH, growth hormone, prolactin, P_4, prostaglandins [PGs], corticoids), TGF-β superfamily members (inhibin, activin, AMH, BMP-15), growth factors (insulin-like growth factor-I [IGF-I], IGF-II, tumor necrosis factor alpha, FGF2), interleukins (IL-1, IL-2, IL-10, IL-12), proteins and peptides (α-fetoprotein, leptin, endothelin, oxytocin, vasopressin, oocyte maturation inhibitor, homocysteine, β-endorphin, lactoferrin, angiotensin II, prorenin), and others.

At ovulation, the cumulus–oocyte complex is released from the ruptured follicle. As the oocyte does not express LH receptors, its maturation is associated with ovulation and mediated by the neighboring GCs and CCs. The LH surge causes a breakdown of cellular communications between the oocyte, CCs and GCs, and because GCs are involved in the maintenance of oocyte arrest, maturation is thereby stimulated [41].

Oocyte Growth

The oocyte, which is present in the ovary of the mammalian female from birth, is arrested at prophase (diplotene stage with four full sets of chromosomes) of the first meiosis. During early follicle development the oocyte grows at the quickest rate, increasing its diameter from approximately 40–70 μm in large primary follicles to around 100 μm in early antral follicles. Next to this stage of development, the oocyte diameter increases at a prolonged rate, reaching approximately 140 μm (120–150 μm) in the preovulatory follicle.

The oocyte can already control follicular growth during early follicle development. Deletion of *Pten* in the oocyte leads to enhanced activation of the primordial follicle, while the deletion of *Pdk1* reduces primordial follicle survival and accelerates ovarian aging [42]. The oocyte, which might possess FSH receptors [43–44], begins to produce factors such as GDF-9 and BMP-15 that are specific regulators of follicle development. Both GDF-9 and BMP-15 bind to specific TGF-β superfamily receptors located on the membrane of GCs or CCs. The oocyte can control its growth through GDF-9, which downregulates KL expression in GCs, which, in turn, regulates BMP-15 expression in the oocyte [45]. Just as the oocyte controls follicular development, follicular cells can also control oocyte growth. Activin secreted from GCs can negatively control oocyte development.

The oocyte is encased by the ZP. The human ZP is a matrix composed of four glycoproteins (ZP1, ZP2, ZP3, and ZPB) [46], which surrounds all mammalian oocytes and mediates several essential roles such as binding sperm in a species-specific manner, inducing the acrosome reaction, preventing polyspermia, and protecting the embryo before implantation. The space formed between the oocyte membrane (oolemma) and the ZP of the oocyte is called the perivitelline space. This space does not develop in the oocyte at the germinal vesicle (GV) stage and could be seen after the oocyte completes its maturation. CCs communicate with the oocyte via transzonal projections (microvilli and cilia), which penetrate the ZP to form oocyte–CC junctions [47].

Small molecules are transferred in both directions and impact both the oocyte and the follicle. To maintain meiotic arrest, GCs produce natriuretic peptide precursor type C (NPPC) that binds NPPC receptors (NPR2) on CCs, resulting in the production of cGMP, which is then transferred to the oocyte via gap junctions to inhibit phosphodiesterase 3A activity, thereby preventing hydrolysis of cAMP, ensuring meiotic arrest. CCs also produce cAMP in response to FSH and LH stimulation. In turn, cAMP activates PKA, which inhibits transition of the oocyte from the GV to prophase of the first meiosis (M I) stage, ensuring the meiotic arrest.

Follicular Steroidogenesis

Steroidogenesis, beginning with the uptake of cholesterol from circulating lipoproteins and storage of cholesterol as esters in cellular lipid droplets, is crucial for the synchronization of follicle growth and oocyte development. The theca interna utilizes cholesterol for *de novo* synthesis of pregnenolone, which is then enzymatically converted into P_4, and then into androstenedione [48]. Androgen secretion by TCs under LH stimulation appears to result from the activity of mitochondrial enzymes, such as cholesterol side-chain cleavage (P450scc), which converts cholesterol to pregnenolone. Then, 3β-hydroxysteroid dehydrogenase (3β-HSD) converts pregnenolone to P_4, which is then converted to androstenedione and testosterone by 17α-hydroxylase/lyase (P450c17α/lyase), respectively. Androgen receptor-mediated events (increased expression of FSH receptor, IGF-I receptor, and IGF-I in GCs) allow the growing follicle to interact with FSH, growth factors, and oocyte-derived factors to promote GC differentiation into mural and cumulus cell layers. The androgens cross the basement membrane into the GC, where they are converted to estrogens by the actions of aromatase (CYP19A1) [49], which is absent in TCs. These changes lead to maximal intrafollicular E_2 concentrations that coincide with the plasma E_2 peak. From the early to late follicular phase, E_2 levels in human FF increase from 658 ng/ml to 2583 ng/ml. At the same time, intrafollicular concentrations of 17α-OH progesterone and P_4 increase; these progestins are mainly produced by TCs, since 3β-HSD is only slightly expressed in GCs [50] and P450c17α/lyase is absent. This two-cell (TC–GC) steroidogenic process, facilitated by GC-derived paracrine factors that promote TC P450c17 activity, ensures adequate aromatizable androgen production for continuous E_2 synthesis, despite declining serum FSH levels with follicle growth (Figure 4.6). E_2 is crucial for proper oocyte development because immature human oocytes have E_2-dependent, calcium-mediated mechanisms of cytoplasmic maturation that are susceptible to inhibition of androgen levels. Immature human oocytes from small, hyperandrogenic polycystic ovary syndrome follicles exhibit lower rates of in vitro maturation, fertilization, and embryo development.

Atretic Follicles

Of the original primordial follicles present at birth, approximately 0.1% mature to the point of ovulation. The remaining 99.9% undergo atresia, a process that begins before birth and continues throughout adolescent and reproductive life, but which is most intense immediately after birth and during puberty and pregnancy [51–52]. Factors that initiate atresia and determine which follicles will ultimately undergo atresia are unknown. Atresia of early follicles (primordial and preantral) begins with degeneration of the oocyte, manifested by nuclear changes. Degeneration of the GCs soon follows and the follicle disappears without a trace. In contrast, atresia of follicles that have reached the antral stage of development is more complex and variable but ultimately leads to obliterative atresia and the formation of scar, corpus fibrosum [53]. The earliest evidence of this process is the mitotic inactivity of

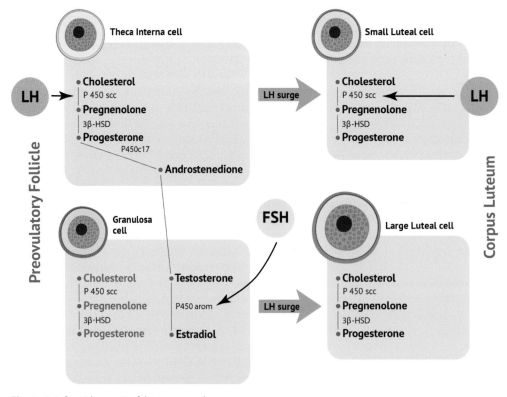

Figure 4.6 Steroidogenesis of the estrous cycle.

the GC. Some follicles may persist as atretic cystic follicles for an indefinite time interval.

Maturation of the Preovulatory Follicle

From the time it is selected, the follicle destined to ovulate enlarges significantly, from 6.9 ± 0.5 mm (diameter, counting from 2 to 5×10^6 GCs) during the early follicular phase, to 18.8 ± 0.5 mm (50 to 100×10^6 GCs) during the late follicular phase, which demands a high growth rate during the early follicular phase. This growth is accompanied by a massive generation of radicals that require protection against free radicals. During this final stage of growth, the GCs are subjected to marked morphological alterations, resulting from modulation of the cytoskeleton organization [54].

From the time it is selected, the follicle destined to ovulate shows marked changes in its steroidogenic activity. On the one hand, the production of androgens by the TCs is enhanced in response to increasing production of inhibin A [55–56], which strongly stimulates P450c17α/lyase. On the other hand, aromatase expression, which is detected only in GCs of follicles $\geq$10 mm [57], is stimulated by increased production of IGF-II [58], while NGF stimulates both FSH receptor synthesis and E_2 production [59]. As the follicle matures, the circulating levels of FSH decline in response to E_2 and inhibin produced by the follicle itself. With the rise in plasma LH levels, the concentration of LH receptors within the GCs, and the binding ability of the preovulatory follicle is elevated [31; 60]. The highest concentrations of LH receptors were found in mural GCs close to the basement membrane, while lower concentrations were measured in GCs located closer to the antrum; CCs and the oocyte lack LH receptors. At this stage, the preovulatory follicle continues to mature under the influence of intrafollicular FSH and E_2 [61–62], thereby maintaining a high E_2:androstenedione ratio [63].

During maturation, the preovulatory follicle becomes a highly vascularized structure [64]. The considerable increase in thecal vascularization occurs as a result of active endothelial cell proliferation in thecal layer blood capillaries, induced by angiogenic factors, such as vascular endothelial growth factor (VEGF) [65].

Shortly before ovulation, the preovulatory follicle reaches a diameter of 15–25 mm [62] and partially protrudes from the ovarian surface at a point that represents the eventual rupture point, or stigma.

Ovulation

Ovulation is the release of an oocyte–cumulus complex from the stigma of the follicle from a single ovary. After the oocyte–cumulus complex is released, it travels down the Fallopian tube, where fertilization by a sperm cell may occur. Ovulation typically occurs in the middle of a woman's menstrual cycle, but the timing of the process varies for each woman, and it may even vary from month to month.

High circulating E_2 levels, released by the dominant follicle, initiate a preovulatory surge of plasma LH [66]. Serum E_2 peaks approximately one day before the LH surge and 37 hours before ovulation. The LH surge generally occurs on days 14–15 of a typical 28-day menstrual cycle (may occur between day 9 and 30 of a cycle). LH surges are extremely variable in configuration (one peak or few peaks), amplitude, and duration (1–10 days) in healthy, contraceptive-free, regularly cycling women with proven fertility [67–69]. The day of the LH surge is believed to be the day of maximum fertility. Ovulation has been estimated to occur 36 ± 5 hours after the onset of the LH surge, 24–36 hours after the E_2 peak, and 10–12 hours after the LH peak [66; 70]. Ovulation is believed to have occurred if the follicle reached a mean diameter of 18 mm to 26 mm and changed in shape or sonographic density [71]. The preovulatory LH rise appears to have a circadian rate, occurring in the early morning in the majority of women. Within 6 hours of the start of the LH surge, the GCs show signs of early luteinization and begin to secrete P_4, initially into the FF, but later into the ovarian vein and general circulation. Circulating P_4 impacts the temperature regulation center of the brain, resulting in a rise in body temperature. The primary reason for this phenomenon is an increase in the production and secretion of norepinephrine, which is a thermogenic neural hormone.

The LH surge induces distinct processes involved in ovulation, which can be split into three components. One component of ovulation is a reactivation of oocyte maturation wherein the oocyte, which has been maintained in the diplotene stage of prophase, progresses to metaphase of the second meiotic division. Another component is GC luteinization, whereupon the GCs develop the enzymatic machinery to synthesize P_4. The third component of the ovulatory response induced by the LH surge is follicular rupture, which is an inflammatory process involving the breakdown of the apical follicular wall (Figure 4.7) [72].

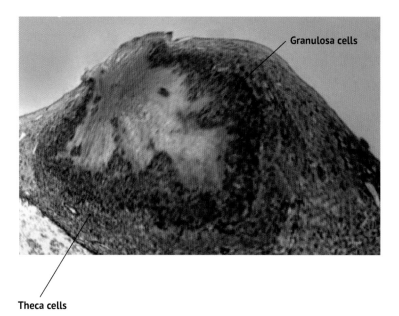

Granulosa cells

Theca cells

Figure 4.7 Ovulation.

The breakdown of the apical follicle wall depends on several events, one of which is constriction [73–74], which can be induced by PGs [75–76]. The LH surge upregulates PG synthesis in GCs, reaching peak concentrations just before ovulation [77]. Oxytocin is another great constrictor and its concentrations are elevated in the FF in response to luteinization [78–79]. Metalloproteinases have also been proposed to be involved in this process [80].

The LH peak induces a significant disruption and decline in gap junctions [54], leading to dissociation of mural GCs and expansion of the cumulus–oocyte complex, which constitutes a highly specialized inflammatory-related process involving activation of a variety of genes, and that is obligatory for successful ovulation [81–82]. LH-induced gap junction gating in ovarian follicles comprises two steps. First, the phosphorylation status of Cx43 protein (gap close/open) is modified immediately upon the LH surge. Later, Cx43 protein concentrations are reduced due to the attenuation of its gene expression at the transcriptional, translational, and post-translational levels [83]. Only gap junctions between GCs and CCs, which are composed of Cx43, are affected, whereas gap junctions between CCs and oocyte remain open because they are formed of Cx37. Gap junction closure between GCs–GCs and GCs–CCs reduces the supply of cGMP to the oocyte, thereby activating intra-oocyte phosphodiesterase that breaks

down intra-oocyte cAMP. Disconnection of the gap junctions reduces the cAMP supply to the oocyte and, therefore, reduces the level of cAMP and switches up maturation-promoting factor, which then reinitiates meiosis and oocyte maturation. LH also inhibits adenylate cyclase and reduces the production of cAMP, which has an added effect on oocyte maturation.

Cumulus–oocyte complex expansion at ovulation requires the action of local factors produced by GCs and the oocyte in response to indirect actions of LH. These include epidermal growth factor (EGF) family members such as amphiregulin, epiregulin [84], and β-cellulin, which are produced by the mural, but not cumulus, GCs in response to LH and are mandatory for CC expansion [85]. Prostaglandin E (PGE) is also involved in this process [86]. Oocyte release of both BMP-15, whose production may be upregulated by FSH [87], and GDF-9, which stimulates, among others, expression of hyaluronan synthase and cyclo-oxygenase 2 [88], is associated with cumulus expansion.

Extragonadal influence on the ovulation process has also been reported. For example, triiodothyronine (T_3) was found to be an important agent of ovulation. It was shown that women with T_3 concentrations >80 ng/dl fail to ovulate [89].

Ruptured released oocyte–cumulus complex at ovulation is transferred to the infundibulum of the Fallopian tube (oviduct), and then moves to the ampulla region through the surface of the ciliated oviductal epithelium and awaits the sperm cells. The FF released by ovulation into the oviduct and peritoneal cavity may have an essential physiological function through its direct stimulatory effect on the oviduct (constriction and epithelial cilia motility) that assists in oocyte–cumulus complex advancement.

Maturation of the Preovulatory Follicle during the Gonadotropin Surge

After the midcycle gonadotropin surge, dramatic metabolic and morphological changes simultaneously occur within the preovulatory and ovulatory follicle that switches from an E_2-producing to a P_4-producing structure. Progesterone receptors appear in GCs, whose proliferation is arrested at this stage [90]. Also, some hours before ovulation and in response to angiogenic factors produced by GCs [65], the granulosa wall, which was avascular before the midcycle gonadotropin surge, appears to be changed after invasion of blood vessels originating from the theca layer.

As a result of the breakdown of the basal lamina during the LH surge, the cholesterol substrate required by GCs to generate progestin, and which is provided to cells in the form of lipoprotein-bound cholesterol, can now reach the follicle via the blood supply [54]. After the gonadotropin surge, both P450scc [57] and 3β-HSD [50; 91] appear in GCs, where the levels of adrenodoxin and steroid acute regulatory (StAR) proteins, which support the entrance of cholesterol into mitochondria, are significantly increased. The production of steroids strongly increases, rising from a mean FF concentration of 4800 ng/ml before the surge, to 11 000 ng/ml after the surge. While follicular progestin production significantly increases, that of androgens and E_2 dramatically declines. The collapsed ovulating follicle develops into a new endocrine gland, called the corpus luteum (CL).

Follicle after the Gonadotropin Surge (Corpus Luteum)

After the LH surge, the postovulatory follicle develops into the CL, or yellow body (the color originated from carotenoids). The ovarian CL was first named by Marcello Malpighi and then described by Regnier de Graaf in the 1600s. The young CL has a cystic center filled with FF and a focally hemorrhagic

coagulum (Figure 4.8). The mature CL (approximately seventh day postovulation) shows increased tissue mass, a smaller cystic center, and varies in size and appearance, but usually measures between 10 mm and 30 mm in diameter [92], and is of a volume of 4.87 cm^3 [93]. Capillaries from the theca interna layer penetrate the granulosa layers and reach its central cavity. Upon potent angiogenesis the theca interna becomes incorporated into the GC layers and forms a new cellular composition, remodeled and different from the layered structure of the preovulatory follicle. The CL is the most active endocrine gland in the body and is essential for the establishment and maintenance of pregnancy in most mammals, including humans. Because of its unique role, CL formation, maintenance, and regression are tightly regulated. Survival and continued function of the CL are both required throughout the first weeks of pregnancy, after which the placenta becomes responsible for the maintenance of gestation. The CL is generally considered to go through three phases during its life cycle: formation, maintenance, and regression. One additional potential phase is rescuing (sustained function) during pregnancy.

The development, maintenance, and steroidogenic function of the CL during the menstrual cycle are generally thought to be LH dependent [94]. During the luteal phase, there is a reduction in the frequency of LH pulses from the pituitary, from a pulse every 100 minutes in the early luteal phase to every 200 minutes in the mid-late luteal phase just before the onset of luteal regression. LH receptors are expressed in the CL [95], and LH is responsible for initiating the differentiation of the somatic cells of the ovarian follicle, TCs and GCs, into the small luteal (SLC) and large luteal (LLC) steroidogenic cells of the CL [96–97]. FSH receptors have also been identified in the early CL, although the role of FSH in luteal function is not clear. After ovulation, peripheral LH, FSH, and E_2 levels fall, but the LH concentration (with pulses approximately every 4 hours) is sufficient to maintain the CL. The newly formed CL is a highly active gland with a marked capacity for steroid synthesis. Opposite to the follicle, CL shifts from E_2 to P_4 production. Progestogenic stimulation provides an intrauterine environment that supports implantation and pregnancy, playing a vital role in the fate of the embryo. The CL of pregnancy may be indistinguishable from the regular CL but is usually larger and bright yellow in contrast to the orange-yellow of the regular late luteal CL.

41

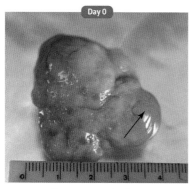

Day 0

Preovulatory follicle

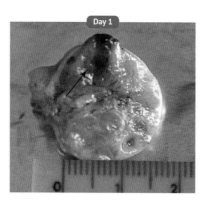

Day 1

Early CL

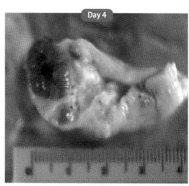

Day 4

Developmental CL

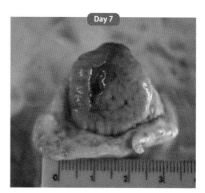

Day 7

Mature CL

Figure 4.8 CL development after ovulation.

P_4 secretion is supported by external LH and internal luteotropic factors (such as prostaglandins PGI_2 and PGE_2) produced by luteal cells. P_4 raises the set-point of the hypothalamic thermoregulatory center, and serum P_4 levels raise the basal body temperature. In contrast to the ovarian follicle, where TCs primarily produce P_4, in the CL both the GC-derived LLC and TC-derived SLC produce P_4. The process includes cholesterol transport into the inner mitochondria, mediated by StAR, conversion of cholesterol to pregnenolone by the P450scc complex, and conversion of pregnenolone to P_4 by 3β-HSD. In most species, aromatase expression is absent throughout the luteal life span, whereas in primates, the CL reacquires the ability to generate moderate amounts of E_2 [98]. Insufficient P_4 secretion early in the first trimester is associated with pregnancy loss and is attributed to premature loss of luteal function.

In the absence of pregnancy, the CL will regress (luteolysis), and the next female cycle will begin. Luteolysis is defined as the loss of steroidogenic function (functional luteolysis) and the subsequent involution of the CL (structural luteolysis). During luteolysis, the CL undergoes dramatic changes in its steroidogenic capacity, vascularization, immune cell activation, extracellular matrix composition, and cell viability. The process of luteolysis is associated with a marked reduction in luteal P_4 production and the loss of luteal steroidogenic cells. Vasoconstriction of small blood vessels in the CL is associated with reduction in blood supply and then with loss of luteal blood supply. The interruption of luteolysis allows the CL to support pregnancy. This CL-supporting agent is human chorionic gonadotropin (hCG) secreted from the developing embryo and which binds to the LH receptors.

The structure and function of the CL are dependent on the development of vasculature via angiogenesis. The establishment of the luteal vascular network begins in the preovulatory follicle and is stimulated by the LH surge. Following ovulation, the CL undergoes extremely rapid growth that is only matched by the fastest-growing tumors [99], alongside intense angiogenesis, higher than that seen in the most aggressive solid tumors. Not surprisingly, the majority of the proliferating cells in the early CL are of vascular origin, with proliferation rates exceeding 25% [100]. Luteal angiogenesis requires highly coordinated interplay between endothelial and steroidogenic cells, as well as fibroblasts and pericytes, to create an extensive and complex vascular network that is essential for luteal function (Figure 4.9). FGF2 and VEGF, which are potent mitogens of vascular endothelial cells (ECs) and stimulators of EC migration and survival [101–102], are the proangiogenic regulators of luteal angiogenesis. Hypoxia inducible factor-1 was found to be the most potent transcription factor of VEGF [103]. However, numerous other factors are expressed by several luteal cell types and also bear important modulatory functions. VEGF is secreted from luteal steroidogenic cells and acts on receptors expressed on ECs [104]. LH-dependent VEGF expression is involved in maintaining the structural and functional integrity of the CL in the normal luteal phase. In simulated early pregnancy, hCG promotes additional VEGF synthesis, and further luteal VEGF secretion, resulting in a second wave of angiogenesis [102]. Regulation of vascular permeability is a key function of the ECs and is important in the supply of nutrients/hormones to the luteal tissue.

Luteolysis occurs in the nongravid uterus and it is inhibited in the presence of embryonic signals [105]. Uterine-derived (or exogenous) prostaglandin $F_{2\alpha}$ ($PGF_{2\alpha}$) initiates luteolysis [106] through a countercurrent system between the uterine vein and the ovarian artery, and rapidly reduces luteal P_4 secretion, within several hours [107]. $PGF_{2\alpha}$ acts directly on luteal steroidogenic and endothelial cells, which express $PGF_{2\alpha}$ receptors (PGFR), or indirectly on immune cells lacking PGFR, which are activated by other cells within the CL. Significant increases in the number of leukocytes [108] and inflammatory cytokines are involved in luteal regression [109]. $PGF_{2\alpha}$ stimulates locally (intra CL) to produce factors such as endothelin-1, angiopoietins, FGF2, thrombospondins, TGF-β1, and plasminogen activator inhibitor-B1, which act sequentially to inhibit P_4 production,

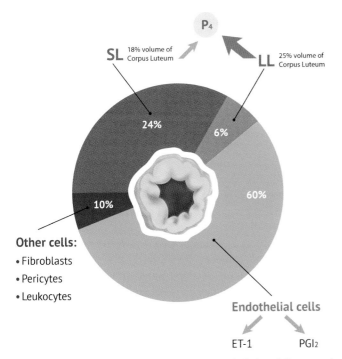

Figure 4.9 Cellular composition of the CL. ET-1, endothelin 1; PGI2, prostaglandin I2 (prostacyclin).

angiogenic support, cell survival, and extracellular matrix remodeling, and induce luteal vasoconstriction to accomplish CL regression [110–114]. There is progressive fibrotic connective tissue replacement of the cellular composition of the CL, shrinkage over a period of several months, and final conversion of the CL to a corpus albicans (white body).

Although LH concentrations and pulse frequency are reduced during the luteal phase, luteolysis occurs in the presence of maintained LH concentrations. Expression of LH receptors is maintained across the luteal phase and luteolysis is initiated in the presence of LH receptors [115]. During luteolysis, there is a decline in luteal hormones, which leads to destabilization of the endometrium and induction of menstruation [116]. The fall in luteal hormones increases pituitary gonadotropin secretion, which stimulates the growth of the small antral follicles present in the ovaries at menstruation, resulting in the initiation of the follicular phase of the ovarian cycle.

Menstruation

During the proliferative phase of the cycle, the cells of the endometrium proliferate. The preovulatory LH surge induces endometrial gland and arteriole growth and development, and coil, both factors that contribute to endometrial thickening. The increasingly coiled endometrial glands begin to secrete nutrient fluid (secretory phase), a process that is obligatory for embryo receptivity.

Physiologically, menstruation is the process whereby the superficial or functional layer of the endometrium lining the uterine cavity degenerates and is removed from the uterine lumen towards the end of the luteal phase of a nonpregnant cycle. Within 5–6 days, the old lining is removed, and a new lining is generated.

Two hypotheses have been proposed for the initiation of menstruation: the vasoconstrictor hypothesis, which emphasizes the actions of PGs and endothelins, and the inflammatory hypothesis, which underscores the role of inflammatory cells and matrix metalloproteinases (MMPs). Intrauterine PGF2α causes constriction of muscle in the walls of the tightly coiled arterioles, yielding endometrial ischemia, menses, and increased uterine contractility. In parallel, lysosomal enzymes can be secreted by macrophages at menstruation. There is also evidence of a critical role of matrix MMPs in tissue breakdown associated with menstruation.

Repair of the endometrium begins as early as 36 hours after the onset of menstrual bleeding, while menstrual desquamation is still in progress, emphasizing the highly focal nature of the degradative and repair processes. During the proliferative phase, it is estrogens that regulate endometrial regeneration, which includes cessation of bleeding, re-epithelialization of the luminal lining, initiation of stromal tissue growth, and vessel repair. Regeneration is completed within 140 hours.

Between the mid-nineteenth and mid-twentieth centuries, the average age of menarche in Europe declined steadily from 17 to 13 years. The average modern woman menstruates between 350 and 400 times. The mean menstrual blood loss per cycle is 43 ml, with 10% of women losing 100 ml blood per month. Therefore, the average woman loses more than 20 liters of menstrual blood during her reproductive life.

Incomplete Meiosis

After the LH surge, the oocyte resumes meiosis and progresses from first meiotic prophase (prophase I) to the second metaphase at the time of ovulation, and regulates both cytoplasmic and nuclear maturation.

The introductory stages of meiosis are similar to those of mitosis; the cell grows during G1, duplicates all of its chromosomes during the S phase, and prepares itself for division during G2. Upon completion of G2, the oocyte enters prophase I of meiosis. Normal gene expression during meiosis (oocyte maturation) and early embryonic development (until the zygotic gene activation) requires well-timed activation of specific maternal mRNA translation. These mRNAs accumulated in the oocyte during the first meiotic arrest at prophase I.

Cytoplasmic polyadenylation element-binding group of proteins (CPEB) is an additional agent important for oocyte meiotic maturation. The CPEB induces cytoplasmic polyadenylation of RNA molecules, thereby promoting translational repression or activation. Deletion of CPEB leads to impaired synaptonemal complex formation, and subsequently to meiotic arrest at the pachytene stage of prophase I. The preovulatory follicle holds the oocyte in a state of arrest at the diplotene stage of prophase I from the moment the fetal gonads form.

Prophase I can occupy 90% or more of the duration of meiosis. The nuclear envelope of the GV oocyte remains intact and only disappears when the meiotic spindle begins to be formed, as prophase I gives way to metaphase I (MI oocyte) (Figure 4.10).

Even the preparatory DNA replication during the first meiotic division tends to take much longer than in an ordinary S phase, and cells can then spend days, months, or even years in prophase I, depending on the species and the gamete being formed.

The extended arrest in meiosis occurs in the primary oocyte (GV-arrested oocyte at prophase I) before birth. Years later, this first division is ended just before ovulation. The ovulated oocyte is then arrested at metaphase II (MII) (incomplete meiosis) until fertilization (which terminates meiosis).

It is clear that the addition of hormones, such as LH and FSH, is essential for the stimulation of oocyte maturation. Furthermore, supplementation of various growth factors (IGF, FGF, GDF, EGF, and many others) is necessary to support the growth of CCs and oocyte maturation.

Two chromosomes (one paternal and one maternal), which are very similar but not identical in a DNA sequence, are called "homologous," and in most cells, they are completely separate and independent chromosomes. After chromosome duplication by DNA replication, the twin copies of the fully replicated chromosome remain tightly connected along their length and are called "sister chromatids." A crossover between homologous chromatids occurs at "hot spots." Regions that are contracted indicate recombination "cold spots," regions where crossovers occur with unusually low frequency. Failed chromosome segregation in oocytes is the most common cause of infertility, natural miscarriage, and birth defects [117].

Meiosis in male gametes significantly differs from female meiosis. Male meiosis does produce four functional gametes during spermatogenesis, from one primary spermatocyte (four sets of DNA) to four late spermatids (yields four sperm cells of one set of DNA each). In females, only one functional egg cell is made (from four sets of DNA in the primary oocyte to two sets of DNA in the MII oocyte, and then to one set of DNA after fertilization). At the end of meiosis I, only one of the two "daughter cells" continues down the oocyte pathway, while the other becomes a non-oocyte called a first "polar body" (PB).

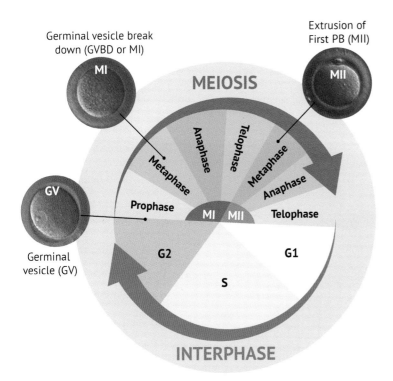

Figure 4.10 Resumption of meiosis. PB, polar body.

Resumption of Oocyte Meiosis

Upon exposure to the LH surge, the GV oocyte passes from prophase I to MI. This step is accompanied by elongation and rotation of the meiotic spindle, with chromosomes oriented on the spindle equator. Then, anaphase I is completed upon the separation of homologous chromosomes to opposite poles. Extrusion of the first PB occurs at the end of telophase I and then initiates MII. However, sister chromatids are not separated until the end of meiosis II (telophase II after fertilization), when the oocyte is already a mature oocyte that can be fertilized by sperm. Thus, completion of nuclear maturation of the oocyte, and release of the first PB, does not mean the oocyte is ready to accept the sperm. During ovulation, the oocyte cytoplasm can be at one of three stages of maturation, i.e., immature, mature, or overmature.

Anaphase II begins when the cohesin proteins that hold the chromatids together are destroyed. The destruction of cohesin enables the sister chromatids to separate to opposite poles of the cell.

The oocyte is a highly sensitive cell. External or internal influences and changes may affect meiosis, such as mutation in the tubulin-β class VIII (*TUBB8*) gene, encoding one of the spindle proteins, which leads to oocyte maturation arrest [118].

Second meiosis is a shorter and simpler process than first meiosis and is completed by extrusion of the second PB (Figure 4.11). Extrusion of the second PB can be visualized 6–9 hours after fertilization.

Female Reproductive Aging

Age is the most important determinant of female fertility potential. Social trends around the world have brought women to delay childbearing into their 30s and, in some cases, their 40s [119–120]. The average age of women giving the first birth has increased from 27 to 29.5 over the last two decades. As women approach their later reproductive years, ovarian natural function declines (the loss of ovarian follicles), and the growing age is associated with lowered fecundity and infertility before the complete cessation of menses [121]. While some research has suggested that a more accelerated process of decline occurs in middle-aged women around the age of 35–38 years [122–123], others suggest that oocyte loss occurs at the same rate through the reproductive lifetime [124]. As the ovarian follicular cohort decreases, women will experience infertility, sterility, cycle shortening, menstrual irregularity, and finally, menopause (or climacteric period). This decline in female fertility brings them to seek the assistance of assisted reproductive technologies (ART). Between 2006 and 2016, the ratio of women over 40 years of age undergoing an autologous in vitro fertilization (IVF) cycle rose from 1:5 to 1:4 [125–126]. While ART may aid some couples who present infertility, it does not compensate for the decline in natural fertility that occurs with age. Also, pregnancy complications increase for both the mother and the offspring with advanced maternal age [127].

The exhaustion of oocytes from the ovaries is a constant process that begins in the embryonic period and continues forward with the majority lost through apoptosis or programmed cell death at the early antral follicle stage [128]. The female fetus ovaries contain 6–7 million oocytes at approximately 20 weeks' gestation. At birth, 1–2 million oocytes remain, and only 300 000–500 000 are present at the onset of puberty [129]. This process carries on until menopause when only a few hundred oocytes remain [130]. The average age of menopause in Western countries is 51, and 1% of women experience premature ovarian failure before age

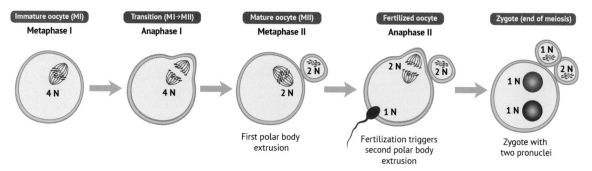

Figure 4.11 Fertilization and culmination of meiosis.

40 (Figure 4.12) [131]. Women who experience menopause have a loss of fertility [132–133]. Cycle irregularity usually occurs 6 to 7 years before menopause [134], regardless of the age of menopause, coinciding with approximately 10 000 remaining follicles [130].

The declining follicular count matches with a decline in inhibin B and E_2, which are produced by the GCs in the early follicular phase [135] and luteal cells of the ovary [136]. There is a feedback correlation between FSH and inhibin B, and the rise in FSH during the early follicular phase is one of the initial marks of ovarian aging-related shortening of the menstrual cycle [137]. This initial sign of ovarian aging may not be clinically apparent or present only as infertility because ovarian hormone production remains, and women continue to ovulate. Also, concentrations of the hypothalamic GnRH are low, perhaps because of prolonged high levels of its release and decreased synthesis. Others claim that the age-related change in the central nervous system is the force that initiates the menopausal transition, i.e., the exhaustion of ovarian follicles is a consequence of the altered temporal organization of neural signals. Gonadotropin secretion in postmenopausal women supports the view that the age-related processes are related to a hypothalamic rather than to a pituitary hypofunction [138].

According to both theories, the shortening of menstrual cycles is due to a shorter follicular phase.

As this transition carries on, menstrual cycles lengthen and become more irregular as women enter the menopause transition, and ovulation is less consistent [130]. Hormonal deficiency is expressed as emotional (frustration, low response to sexual stimuli) and physical (vaginal dryness, thinning of vaginal walls) symptoms. In some cases, hormonal replacement therapy may be used to relieve menopause symptoms. Once women start to notice clinical signs of ovarian aging (such as cycle shortening or irregularity), their fertility may be greatly reduced. Markers of the ovarian reserve (AMH and AFC levels) may be useful to predict earlier menopause for women who do not yet have clinical signs or symptoms of ovarian aging but who may already have decreased fertility. Menopausal onset has a strong genetic component to age at onset, and associations in menopausal age are demonstrated in mother–daughter and sister pairs [139–140]. Telomeres cap the chromosome ends, preventing the exposure of the DNA end, which resembles a DNA break and prompts a DNA damage response. Studies in mice and women show that telomere shortening in oocytes provides a parsimonious explanation for the effects of reproductive aging on oocyte quality [141]. It was proposed that the shortening of oocyte telomeres associated with increasing oocyte fragmentation and aneuploidy is an evolutionary mechanism [142–143]

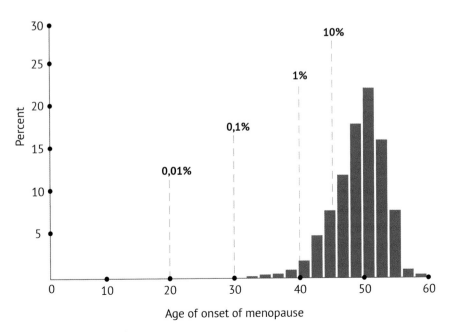

Figure 4.12 The onset of menopause.

to prevent women of advanced maternal age from carrying a pregnancy that would risk their health [144]. Other factors, such as smoking, alcohol use, and night work, have been associated with a decreased follicular pool and earlier menopause [134; 144–145].

The quality of the oocyte also appears to be affected by age. Studies on IVF oocytes have shown that the rate of oocyte aneuploidy increases with age [146]. The aneuploidy rate is low in women below the age of 35 (10%), but increases to 30% by the age of 40, to 40% by the age of 43, and to 100% in women older than 45 years of age [146]. However, the evaluations were performed in gonadotropin-stimulated oocytes, and therefore may not imitate the rate of aneuploidy in oocytes from a dominant follicle recruited during a non-stimulated or natural cycle. Nevertheless, at the same time, these observations correlate with the increase in chromosomally abnormal pregnancies and spontaneous abortions with age [147]. The deterioration in oocyte quality may be in the formation and function of the spindles, which appear to be more diffuse [148], and loss of kinetochore spindle assembly checkpoint proteins [149]. This may result in less tightly arranged chromosomes, which may lead to meiotic errors, abnormal fertilization, and termination of embryo development. The frequency of trisomy increases with maternal age [150]. Loss of cohesion between sisters chromatids close to the centromeres is an age-related dysfunction which may cause chromosomal missegregation, and ultimately lead to trisomy [151]. Cohesins form a complex of proteins that holds sister chromatids together after DNA replication and is responsible for maintaining the bivalent structure throughout the extended period of quiescence. Only at anaphase, the cohesins are removed to trigger the separation of sister chromatids. Accumulating evidence has suggested an age-related disruption of cohesin function, leading to missegregation within the oocyte, especially in the presence of a low recombination rate of chromosomes [152]. The levels of Aurora kinase, which destabilizes incorrect kinetochore–microtubule attachment, reduce with maternal age, and this leads to reduced levels of spindle assembly checkpoint of the oocyte [149], affecting chromosomal separation. All these events lead to defective oocytes, sharply decreased fertility, and miscarriages.

Women mostly aged 35 years and older show chromosomal abnormalities originating from errors of first meiosis, second meiosis, or both [153]. Reverse segregation, i.e., split of all sister chromatids at meiosis I, and precocious separation of sister chromatids are the underlying causes of the majority of aneuploidy in oocytes [154]. The frequencies of trisomy change from 5% at 28 years of age to 40–50% at 43 years of age [150].

Age-related instability in mitochondrial DNA (mtDNA) may also affect oocyte competence and transmission of mitochondrial abnormalities to the offspring. Lower levels of mtDNA are predictive of poor oocyte quality and result in abnormal, premature mitochondrial biogenesis in early embryonic development [155].

Population studies have consistently noted that the decline in birth rates begins when women reach the age of 35. Typically, women deliver their last child at age 41 (range: 23–51 years) [156]. However, natural population studies may not take into account nonreproductive factors, such as contraception, coital frequency, aging partners, and other medical conditions that may affect live birth rates. Also, pathological conditions such as fibroids and endometriosis that are noted to prevent pregnancy rates are more frequent in later reproductive years. Natural fertility studies of patients who had recently stopped contraception have shown that younger women have a higher fecundity rate, and therefore conceive sooner than older women [157]. Although social changes have brought women to delay their reproduction, concomitant advances in reproductive sciences have led to increased options for fertility treatment and ART. However, this may give women a false sense of security in delaying pregnancy while pursuing their education and careers, with the belief that ART will help them to conceive if they have difficulty conceiving later. However, ART success rates in women using their oocytes are directly linked to the age of the women [158], and many women may not realize that successful ART in older women is often only with donor oocytes.

The uterine endometrium can maintain a pregnancy throughout a woman's reproductive years and even further than the natural reproductive years. Age does not affect the endometrium's response to hormonal stimulation [159]. Pregnancy rates from donor oocyte cycles also confirm that the age of the recipient does not affect pregnancy rates [160].

Although chronological age alone serves as a good marker of ovarian reserve, some women have a decrease in their natural fertility earlier than average, while some older women may maintain above-average ovarian function. Many attempts to assess ovarian reserve have been made. However, testing has mainly been performed on infertile women, with little data on the distribution of the normal fertile women. The most commonly used ovarian reserve test is the measurement of cycle day 3 or basal FSH levels. An elevated basal FSH level (higher than 14 IU/L) is the first detectable sign of ovarian aging and usually occurs in women aged 35 to 40 [161]. Elevated basal FSH levels are less predictive of pregnancy potential in women less than age 35 [162]. An ovarian AFC can be performed early in the menstrual cycle using transvaginal ultrasound, which can identify antral follicles between 2 mm and 10 mm in diameter [163]. AFC is considered to be representative of the available follicle pool. However, although a decline in AFC is correlated with both the onset of menopause and reduced ovarian response to stimulation, AFC alone is not a good predictor of fertility potency [164]. AMH is produced by the GCs of preantral and small antral follicles, but not dominant follicles [132] and is therefore reflective of the size of the antral follicle pool. AMH level decreases with decreasing AFC, which, in turn, is a marker of the antral follicle cohort predicting the live birth rate [165–166]. Levels remain consistent throughout the menstrual cycle [167] and become undetectable in women after menopause [168]. Taken together, AFC and AMH are ovarian reserve markers and can be useful for the prediction of poor ovarian response to IVF [169].

References

1. Gottsch ML, Cunningham MJ, Smith JT, et al. A role for kisspeptins in the regulation of gonadotropin secretion in the mouse. *Endocrinology* 2004; **145**:4073–4077.

2. Moreno I, Codoñer FM, Vilella F, et al. Evidence that the endometrial microbiota has an effect on implantation success or failure. *Am. J. Obstet. Gynecol.* 2016; **215**:684–703.

3. Ravel J, Gajer P, Abdo Z, et al. Vaginal microbiome of reproductive-age women. *Proc. Natl. Acad. Sci. U. S. A.* 2011; **108**(Suppl. 1):4680–4687.

4. Gougeon A. Regulation of ovarian follicular development in primates: facts and hypotheses. *Endocr. Rev.* 1996; **17**:121–155.

5. Ng EH, Yeung WS, Fong DY, Ho PC. Effects of age on hormonal and ultrasound markers of ovarian reserve in Chinese women with proven fertility. *Hum. Reprod.* 2003; **18**:2169–2174.

6. Dierich A, Sairam MR, Monaco L, et al. Impairing follicle-stimulating hormone (FSH) signaling in vivo: targeted disruption of the FSH receptor leads to aberrant gametogenesis and hormonal imbalance. *Proc. Natl. Acad. Sci. U. S. A.* 1998; **95**:13612–13617.

7. Jayaprakasan K, Hilwah N, Kendall NR, et al. Does 3D ultrasound offer any advantage in the pretreatment assessment of ovarian reserve and prediction of outcome after assisted reproduction treatment? *Hum. Reprod.* 2007; **22**:1932–1941.

8. Kumar TR, Wang Y, Lu N, Matzuk MM. Follicle stimulating hormone is required for ovarian follicle maturation but not for male fertility. *Nat. Genet.* 1997; **15**:201–204.

9. Matthews CH, Borgato S, Beck-Peccoz P, et al. Primary amenorrhoea and infertility due to a mutation in the beta-subunit of follicle-stimulating hormone. *Nat. Genet.* 1993; **5**:83–86.

10. Eppig J. Oocyte control of ovarian follicular development and function in mammals. *Reproduction* 2001; **122**:829–838.

11. Kidder GM, Mhawi AA. Gap junctions and ovarian folliculogenesis. *Reproduction* 2002; **123**:613–620.

12. Eppig JJ, Wigglesworth K, Pendola FL. The mammalian oocyte orchestrates the rate of ovarian follicular development. *Proc. Natl. Acad. Sci. U. S. A.* 2002; **99**:2890–2894.

13. Vitt UA, Hayashi M, Klein C, Hsueh AJW. Growth differentiation factor-9 stimulates proliferation but suppresses the follicle stimulating hormone-induced differentiation of cultured granulosa cells from small antral and preovulatory rat follicles. *Biol. Reprod.* 2000; **62**:370–377.

14. Parrott JA, Skinner MK. Kit-ligand/stem cell factor induces primordial follicle development and initiates folliculogenesis. *Endocrinology* 1999; **140**:4262–4271.

15. Nilsson E, Parrott JA, Skinner MK. Basic fibroblast growth factor induces primordial follicle development and initiates folliculogenesis. *Mol. Cell. Endocrinol.* 2001; **25**:123–130.

16. Dissen GA, Garcia-Rudaz C, Ojeda SR. Role of neurotrophic factors in early ovarian development. *Semin. Reprod. Med.* 2009; **27**:24–31.

17. Nilsson E, Dole G, Skinner MK. Neurotrophin NT3 promotes ovarian primordial to primary follicle transition. *Reproduction* 2009; **138**:697–707.

18. Abir R, Fisch B, Jin S, et al. Presence of NGF and its receptors in ovaries from human fetuses and adults. *Mol. Hum. Reprod.* 2005; **11**:229–236.

19. El-Fouly MA, Cook B, Nekola M, Nalbandov AV. Role of the ovum in follicular luteinization. *Endocrinology* 1970; **87**:286–293.

20. Nekola MV, Nalbandov AV. Morphological changes of rat follicular cells as influenced by oocytes. *Biol. Reprod.* 1971; **4**:154–160.

21. Weenen C, Laven JSE, von Bergh ARM, et al. Anti-Müllerian hormone expression pattern in the human ovary: potential implications for initial and cyclic follicle recruitment. *Mol. Hum. Reprod.* 2004; **10**:77–83.

22. Jeppesen JV, Anderson RA, Kelsey TW, et al. Which follicles make the most anti-Müllerian hormone in humans? Evidence for an abrupt decline in AMH production at the time of follicle selection. *Mol. Hum. Reprod.* 2013; **19**:519–527.

23. Amsterdam A, Koch Y, Lieberman ME, Lindner HR. Distribution of binding sites for human chorionic gonadotropin in the preovulatory follicle of the rat. *J. Cell. Biol.* 1975; **67**:894–900.

24. Lawrence TS, Dekel N, Beers WH. Binding of human chorionic gonadotropin by rat cumuli oophori and granulosa cells: a comparative study. *Endocrinology* 1980; **106**:1114–1118.

25. Chen L, Russell PT, Larsen WJ. Functional significance of cumulus expansion in the mouse: roles for the preovulatory synthesis of hyaluronic acid within the cumulus mass. *Mol. Reprod. Dev.* 1993; **34**:87–93.

26. Peng XR, Hsueh AJ, LaPolt PS, Bjersing L, Ny T. Localization of luteinizing hormone receptor messenger ribonucleic acid expression in ovarian cell types during follicle development and ovulation. *Endocrinology* 1991; **129**:3200–3207.

27. Gougeon A. Rate of follicular growth in the human ovary. In: Rolland R, Van Hall EV, Hillier SG, McNatty KP, Schoemaker JS, eds., *Follicular Maturation and Ovulation*. Amsterdam: Excerpta Medica. 1982; 155–163.

28. McNatty KP, Hillier SG, van den Boogaard AMJ, et al. Follicular development during the luteal phase of the human menstrual cycle. *J. Clin. Endocrinol. Metab.* 1983; **56**:1022–1031.

29. Pache TD, Wladimiroff JW, de Jong FH, Hop WC, Fauser BCJM. Growth patterns of non dominant ovarian follicles during the normal menstrual cycle. *Fertil. Steril.* 1990; **54**:638–642.

30. Gougeon A, Lefèvre B. Evolution of the diameters of the largest healthy and atretic follicles during the human menstrual cycle. *J. Reprod. Fert.* 1983; **69**:497–502.

31. Kobayashi M, Nakano R, Ooshima A. Immunocytochemical localization of pituitary gonadotrophins and gonadal steroids confirms the 'two-cell, two-gonadotrophin' hypothesis of steroidogenesis in the human ovary. *J. Endocrinol.* 1990; **126**:483–488.

32. Soules MR, Steiner RA, Clifton DK, et al. Progesterone modulation of pulsatile luteinizing hormone secretion in normal women. *J. Clin. Endocrinol. Metab.* 1984; **58**:378–383.

33. Crowley WF, McArthur JW. Simulations of the normal menstrual cycle in Kallmann's syndrome by pulsatile administration of luteinizing hormone-releasing hormone (LHRH). *J. Clin. Endocrinol. Metab.* 1980; **51**:173–175.

34. Solovyeva EV, Hayashi M, Margi K, et al. Growth differentiation factor-9 stimulates rat theca-interstitial cell androgen biosynthesis. *Biol. Reprod.* 2000; **63**:1214–1218.

35. Dunlop CE, Anderson RA. The regulation and assessment of follicular growth. *Scand. J. Clin. Lab. Invest. Suppl.* 2014; **244**:13–17.

36. Donez J, Squifflet J, Jadoul P, et al. Pregnancy and live birth after autotransplantation of frozen-thawed ovarian tissue in a patient with metastatic disease undergoing chemotherapy and hematopoietic stem cell transplantation. *Fertil. Steril.* 1987; **2011**:e1-e4.

37. Choi J. Smitz J. Luteinizing hormone and human chorionic gonadotropin: origins of difference. *Mol. Cell. Endocrinol.* 2014; **383**:203–213.

38. CasariniL, LispiM, Longobardi S, et al. LH and hCG action on the same receptor results in quantitatively and qualitatively different intracellular signaling. *PLoS One* 2012; 7, e46682.

39. Wide L, Bakos O. More basic forms of both human follicle-stimulating hormone and luteinizing hormone in serum at midcycle compared with the follicular or luteal phase. *J. Clin. Endocrinol. Metab.* 1993; **76**:885–889.

40. McNatty KP. Ovarian follicular development from the onset of luteal regression in humans and sheep. In: Rolland R, Van Hall EV, Hillier SG, McNatty KP, Schoemaker JS, eds., *Follicular Maturation and Ovulation*. Amsterdam: Excerpta Medica. 1982; 1–18.

41. Liu L, Kong N, Xia G, Zhang M. Molecular control of oocyte meiotic arrest and resumption. *Reprod. Fertil. Dev.* 2013; **25**:463–471.

42. Reddy P, Adhikari D, Zheng W, et al. PDK1 signaling in oocytes controls reproductive aging and lifespan by manipulating the survival of primordial follicles. *Hum. Mol. Genet.* 2009; **18**:2813–2824.

43. Meduri G, Charnaux N, Driancourt MA, et al. Follicle-stimulating hormone receptors in oocytes? *J. Clin. Endocrinol. Metab.* 2002; **87**:2266–2276.

44. Patsoula E, Loutradis D, Drakakis P, et al. Messenger RNA expression for the follicle-stimulating hormone

receptor and luteinizing hormone receptor in human oocytes and pre-implantation-stage embryos. *Fertil. Steril.* 2003; **79**:1187–1193.

45. Otsuka F, Shimasaki S. A negative feedback system between oocyte bone morphogenetic protein 15 and granulosa cell kit ligand: its role in regulating granulosa cell mitosis. *Proc. Natl. Acad. Sci. U. S. A.* 2002; **99**:8060–8065.

46. Lefievre L, Conner SJ, Salpekar A, et al. Four zona pellucida glycoproteins are expressed in the human. *Hum. Reprod.* 2004; **19**:1580–1586.

47. Motta PM, Makabe S, Naguro T, Correr S. Oocyte follicle cells association during development of human ovarian follicle. A study by high resolution scanning and transmission electron microscopy. *Arch. Histol. Cytol.* 1994; **57**:369–394.

48. Bergh C, Olsson JH, Selleskog U, Hillensjo T. Steroid production in cultured thecal cell obtained from human ovarian follicles. *Hum. Reprod.* 1993; **8**:519–524.

49. Gilling-Smith C, Franks S. Ovarian function in assisted reproduction. In: Leung PC, Adashi EY, eds., *The Ovary*, 2nd ed. San Diego: Elsevier Academic Press. 2004; 473–488.

50. Gougeon A. Steroid 3β-ol-dehydrogenase activity in the largest healthy and atretic follicles in the human ovary during the menstrual cycle. *Ann. Biol. Anim. Biochim. Biophys.* 1977; **17**:1087–1094.

51. Curtis EM. Normal ovarian histology in infancy and childhood. *Obstet. Gynecol.* 1962; **19**:444–454.

52. Dekel N, David MP, Yedwab GA, Kraicer PF. Follicular development during late pregnancy. *Int. J. Fertil.* 1977; **22**:24–29.

53. Bloom W, Fawcett DW. *A Textbook of Histology*, 10th ed. Philadelphia: Saunders. 1975.

54. Amsterdam A, Rotmensch S. Structure-function relationships during granulosa cell differentiation. *Endocr. Rev.* 1987; **8**:309–337.

55. Hillier SG, Yong EL, Illingworth PJ, et al. Effect of recombinant inhibin on androgen synthesis in cultured human thecal cells. *Mol. Cell. Endocrinol.* 1991; **75**:R1–R6.

56. Roberts VJ, Barth S, El-Roeiy A, Yen SSC. Expression of inhibin/activin subunits and follistatin messenger ribonucleic acids and proteins in ovarian follicles and the corpus luteum during the human menstrual cycle. *J. Clin. Endocrinol. Metab.* 1993; **77**:1402–1410.

57. Sasano H, Okamoto M, Mason JI, et al. Immunolocalization of aromatase, 17α-hydroxylase and side-chain cleavage cytochrome P-450 in the human ovary. *J. Reprod. Fertil.* 1989; **85**:163–169.

58. Hernandez ER, Hurwitz A, Vera A, et al. Expression of the genes encoding the insulin-like growth factors and their receptors in the human ovary. *J. Clin. Endocrinol. Metab.* 1992; **74**:419–425.

59. Salas C, Julio-Pieper M, Valladares M, et al. Nerve growth factor-dependent activation of trkA receptors in the human ovary results in synthesis of follicle-stimulating hormone receptors and estrogen secretion. *J. Clin. Endocrinol. Metab.* 2006; **91**:2396–2403.

60. Shima K, Kitayama S, Nakano R. Gonadotropin binding sites in human ovarian follicles and corpora lutea during the menstrual cycle. *Obstet. Gynecol.* 1987; **69**:800–806.

61. McNatty KP, Makris A, DeGrazia C, Osathanondh R, Rayan KJ. The production of progesterone, androgens, and estrogens by granulosa cells, thecal tissue, and stromal tissue from human ovaries in vitro. *J. Clin. Endocrinol. Metab.* 1979; **49**:687–699.

62. McNatty KP, Smith DM, Makris A, Osathanondh R, Ryan KJ. The microenvironment of the human antral follicle: interrelationship among the steroid levels in antral fluid, the population of granulosa cells and the status of the oocyte in vivo and in vitro. *J. Clin. Endocrinol. Metab.* 1979; **49**:851–860.

63. Hillier SG. Intrafollicular paracrine function of ovarian androgen. *J. Steroid. Biochem.* 1987; **27**:351–357.

64. Zeleznik AJ, Schuler HM, Reichert LE. Gonadotropin-binding sites in the rhesus monkey ovary: role of the vasculature in the selective distribution of human chorionic gonadotropin to the preovulatory follicle. *Endocrinology* 1981; **109**:356–362.

65. Wulff C, Wiegand SJ, Saunders PT, Scobie GA, Fraser HM. Angiogenesis during follicular development in the primate and its inhibition by treatment with truncated Flt-1-Fc (vascular endothelial growth factor Trap[A40]). *Endocrinology* 2001; **142**:3244–3254.

66. Pauerstein CJ, Eddy CA, Croxatto HD, et al. Temporal relationships of estrogen, progesterone, and luteinizing hormone levels to ovulation in women and infra-human primates. *Am. J. Obstet. Gynecol.* 1978; **130**:876–886.

67. Park SJ, Goldsmith LT, Skurnick JH, Wojtczuk A, Weiss G. Characteristics of the urinary luteinizing hormone surge in young ovulatory women. *Fertil. Steril.* 2007; **88**:684–690.

68. Direito A, Bailly S, Mariani A, Ecochard R. Relationships between the luteinizing hormone surge and other characteristics of the menstrual cycle in normally ovulating women. *Fertil. Steril.* 2012; **99**:279–285.

69. Alliende ME. Luteinizing hormone surge in normally ovulating women. *Fertil. Steril.* 2013; **99**:e14–e15.

70. Yussman MA, Taymor MI, Miyata J, Pheteplace C. Serum levels of follicle-stimulating hormone, luteinizing hormone, and plasma progestins correlated with human ovulation. *Fertil. Steril.* 1970; **21**:119–125.

71. Kerin J. Ovulation detection in the human. *Clin. Reprod. Fertil.* 1982; **1**:27–54.

72. Richards JS, Russell DL, Ochsner S, Espey LL. Ovulation: new dimensions and new regulators of the inflammatory-like response. *Ann. Rev. Physiol.* 2002; **64**:69–92.

73. Okamura H, Okazaki T, Nakajima A. Effects of electrical stimulation on human ovarian contractility. *Obstet. Gynecol.* 1975; **45**:557–561.

74. Okamura H, Takenaka A, Yajima Y, Nishimura T. Ovulatory changes in the wall at the apex of the human Graafian follicle. *J. Reprod. Fertil.* 1980; **58**:153–155.

75. Duffy DM. Novel contraceptive targets to inhibit ovulation: the prostaglandin E2 pathway. *Hum. Reprod. Update* 2015; **21**:652–670.

76. Priddy AR, Killick SR, Elstein M, et al. Ovarian follicular fluid eicosanoid concentrations during the pre-ovulatory period in humans. *Prostaglandins* 1989; **38**:197–202.

77. Duffy DM, Stouffer RL. The ovulatory gonadotrophin surge stimulates cyclooxygenase expression and prostaglandin production by the monkey follicle. *Mol. Hum. Reprod.* 2001; **7**:731–739.

78. Tjugum J, Norström A, Dennefors B, Lundin S. Oxytocin in human follicular fluid and its possible role in the ovulatory process as studied in vitro. *Hum. Reprod.* 1986; **1**:283286.

79. Meidan R, Altstein M, Girsh E. Biosynthesis and release of oxytocin by granulosa cells derived from preovulatory bovine follicles: effects of forskolin and insulin-like growth factor-I. *Biol. Reprod.* 1992; **46**:715–720.

80. Horka P, Malickova K, Jarosova R, et al. Matrix metalloproteinases in serum and the follicular fluid of women treated by in vitro fertilization. *J. Assist. Reprod. Genet.* 2012; **29**:1207–1212.

81. Hernandez-Gonzalez I, Gonzalez-Robayna I, Shimada M, et al. Gene expression profiles of cumulus cell oocyte complexes during ovulation reveal cumulus cells express neuronal and immune-related genes: does this expand their role in the ovulation process? *Mol. Endocrinol.* 2006; **20**:1300–1321.

82. Edson MA, Nagaraja AK, Matzuk MM. The mammalian ovary from genesis to revelation. *Endocr. Rev.* 2009; **30**:624–712.

83. Gershon E, Plaks V, Dekel N. Gap junctions in the ovary: expression, localization and function. *Mol. Cell. Endocrinol.* 2008; **282**:18–25.

84. Freimann S, Ben-Ami I, Dantes A, Ron-El R, Amsterdam A. EGF-like factor epiregulin and amphiregulin expression is regulated by gonadotropins/cAMP in human ovarian follicular cells. *Biochem. Biophys. Res. Commun.* 2004; **324**:829–834.

85. Park JY, Su YQ, Ariga M, et al. EGF-like growth factors as mediators of LH action in the ovulatory follicle. *Science* 2004; **303**:682–684.

86. Hizaki H, Segi E, Sugimoto Y, et al. Abortive expansion of the cumulus and impaired fertility in mice lacking the prostaglandin E receptor subtype EP(2). *Proc. Natl. Acad. Sci. U. S. A.* 1999; **96**:10501–10506.

87. Gueripel X, Brun V, Gougeon A. Oocyte bone morphogenetic protein 15, but not growth differentiation factor 9, is increased during gonadotropin-induced follicular development in the immature mouse and is associated with cumulus oophorus expansion. *Biol. Reprod.* 2006; **75**:836–843.

88. Elvin JA, Yan C, Matzuk MM. Oocyte-expressed TGF-beta superfamily members in female fertility. *Mol. Cell. Endocrinol.* 2000; **159**:1–5.

89. Maruo T, Katayama K, Barnea ER, Mochizuki M. A role for thyroid hormone in the induction of ovulation and corpus luteum function. *Horm. Res.* 1992; **37** (Suppl. 1):12–18.

90. Chaffkin LM, Luciano AA, Peluso JJ. Progesterone as an autocrine/paracrine regulator of human granulosa cell proliferation. *J. Clin. Endocrinol. Metab.* 1992; **75**:1404–1408.

91. Sasano H, Mori T, Sasano N, Nagura H, Mason JI. Immunolocalization of 3beta-hydroxysteroid dehydrogenase in human ovary. *J. Reprod. Fertil.* 1990; **89**:743–751.

92. Brezinka C. 3D ultrasound imaging of the human corpus luteum. *Reprod. Biol.* 2014; **14**:110–114.

93. Jokubkiene L, Sladkevičius P, Rovas L, Valentin L. Assessment of changes in volume and vascularity of the ovaries during the normal menstrual cycle using three dimentional power Doppler ultrasound. *Hum. Reprod.* 2006; **21**:2661–2668.

94. Stouffer RL, Bishop CV, Bogan RL, Xu F, Hennebold JD. Endocrine and local control of the primate corpus luteum. *Reprod. Biol.* 2013; **13**:259–271.

95. Nishimori K, Dunkel L, Hsueh A, Yamoto M, Nakano R. Expression of luteinizing hormone and chorionic gonadotropin receptor messenger ribonucleic acid in human corpora lutea during menstrual cycle and pregnancy. *J. Clin. Endocrinol. Metab.* 1995; **80**:1444–1448.

96. Crisp TM, Dessouky DA, Denys FR. The fine structure of the human corpus luteum of early pregnancy and during the progestational phase of menstrual cycle. *Am. J. Anat.* 1970; **127**:37–69.

97. Meidan R, Girsh E, Blum O, Aberdam E. In vitro differentiation of bovine theca and granulosa cells into small and large luteal-like cells: morphological and functional characteristics. *Biol. Reprod.* 1990; **43**:913–921.

98. Sanders SL, Stouffer RL. Localization of steroidogenic enzymes in macaque luteal tissue during the menstrual cycle and simulated early pregnancy: immunohistochemical evidence supporting the two-cell model for estrogen production in the primate corpus luteum. *Biol. Reprod.* 1997; **56**:1077–1087.

99. Reynolds L, Redmer D. Growth and development of the corpus luteum. *J. Reprod. Fertil. Suppl.* 1999; **54**:181–191.

100. Robinson RS, Woad KJ, Hammond AJ, et al. Angiogenesis and vascular function in the ovary. *Reproduction* 2009; **138**:869–881.

101. Ferrara N, Chen H, Davis-Smyth T, et al. Vascular endothelial growth factor is essential for corpus luteum angiogenesis. *Nat. Med.* 1998; **4**:336–340.

102. Wulff C, Dickson SE, Duncan WC, Fraser HM. Angiogenesis in the human corpus luteum: simulated early pregnancy by hCG treatment is associated with both angiogenesis and vessel stabilization. *Hum. Reprod.* 2001; **16**:2515–2524.

103. Forsythe JA, Jiang BH, Iyer NV, et al. Activation of vascular endothelial growth factor gene transcription by hypoxia-inducible factor 1. *Mol. Cell. Biol.* 1996; **16**:4604–4613.

104. Fraser HM, Duncan WC. Regulation and manipulation of angiogenesis in the ovary and endometrium. *Reprod. Fertil. Dev.* 2009; **21**:277–392.

105. Spencer TE, Bazer FW. Conceptus signals for establishment and maintenance of pregnancy. *Reprod. Biol. Endocrinol.* 2004; **2**:49.

106. Horton EW, Poyser NL. Uterine luteolytic hormone: a physiological role of prostaglandin F2α. *Physiol. Rev.* 1976; **56**:595–651.

107. Miyamoto A, Shirasuna K, Shimizu T, Bollwein H, Schams D. Regulation of corpus luteum development and maintenance: specific roles of angiogenesis and action of prostaglandin F2α. *Soc. Reprod. Fertil. Suppl.* 2010; **67**:289–304.

108. Best CL, Pudney J, Welch WR, Burger N, Hill JA. Localization and characterization of white blood cell populations within the human ovary throughout the menstrual cycle and menopause. *Hum. Reprod.* 1996; **11**:790–797.

109. Townson DH, Liptak AR. Chemokines in the corpus luteum: implications of leukocyte chemotaxis. *Reprod. Biol. Endocrinol.* 2003; **1**:94.

110. Girsh E, Milvae RA, Wang W, Meidan R. Effect of endothelin-1 on bovine luteal cell function: role in prostaglandin F2a-induced antisteroidogenic action. *Endocrinology* 1996; **137**:1306–1312.

111. Wulff C, Wilson H, Largue P, et al. Angiogenesis in the human corpus luteum: localization and changes in angiopoietins, tie-2, and vascular endothelial growth factor messenger ribonucleic acid. *J. Clin. Endocrinol. Metab.* 2000; **85**:4302–4309.

112. Zalman Y, Klipper E, Farberov S, et al. Regulation of angiogenesis-related prostaglandin F2α-induced genes in the bovine corpus luteum. *Biol. Reprod.* 2012; **86**:92.

113. Farberov S, Meidan R. Thrombospondin-1 affects bovine luteal function via transforming growth factor β1-dependent and independent actions. *Biol. Reprod.* 2016; **94**:25.

114. Yadav VK, Lakshmi G, Medhamurthy R. Prostaglandin F2α-mediated activation of apoptotic signaling cascades in the corpus luteum during apoptosis: involvement of caspase-activated DNase. *J. Biol. Chem.* 2005; **280**:10357–10367.

115. Duncan WC, McNeilly AS, Fraser HM, Illingworth PJ. Luteinizing hormone receptor in the human corpus luteum: lack of down regulation during maternal recognition of pregnancy. *Hum. Reprod.* 1996; **11**:2291–2297.

116. Jabbour HN, Kelly RW, Fraser HM, Critchley HO. Endocrine regulation of menstruation. Endocr. Rev. 2006; **27**:17–46.

117. Nagaoka SI, Hassold TJ, Hunt PA. Human aneuploidy: mechanisms and new insights into an age-old problem. *Nat. Rev. Genet.* 2012; **13**:493–504.

118. Huang L, Tong X, Luo L, et al. Mutation analysis of the TUBB8 gene in nine infertile women with oocyte maturation arrest. *RBM Online* 2017; **35**:305–310.

119. American College of Obstetricians and Gynecologists. ACOG Committee Opinion. Age-related fertility decline. *Obstet. Gynecol.* 2008; **112**:409–411.

120. Ziebe S, Devroey P. Assisted reproductive technologies are an integrated part of national strategies addressing demographic and reproductive challenges. *Hum. Reprod. Update.* 2008; **14**:583–592.

121. Menken J, Trussell J, Larsen U. Age and infertility. Science 1986; **233**:1389–1394.

122. Faddy MJ, Gosden RG, Gougeon A, Richardson SJ, Nelson JF. Accelerated disappearance of ovarian follicles in mid-life: implications for forecasting menopause. *Hum. Reprod.* 1992; **7**:1342–1346.

123. Rosen MP, Johnstone E, McCulloch CE, et al. A characterization of the relationship of ovarian reserve markers with age. *Fertil. Steril.* 2012; **97**:238–243.

124. Hansen KR, Knowlton NS, Thyer AC, et al. A new model of reproductive aging: the decline in ovarian non-growing follicle number from birth to menopause. *Hum. Reprod.* 2008; **23**:699–708.

125. Wang YA, Dean J, Badgery-Parker T, Sullivan EA. *Assisted Reproduction Technology in Australia and New Zealand 2006.* Sydney: AIHW National Peritnatal Statistics Unit. 2008.

126. Fitzgerald O, Paul RC, Harris K, Chambers GM. *Assisted Reproductive Technology in Australia and New Zealand 2016.* Sydney: National Perinatal Epidemiology and Statistics Unit, the Univeristy of New South Wales Sydney. 2018.

127. Gilbert WM, Nesbitt TS, Danielsen B. Childbearing beyond age 40: pregnancy outcome in 24,032 cases. *Obstet. Gynecol.* 1999; **93**:9–14.

128. Meng L, Jan SZ, Hamer G, et al. Preantral follicular atresia occurs mainly through autophagy, while antral follicles degenerate mostly through apoptosis. *Biol. Reprod.* 2018; **99**:853–863.

129. Baker TG. A quantitative and cytological study of germ cells in human ovaries. *Proc. R. Soc. Lond. B. Biol. Sci.* 1963;**158**:417–433.

130. Richardson SJ, Senikas V, Nelson JF. Follicular depletion during the menopausal transition: evidence for accelerated loss and ultimate exhaustion. *J. Clin. Endocrinol. Metab.* 1987; **65**:1231–1237.

131. Murray A, Schoemaker MJ, Bennett CE, et al. Population-based estimates of the prevalence of FMR1 expansion mutations in women with early menopause and primary ovarian insufficiency. *Genet. Med.* 2014; **16**:19–24.

132. Broekmans FJ, Soules MR, Fauser BC. Ovarian aging: mechanisms and clinical consequences. *Endocr. Rev.* 2009; **30**:465–493.

133. Johnson NP, Bagrie EM, Coomarasamy A, et al. Ovarian reserve tests for predicting fertility outcomes for assisted reproductive technology: the International Systematic Collaboration of Ovarian Reserve Evaluation protocol for a systematic review of ovarian reserve test accuracy. *BJOG* 2006; **113**:1472–1480.

134. te Velde ER, Pearson PL. The variability of female reproductive ageing. *Hum. Reprod. Update* 2002; **8**:141–154.

135. Klein NA, Battaglia DE, Miller PB, et al. Ovarian follicular development and the follicular fluid hormones and growth factors in normal women of advanced reproductive age. *J. Clin. Endocrinol. Metab.* 1996; **81**:1946–1951.

136. Burger HG, Hale GE, Dennerstein L, Robertson DM. Cycle and hormone changes during perimenopause: the key role of ovarian function. *Menopause* 2008; **15**:603–612.

137. Klein NA, Battaglia DE, Fujimoto VY, et al. Reproductive aging: accelerated ovarian follicular development associated with a monotropic follicle-stimulating hormone rise in normal older women. *J. Clin. Endocrinol. Metab.* 1996; **81**:1038–1045.

138. Rossmanith WG. Gonadotropin secretion during aging in women. *Exp. Gerontology* 1995; **30**:369–381.

139. de Bruin JP, Bovenhuis H, van Noord PA, et al. The role of genetic factors in age at natural menopause. *Hum. Reprod.* 2001; **16**:2014–2018.

140. van Asselt KM, Kok HS, Pearson PL, et al. Heritability of menopausal age in mothers and daughters. *Fertil. Steril.* 2004; **82**:1348–1351.

141. Kalmbach KH, Antunes DM, Kohlrausch F, Keefe DL. Telomeres and female reproductive aging. *Semin. Reprod. Med.* 2015; **33**:389–395.

142. Keefe DL, Marquard K, Liu L. The telomere theory of reproductive senescence in women. *Curr. Opin. Obstet. Gynecol.* 2006; **18**:280–285.

143. Keefe DL. Telomeres, reproductive aging, and genomic instability during early development. *Reprod. Sci.* 2016; **23**:1612–1615.

144. Westhoff C, Murphy P, Heller D. Predictors of ovarian follicle number. *Fertil. Steril.* 2000; **74**:624–628.

145. Stock D, Knight JA, Raboud J, et al. Rotating night shift work and menopausal age. *Hum. Reprod.* 2019; **34**:539–548.

146. Pellestor F, Andreo B, Arnal F, Humeau C, Demaille J. Maternal aging and chromosomal abnormalities: new data drawn from in vitro unfertilized human oocytes. *Hum. Genet.* 2003; **112**:195–203.

147. Alberman E, Creasy M, Elleott M, Spicier C. Maternal factors associated with fetal chromosomal anomalies in spontaneous abortions. *Br. J. Obstet. Gynecol.* 1976; **83**:621–627.

148. Volarcik K, Sheean L, Goldfarb J, et al. The meiotic competence of in-vitro matured human oocytes is influenced by donor age: evidence that folliculogenesis is compromised in the reproductively aged ovary. *Hum. Reprod.* 1998; **13**:154–160.

149. Yun Y, Holt JE, Lane SI, et al. Reduced ability to recover from spindle disruption and loss of kinetochore spindle assembly checkpoint proteins in oocytes from aged mice. *Cell Cycle* 2014; **13**:1938–1947.

150. Hassold T, Hunt P. To err (meiotically) is human: the genesis of human aneuploidy. *Nat. Rev. Genet.* 2001; **2**:280–291.

151. Chiang T, Duncan FE, Schindler K, Schultz RM, Lampson MA. Evidence that weakened centromere cohesion is a leading cause of age-related aneuploidy in oocytes. *Curr. Biol.* 2010; **20**:1522–1528.

152. Cheng JM, Liu YX. Age-related loss of cohesion: causes and effects. *Int. J. Mol. Sci.* 2017; **18**. doi:10.3390/ijms18071578.

153. Kuliev A, Verlinsky Y. Meiotic and mitotic nondisjunction: lessons from preimplantation genetic diagnosis. *Hum. Reprod. Update* 2004; **10**:401–407.

154. Nagaoka SI, Hassold TJ, Hunt PA. Human aneuploidy: mechanisms and new insights into an age-old problem. *Nat. Rev. Genet.* 2012; **13**:493–504.

155. May-Panloup P, Boucret L, Chao de la Barca JM, et al. Ovarian ageing: the role of mitochondria in oocytes and follicles. *Hum. Reprod. Update* 2016; **22**:725–743.

156. Broekmans FJ, Faddy MJ, Scheffer G, te Velde ER. Antral follicle counts are related to age at natural fertility loss and age at menopause. *Menopause* 2004; **11**:607–614.

157. Tietze C. Fertility after discontinuation of intrauterine and oral contraception. *Int. J. Fertil.* 1968; **13**:385–389.

158. Gunby J, Bissonnette F, Librach C, Cowan L; IVF Directors Group of the Canadian Fertility and Andrology Society. Assisted reproductive technologies (ART) in Canada: 2006 results from the Canadian ART Register. *Fertil. Steril.* 2010; **93**:2189–2201.

159. Noci I, Borri P, Chieffi O, et al. Aging of the human endometrium: a basic morphological and immunohistochemical study. *Eur. J. Obstet. Gynecol. Reprod. Biol.* 1995; **63**:181–185.

160. Wang YA, Farquhar C, Sullivan EA. Donor age is a major determinant of success of oocyte donation/recipient programme. *Hum. Reprod.* 2012; **27**:118-125.

161. Sherman BM, West JH, Korenman SG. The menopausal transition: analysis of LH, FSH, estradiol, and progesterone concentrations during menstrual cycles of older women. *J. Clin. Endocrinol. Metab.* 1976; **42**:629–636.

162. Sabatini L, Zosmer A, Hennessy EM, Tozer A, Al-Shawaf T. Relevance of basal serum FSH to IVF outcome varies with patient age. *RBM Online* 2008; **17**:10–19.

163. Broekmans FJ, de Ziegler D, Howles CM, et al. The antral follicle count: practical recommendations for better standardization. *Fertil. Steril.* 2010; **94**:1044–1051.

164. Broekmans FJ, Kwee J, Hendriks DJ, Mol BW, Lambalk CB. A systematic review of tests predicting ovarian reserve and IVF outcome. *Hum. Reprod. Update* 2006; **12**:685–718.

165. La Marca A, Volpe A. Anti-Mullerian hormone (AMH) in female reproduction: is measurement of circulating AMH a useful tool? *Clin. Endocrinol.* 2006; **64**:603–610.

166. Li HWR, Yeung WSB, Lau EYL, Ho PC, Ng EHY. Evaluating the performance of serum antimullerian hormone concentration in predicting the live birth rate of controlled ovarian stimulation and intrauterine insemination. *Fertil. Steril.* 2010; **94**:2177–2181.

167. Hehenkamp WJ, Looman CW, Themmen AP, et al. Anti-Mullerian hormone levels in the spontaneous menstrual cycle do not show substantial fluctuation. *J. Clin. Endocrinol. Metab.* 2006; **91**:4057–4063.

168. Sowers MR, Eyvazzadeh AD, McConnell D, et al. Anti-mullerian hormone and inhibin B in the definition of ovarian aging and the menopause transition. *J. Clin. Endocrinol. Metab.* 2008; **93**:3478–3483.

169. Broekmans FJ. Testing for ovarian reserve in assisted reproduction programs: the current point of view. *Fact Views Vis. Obgin.* 2009; **1**:79–81.

Chapter 5

Conception

Conception is the process of becoming pregnant, which involves fertilization of the oocyte by a sperm cell and implantation of the formed embryo in the uterus.

Fertilization

Cervical mucus is a regulator of the sperm transfer from the vagina to the uterine cavity. Estradiol (E_2) stimulates the production of large amounts of thin, watery, alkaline acellular cervical mucus with ferning, spinnbarkeit (crystallization), and sperm receptivity. Progesterone (P_4) inhibits the secretory activity of cellular mucus and produces low spinnbarkeit and absence of ferning, which is impenetrable by spermatozoa. In midcycle, the cervix softens progressively, the os of the cervical canal dilates, and clear, profuse mucus exudes from the external os. In a few days after ovulation, the cervix becomes firm, and the os closes. The cervix is the first barrier for the sperm to overcome.

After ejaculation, within minutes of vaginal deposition, human sperm cells begin to leave the seminal pool and swim into the cervical canal (22 mm in length) where they could be found in 1.5–3 minutes post-ejaculation [1]. The sperm cells make their way through the uterine cavity (could be less than 10 minutes) into the Fallopian tubes, which have increased secretory activity. The Fallopian tube secretes mucus that results in the sticking of spermatozoa to the epithelium of the tube. Sperm binding occurs at the microvilli of the secretory cells [2]. There is chemotaxis of sperm cells to the cumulus–oocyte complex within the Fallopian tube, due to chemoattractants in the follicular fluid at ovulation time [3], which continue to be secreted by the cumulus-oocyte complex [4]. Peristaltic contractions of the female reproductive tract and cilia movement along the lining of the Fallopian tubes also assist the movement of sperm. Spermatozoa "swim" up the tube (extends about 10 cm) toward the ovum. Despite all this, however, only a small number of the sperm deposited in the vagina ever reach the ovum. Only 25–50 sperm cells out of 250–500 million spermatozoa reach their target.

Fertilization most often occurs in the outer one-third part of the oviduct, named "ampulla." Sperm cells penetrate the cumulus layer (of approximately 5000 cumulus cells) by cleavage of the extracellular matrix (mostly composed of hyaluronic acid) under acrosomal hyaluronidase and reach the zona pellucida (ZP). Spermatozoa that have completed their acrosome reaction before meeting the cumulus cannot penetrate [5–6]. Receptor molecules on the layer of ZP that surround the ovum bind sperm attracted to the area. Once bound to a ZP2 (sperm-binding ligand), the sperm cell releases enzymes from the acrosome (acrosome exocytosis), becomes incorporated into the ZP, and penetrates ZP rapidly by acrosin, a trypsin-like proteinase of the sperm. Once the spermatozoon reaches the surface of the ovum, the two plasma membranes fuse, and the nucleus of the sperm moves inside the oocyte.

The fusion between sperm and oocyte membranes leads the sperm cell to deliver a putative oocyte activation factor – phospholipase C zeta (PLCζ) – to the oocyte [7]. In addition to that, the sperm cell donates to the oocyte its DNA and centrosome, which contains a pair of centrioles (the oocyte has none). The sperm's centrioles are essential to organize a centrosome, which will form a spindle enabling the mitotic division of the zygote.

At the moment of sperm and oocyte membrane fusion, PLCζ hydrolyzes phosphatidylinositol biphosphate from the oocyte membrane into inositol triphosphate (IP_3) and diacylglycerol (DAG) (Figure 5.1). IP_3 interacts with its receptor on the membrane of the endoplasmic reticulum (ER), which allows Ca^{2+} release from the ER. Mutations in sperm PLCζ may prevent calcium signaling. The rise in Ca^{2+} increases the action of calcium-dependent protein kinase (PKC), activated by DAG, thus leading to the cortical reaction of the

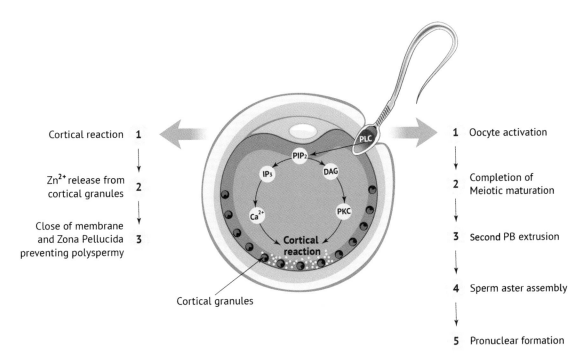

Figure 5.1 The fertilization process includes cortical reaction preventing polyspermy and completion of the meiotic oocyte division. PIP$_2$, phosphatidylinositol 4,5-bisphosphate.

oocyte (activation of peripheral cortical granules; estimated ~8000 granules in the oocyte). The content of these granules is released into the perivitelline space immediately after fertilization (exocytosis) for the establishment of the polyspermy block. Zink sparks from peripheral cortical granules last ~10–15 seconds after cortical granule exocytosis. Cortical granules also release ovastacin, a Zn^{2+}-related metallopeptidase that cleaves ZP proteins (closing of ZP) and membrane to provide a definitive block to the polyspermy. Cortical granules developed from Golgi complexes during oocyte development; however, their total number could be more related to the cytoplasmic maturation rather than nuclear maturation.

Reinitiated meiosis continues events, which lead to extrusion of the second polar body and zygote formation (male and female pronuclear).

A human oocyte contains an estimated ~100 000 – 200 000 copies of mitochondrial DNA (mtDNA), whereas a sperm cell delivers its ~25–75 copies of mtDNA. Paternal mitochondria are rapidly eliminated after fertilization as they are separated from the axoneme and degraded in lysosomes. A sharp reduction in paternal mtDNA content, together with the action of a specific ubiquitination mechanism of

mitochondria destruction in the early embryo, explains the absence of paternal transmission of mtDNA to the developing embryo [8].

In as much as the oocyte lives only a short time (probably a day only) after leaving the ruptured follicle, the "fertilization window" occurs around the time of ovulation. Spermatozoa may live up to a few days after entering the female tract, therefore sexual intercourse any time from about 3 days before ovulation to a day or so after ovulation may result in fertilization.

Implantation

Implantation is the process by which the embryo attaches to the endometrium, first invading the epithelium and then forming the placenta. This process is commonly seen as one of the strongest connections in nature (Figure 5.2). Conceptus (embryo/fetus and associated extraembryonic membranes) growth and development require P_4 and placental hormone actions on the uterus that regulate endometrial differentiation, uterine receptivity for blastocyst implantation, and conceptus–uterine interactions for implantation. Successful implantation depends on embryo quality and endometrial receptivity. There are three major stages in implantation of the embryo: apposition,

57

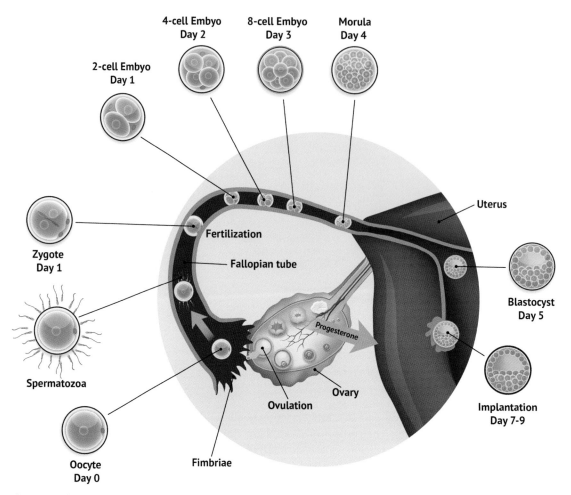

Figure 5.2 The early development of the embryo and its journey throughout a reproductive tract.

attachment (adhesion), and invasion, which are only implemented if three major conditions are fulfilled: a receptive endometrium, a functional embryo, and a functional embryo–endometrial dialog (secretions). The basic characteristics of the processes of attachment and invasion of the embryo to the uterine epithelial surface are common to many species. For the achievement of a successful pregnancy, perfect synchronism between the embryo development stage, changes in the endometrial environment, and conceptus–uterine interaction are necessary [9].

The implantation period is associated with changes in endometrial epithelial morphology and receptivity. The epithelial cells of the uterus are of two varieties. The luminal epithelial cells face the lumen of the uterus, while others radiate into the endometrial stroma toward the base of the myometrium to form

the uterine glands. These glands secrete a fluid rich in mucins, proteins, enzymes, growth factors, cytokines, and integrins, which all together play the role of an orchestra in implantation. The endometrial epithelium and uterine glands cyclically undergo dynamic remodeling, which is dictated by hormone-driven modification of the endometrium. The human endometrium is receptive to blastocyst implantation only during a very narrow time window in the luteal phase, which begins approximately 7 days after ovulation and lasts less than 2 days. This period, known as the "implantation window," is the time of maximum endometrial receptivity for implantation [10], which is manifested by the expression of peptides and proteins that can serve as biomarkers of uterine receptivity [11]. Impaired uterine receptivity and embryo invasion are currently considered the major limiting factor for the establishment of pregnancy. It is estimated that suboptimal embryo quality accounts for one-third of implantation failures, while suboptimal endometrial receptivity and altered embryo–endometrial dialog are responsible for the remaining two-thirds [12–13].

The implantation window is characterized by the appearance of membrane apical protrusions, called pinopodes or uterodomes [14], on the cells of the luminal epithelium [15] and expression of full-length luteinizing hormone/human chorionic gonadotropin (LH/hCG) receptor [16]. Pinopodes are P_4-dependent organelles that become visible between days 20 and 21 of the natural menstrual cycle [15; 17], persist for 24–48 hours [11; 18], and are observed between days 8 and 10 after the LH surge [19], with variation in the cycle days, on which these organelles form, of up to 5 days between different individuals [17; 20]. The apical surface of endometrial pinopodes participates in the adhesion process of the blastocyst, through mechanisms that are still unclear (Figure 5.3) [20].

The embryo must recognize a site susceptible to anchoring and does so by rolling itself over the uterine lumen. The apical cell surfaces of the epithelia contain numerous microvilli, which are covered by a thick layer of glycocalyx (Figure 5.4); the embryo contains several complementary receptors and/or ligands, and these receptor–ligand interactions aid in initial adhesion [21–22]. The attachment–detachment events between the endometrial epithelium and the embryo have very localized effects. The embryo initially attaches to the wall of the uterus via its surface L-selectin, which binds carbohydrates on the uterine wall until it gradually slows to a complete stop. This embryo–uterine interaction was described as "a tennis ball rolling across a surface covered in syrup" [23]. Trophectoderm cells secrete syncytin-1, which may help the embryo stick to the endometrium and which plays a role in implantation and early placental development [24]. At the same time, the endometrium expresses binding proteins, i.e., integrin β3 and cadherin. The embryo is not always successful in attachment but continues making attempts until it locates a site that ultimately allows docking. Once the embryo adheres, it anchors and breaches the

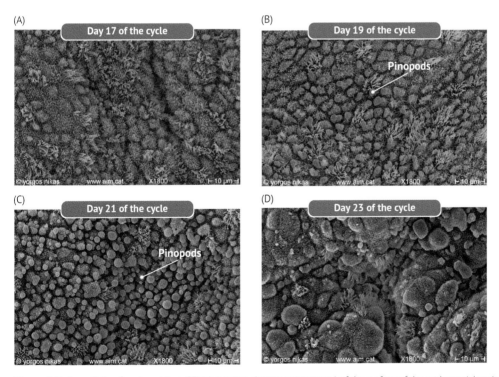

Figure 5.3 Receptivity of endometrium. SEM (scanning electron microscopy) of the surface of the endometrial cavity at sequential days of a 28-day menstrual cycle. (A) Day 17: the apical membranes of the endometrial epithelial cells are covered by dense microvilli. (B) Day 19: smooth membranes develop and protrude towards the lumen (developing pinopodes). (C) Day 21: smooth membranes replace microvilli and protrude maximally (fully developed pinopodes). (D) Day 23: short microvilli reappear on the apices and the visible cell size increases (regressing pinopodes). The photocopies are generously provided by Dr. Yorgos Nikas.

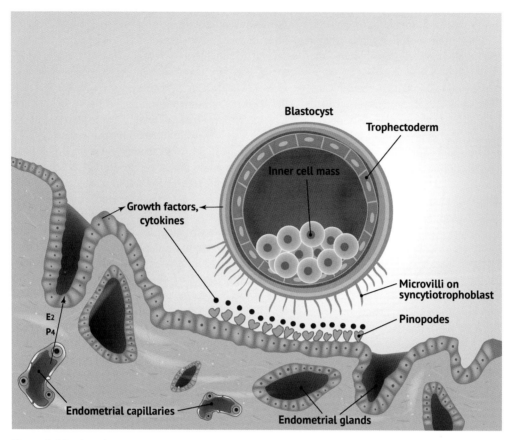

Figure 5.4 Implantation.

luminal epithelium to gain entry. Once the embryo breaches the luminal epithelium, the uterus transforms itself completely into a decidua by a process called decidualization, which involves remodeling of the endometrium that includes secretory transformation of the uterine stroma, an influx of specialized uterine natural killer (NK) cells, the exclusion of maternal T and B cells, and finally vascular remodeling [25]. The decidua is a highly vascularized environment created to house and nourish the embryo. In the decidua, the NK cells, which are generally cytotoxic to major histocompatibility complex (MHC)-null target cells, switch to a molecular phenotype that is less cytotoxic [26], and the numbers of T and B cells are kept to a minimum to avoid inflammation and fetal rejection [26].

hCG is an autocrine and paracrine regulator and its interaction with LH/hCG endometrial receptors has been implicated in decidualization [27–28]. hCG is a heterodimeric glycoprotein composed of two subunits, α and β, and shares a common α-subunit with all three pituitary glycoprotein hormones. Their specific bioactivity relates to differences in their β-subunits. LHβ and hCGβ are very similar (82% homology), but differ in terms of receptor affinity and half-life, with that of LH being much shorter, i.e., 21 minutes compared with 12 hours for hCG [29]. Circulating hCG, as well as LH, exists as a mix of isoforms. The sources of the various isoforms appear to differ, produced by the forming blastocyst, chorionic villi, and extravillous cytotrophoblast [30]. In clinical practice, hCG dynamics are used to investigate the early stages of pregnancy, as concentrations normally double every 48 hours in the first 6 weeks of pregnancy [31]. Pregnancy tests detect the presence of the hCG that is excreted in the urine of pregnant women as early as 1–2 days after implantation occurs. One of the major functions of hCG is a luteal rescue from luteolysis [32].

hCG maintains the weight of the corpus luteum (CL) [33], whereas, at the cellular level, hCG also preserves luteal cell size, morphology, and luteal secretions [34]. The steroidogenic function of the CL during early gestation is similar to its function during the menstrual cycle, inducing an increase in circulating P_4 and E_2. Despite the stimulus of exponentially increasing levels of hCG, the production of P_4 by the CL appears to be maintained at a relatively constant level [35]. Increasing trophoblastic production of P_4 allows pregnancy to progress independently of the CL [36]. CL peptidergic function, as indicated by relaxin and inhibin A luteal production, is also markedly enhanced and is dependent on hCG stimulation [37]. Relaxin acts on several tissues, including the embryo and uterus, and may optimize maternal–fetal function and maternal adaptations to pregnancy [38].

Endometrial thickness is the most investigated marker of endometrial receptivity and has become a classic example of the limited benefit of means in the context of endometrial receptivity. Endometrial thickness greater than 7 mm (7–14 mm) and endometrial volume greater than 2 ml, with triple line pattern and endometrial blood flow, all measured on the day of hCG trigger injection, is the prognostic profile for endometrial receptivity in in vitro fertilization (IVF) treatment [39]. Histological criteria for endometrial dating can observe a delay in the secretory phase and detect receptivity [40]. Higher clinical pregnancy and live birth rates were observed in women with delayed embryo transfer as manifested by pinopodes formation, compared with women with standard IVF embryo transfer [41]. A higher score of pinopode formation was associated with higher clinical pregnancy rates compared to lower scores [42]. Endometrial receptivity array (ERA) is a molecular diagnostic test based on microarray technology that classifies endometrial biopsies into receptive, pre-receptive or proliferative, based on the expression of 238 selected genes from a tissue sample accepted after endometrial biopsy [43]. Women then undergo personalized embryo transfer (pET), with the frozen–thawed embryo transfer timed according to the receptive status as identified by ERA, however inconvenient the results, for now a day, accepted with ERA and pET [44–45]. A significant association between various Doppler signals in the endometrium and pregnancy rates has been reported; however, its clinical relevance remains uncertain [46].

For endometrial receptivity and implantation, a cross-talk between the blastocyst and the endometrium is essential. This cross-talk is based on the secretion of cytokines and growth factors, cell-derived polypeptides, and proteins that have the capacity to bind to specific cell surface receptors and may act as potent intercellular signals regulating functions of endometrial cells. They regulate cell proliferation, differentiation, and apoptosis, by autocrine, paracrine, and endocrine mechanisms. Cytokines produced by the uterine mucosa and the embryo may play a role in maternal–embryonic interactions, augmenting endometrial receptivity by regulation of the expression of adhesion and anti-adhesion proteins [47]. Among the main cytokines and growth factors that have been implicated in implantation by facilitating endometrial receptivity are: leukemia inhibitory factor, interleukin-1 (IL-1), heparin binding-epidermal growth factor, granulocyte-macrophage colony-stimulating factor-1 (GM-CSF-1), insulin-like growth factor (IGF) binding protein-1, and keratinocyte growth factor [48–54]. Trophoblast invasion is an active enzymatic process. Human cytotrophoblastic cells are invasive because of their capacity to secrete metalloproteinases [55] and collagenase (type IV) that allow the blastocyst to penetrate the wall of the uterus, usually the posterior wall [56]. Embryo cross-talk secretions include interleukins (IL-1, IL-6, IL-10), GM-CSF, IGF-II, and interferon. The embryo/trophoblastic extracellular vesicles contain a variety of RNA and miRNA species that have diverse targets on both epithelial and stromal endometrial cells [57–58]. The target genes of these miRNAs are predicted to mediate cellular activities, such as adhesion and migration, suggesting that embryos could potentially modify the expression of the endometrial genome so that it improves trophoblast adhesion. The cytokine GM-CSF is expressed by epithelial cells of the uterus, reaching a maximum during the mid-secretory phase [59], and promotes implantation competence. The secretion of uterine GM-CSF is induced by hCG [60]; however, the embryonic origin of GM-CSF also exists [61]. GM-CSF deficiency is associated with altered implantation and placental development, elevated intrauterine growth retardation, preeclampsia, and increased miscarriage [62].

Does implantation exist in the uterus only? The embryo can implant outside of the endometrium, including in the Fallopian tube, or peritoneum wall, liver, or other places reached by intensive blood supply needed for implantation. Implantation of the embryo in a location other than the uterus is referred to as an ectopic pregnancy (from the Greek *ectopos* – "displaced").

Chronologically, one of the earliest promoters of trophoblast invasion seems to be the inner cell mass (ICM) of the embryo itself. Extracellular vesicles produced by the embryonic stem cell of the ICM can trigger trophoblast invasion. As the blastocyst further develops, with gastrulation, the ICM forms a structure of epiblast (forms the allantois) and primitive endoderm, with two cavities called the amniotic cavity (visualization of amniotic sac by ultrasound at ~5 weeks of pregnancy) and yolk sac (visualization at ~6 weeks of pregnancy). The yolk sac is most important in animals such as birds that depend heavily on yolk as a nutrient for the developing embryo. Because the uterine lining provides nutrients to the developing embryo in humans, the function of the yolk sac is not nutritive. Instead, it has other functions, including the production of blood cells. The amniotic cavity becomes a fluid-filled, shock-absorbing sac in which the embryo floats during development. It is the ICM that eventually forms the tissues of the offspring's body. The trophectoderm (also known as the trophoblast) forms the support structures. The chorion develops from the trophoblast to become a fetal membrane in the placenta. The chorionic villi are extensions of the blood vessels of the chorion that bring the embryonic circulation to the placenta. The placenta anchors the developing embryo to the uterus and provides a "bridge" for the exchange of nutrients and waste products between the mother and embryo.

Placenta

The placenta is a highly specialized structure that has transient, but very important functions during pregnancy. It is composed of tissues from mother and embryo and functions as an excretory, respiratory, and endocrine organ. During early development, the capacity of trophoblast cells (primitive syncytium) to invade deeply into the maternal uterine tissue, reaching as far as the myometrium, and their ability to remodel the maternal vasculature are a key to ensuring the formation of a functional placenta. The primitive syncytium secretes enzymes that digest and loosen the surrounding decidua, thereby allowing expansion of the primitive syncytium into the ensuing spaces.

Placental tissue normally separates the maternal and fetal blood supplies so that no intermixing occurs, and serves as an effective barrier that protects the developing embryo from many harmful substances. Unfortunately, toxic substances such as alcohol and some infectious organisms can penetrate this protective placental barrier. The nutrient-supplying function of the placenta is its most appreciated role. Defects in placental nutrient transport capacity usually manifest relatively late in gestation, i.e., in the second or third trimester in humans, and result in fetal growth retardation, which is often accompanied by other complications such as preeclampsia. Gene knockouts causing placental abnormalities in mouse models are significantly more likely to exhibit brain, heart, and vascular system defects compared with knockouts that do not affect placentation [63]. This mouse model revealed that the placenta is morphologically abnormal in about two-thirds of embryonic lethal mutant mouse lines [64]. The causative reasons for this developmental co-association remain unknown.

The placenta is embedded within the decidua, the maternal component of the maternal–fetal interface (the endometrium). At predecidualization differentiation of endometrial fibroblast-like cells into enlarged and granulated decidual stromal cells, and an influx of leukocytes can be observed [65]. During decidualization, there is both fetally and maternally mediated remodeling of the spiral arteries so that the placenta becomes bathed in maternal blood, which facilitates the exchange of nutrients, gases, and waste. Remodeling by fetal trophoblasts and maternal leukocytes results in the dilation of the spiral arteries; this decreases the force and maximizes the volume of the maternal blood bathing the placenta [66]. This remodeling can be divided into stages of trophoblast invasion-independent vascular changes (maternal activation of local decidual artery renin–angiotensin system), vascular remodeling induced by perivascular interstitial trophoblasts (uteroplacental arteries within the implantation region are invaded by extravillous trophoblast cells), and trophoblast infiltration of vessel walls (infiltration of the arterial wall by endovascular trophoblast). The utero-placental arteries undergo further dilation, reaching up to several times the original diameter of the lumen. Trophoblast infiltration of the media smooth muscle coincides with a loss of elastic fibers. At the same time, angiogenesis is induced by cytotrophoblasts (via vascular endothelial growth factor and proliferation) and vasodilation is induced by NK cells. The stromal cells of the endometrium respond to all these signals and transform into decidual cells.

The definitive structure of the placenta is composed of villous trees and is established by the third week of gestation. A single layer of contiguous multinucleated syncytiotrophoblasts lines the outermost surface of the human placental villous trees and acts as the major cellular barrier between the fetal compartment and maternal blood. Underlying the syncytiotrophoblast layer are undifferentiated, mononucleated cytotrophoblasts, which are progenitor trophoblast cells which can fuse to replenish the syncytiotrophoblast layer or differentiate into mononucleated extravillous trophoblasts, which are located at the tips of the anchoring villi. During the first trimester, the human placenta is hemodichorial, with two layers of trophoblasts separating the fetal and maternal bloodstreams. As the placenta grows, the underlying cytotrophoblast layer thins and becomes dispersed; thus, the human placenta of the second and third trimesters is essentially hemomonochorial, with only a single layer of syncytiotrophoblasts. The syncytiotrophoblasts also function as the main endocrine cells of the placenta, producing hCG and P_4 that support pregnancy [67]. During the first 8 weeks of gestation, syncytiotrophoblast secretion of hCG is required to "rescue" the CL from its impending demise and hCG extends the functional life span of the CL in early pregnancy by the production of P_4 [32]. At around 8 weeks of gestation, the luteo-placental shift occurs, as the placenta is producing enough hormones to support pregnancy. At this time, the volume of the CL decreases, and rising concentrations of the placental pregnancy-associated plasma protein-A can be detected in the serum, suggesting increasing placental function [68]. The CL loses its functional integrity between 8 and 10 weeks of gestation.

Extravillous trophoblasts physically anchor the human placenta to the decidua. In the first trimester, extravillous trophoblasts act as a plug for the spiral arteries, thus creating a hypoxic environment by excluding the oxygen-rich maternal blood. During the transition from the first to the second trimester, the extravillous trophoblast plug is eroded, and the intervillous space becomes flooded with maternal blood. The direct contact between maternal blood and syncytiotrophoblasts allows for efficient gas, nutrient, and waste exchange, which is maintained throughout the rest of pregnancy. Because direct contact between the maternal blood and the placenta does not occur until the end of the first trimester, this event distinguishes the early (first trimester) from the later (second and third trimesters) stages of pregnancy.

Placental tissue also has endocrine functions, as it secretes large amounts of hCG produced already in the blastocyst stage. hCG secretion peaks at about 8–9 weeks after fertilization, then drops to a steady low level by about week 16. The function of hCG, in general, is to act as a gonadotropin and stimulate the CL to continue its secretion of E_2 and P_4. As the placenta develops, it begins to secrete its own E_2 and P_4, corresponding with a decrease in hCG secretion, which reduces luteal secretion of these hormones. After about 3 months of pregnancy, the CL has degenerated, and the placenta has completely taken over the work of secreting the hormones needed to sustain the pregnancy.

Placental immune system. In addition to stromal cells, a remarkably large portion (~40%) of the decidua is composed of maternal leukocytes. In the first-trimester decidua basalis (the site of implantation and trophoblast invasion) decidual NK (dNK) cells comprise the majority (~70%) of immune cells, followed by decidual macrophages (20–25%) and T cells (3–10%) [26]. Most of our understanding of maternal leukocytes at the maternal–fetal interface has been determined in mouse studies and correlated to observations in human patient samples. dNK cells are the largest population of maternal leukocytes and a unique tissue-specific population that accumulates at the maternal–fetal interface, where they contribute to decidualization and implantation [69]. The dNK cells of pregnancy are phenotypically distinct from peripherally circulating NK cells. There is a cyclic enrichment of NK cells in the uterus after ovulation, which is sustained during pregnancy. dNK cells produce a vast array of growth factors, angiogenic factors, and cytokines [70]. Through these secretions, they help remodel the decidua and spiral arteries, promote trophoblast invasion, and increase the availability of maternal blood at the implantation site [71]. In patients with unexplained infertility, endometrial biopsies have found substantially fewer NK cells than in fertile women [72].

Decidual macrophages are the primary antigen-presenting cells at the maternal–fetal interface in early pregnancy [26]. Like uterine NK cells, levels of uterine macrophages rise and fall with the menstrual cycle and then increase upon fertilization [73]. Decidual macrophages have many functions during pregnancy. Like dNK cells, they aid in remodeling the spiral arteries and trophoblast invasion [74]. Decidual macrophages are proposed to perform "cleanup" functions by phagocytosing apoptotic trophoblasts, which prevents activation of pro-inflammatory pathways in the decidua [75].

Observational experiments have identified regulatory T (Treg) cells in the human decidua, and cases of

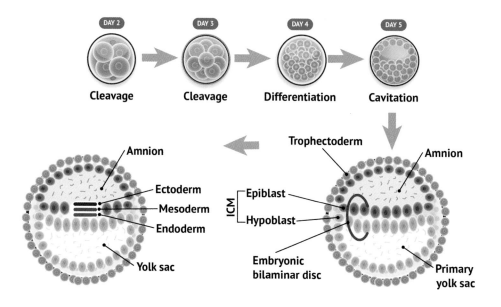

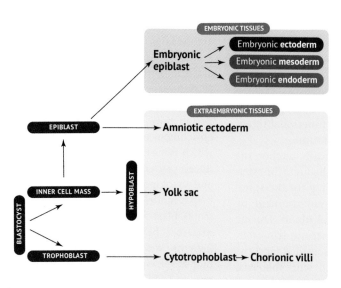

Figure 5.5 Implanted embryo development and early formation of the embryonic tissues.

human infertility, recurrent spontaneous abortions, and other pregnancy complications have been inversely correlated with Treg cell frequencies or functionality [76].

Maternal tolerance, which permits a mother to carry the fetus to term despite the presence of foreign fetal antigen, is a poorly understood phenomenon that seems to defy some of the basic tenets of immunology. For a successful pregnancy, maternal tolerance must be established, and the failure of maternal tolerance is correlated with preeclampsia and miscarriage [77]. In general, tolerance is mediated by the restriction and modulation of leukocytes that permeate the maternal–fetal interface. Maternal tolerance may occur through species-specific mechanisms. In humans, placental extravillous trophoblasts express human leukocyte antigen-G (HLA-G), a nonclassical MHC molecule, which has been suggested to have a role in the escape of the cells from immune recognition and destruction. HLA-G interacts directly or indirectly, via HLA-E, with specific killer inhibitory receptors (Fas) present on the surface

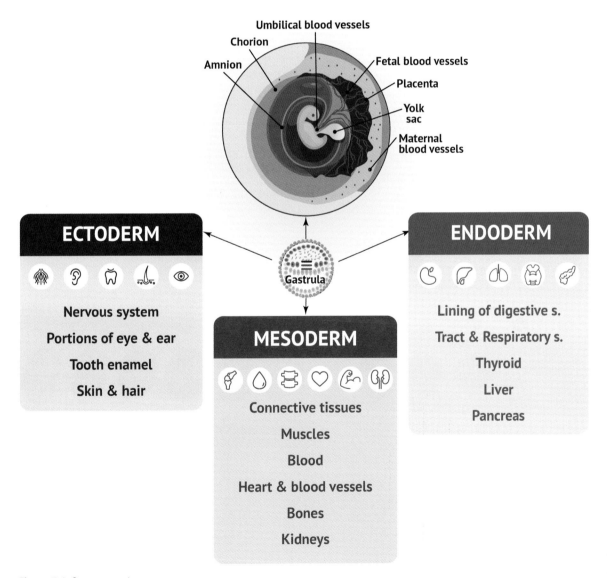

Figure 5.6 Organogenesis.

of leukocytes, thereby protecting the fetal cells from maternal immune attacks [78]. dNK cells interact with HLA-G$^+$ invasive trophoblastic cells, which may result in apoptosis of leukocytes [79].

The placenta secretes antiviral molecules that broadly function to restrict viral infections. The human placenta can also actively transport protective antibodies to the fetus. Transplacental passage of maternal humoral immunity in humans begins at week 16 of gestation and increases during the course of pregnancy so that, at term, the fetus has a greater serum concentration of maternally derived IgG than its mother [80].

Periods of Pregnancy

The length of pregnancy (about 39 weeks) is called the gestation period, which is divided into 3-month segments, called trimesters. The first trimester extends from the first day of the last menstrual period to the end of the twelfth week. The second trimester extends from the twelfth to the twenty-eighth week of pregnancy. The third trimester extends from the twenty-eighth week until delivery. The embryonic period of development extends from fertilization until the end of week 8 of gestation. After week 8, the term "embryo" is replaced by the term "fetus" until delivery.

Formation of the Embryonic Germ Layers

The chorion arises from the trophoblast and forms the fetal membrane in the placenta. Extraembryonic cells derived from the chorionic villi form a layer around the external surfaces of the amnion and yolk sac (Figure 5.5). The embryonic disc gives rise to the fetus itself. There are three layers of specialized cells called primary germ layers: endoderm (or inside layer), ectoderm (or outside layer), and mesoderm (or middle layer), which give rise to all parts of the body by a process called morphogenesis (Figures 5.6 and 5.7).

Endoderm. The inner germ layer forms the lining of various tracts, as well as several glands, e.g., the lining of the respiratory tract and gastrointestinal tract, including some of the accessory structures such as tonsils. The linings of the pancreatic ducts, hepatic ducts, and urinary tract also have an endodermal origin, as do the glandular epithelium of the thymus, thyroid, and parathyroid.

Ectoderm. The outer germ layer forms many of the structures around the periphery of the body, e.g., the epidermis of the skin, enamel of the teeth, cornea, and lens of the eye. Besides these peripheral structures, various components of the nervous system, including the brain and the spinal cord, have an ectodermal origin.

Mesoderm. The middle germ layer forms most of the organs and other structures between those formed by the endoderm and ectoderm, e.g., the dermis of the skin, bones, skeletal muscles, many of the glands of the body, kidneys, gonads, and components of the circulatory system.

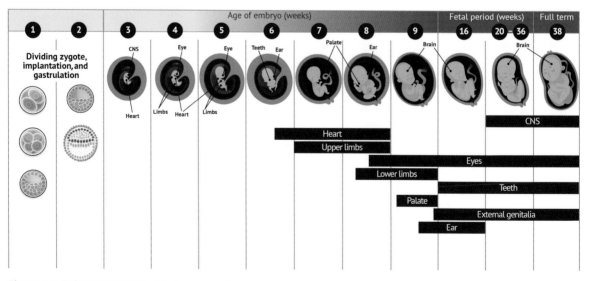

Figure 5.7 Embryogenesis. CNS, central nervous system.

Anomalies in or failure of embryo or endometrium development lead to miscarriages. Most miscarriages in the first trimester are sporadic, with chromosomal or morphological abnormalities of the developing embryo [81]. Endometrial stem cell deficiency and stromal senescence limit the differentiation capacity of the endometrium and predispose for pregnancy failure, which is associated with recurrent pregnancy loss [82]. It was suggested that women who carry the genes for inherited thrombophilia are more likely to have a clotting problem leading to miscarriage. The three major gene mutations which lead to inherited thrombophilias are factor V Leiden mutation, factor II (prothrombin) G20210 gene mutation, and methylenetetrahydrofolate reductase (*MTHFR*) mutation (leading to hyperhomocysteinemia). However, the evidence that clotting problems lead to a miscarriage is still weak [83].

References

1. Sobrero AJ, Macleod J. The immediate postcoital test. *Fertil. Steril.* 1962; **13**:184–189.

2. Pacey AA, Hill CJ, Scudamore IW, et al. The interaction in vitro of human spermatozoa with epithelial cells from the human uterine (fallopian) tube. *Hum. Reprod.* 1995; **10**:360–366.

3. Hunter RHF, Petersen HH, Greve T. Ovarian follicular fluid, progesterone and Ca^{2+} ion influences on sperm release from the Fallopian tube reservoir. *Mol. Reprod. Dev.* 1999; **54**:283–291.

4. Sun F, Bahat A, Gakamsky A, et al. Human sperm chemotaxis: both the oocyte and its surrounding cumulus cells secrete sperm attractants. *Hum. Reprod.* 2005; **20**:761–767.

5. Talbot P. Sperm penetration through oocyte investments in mammals. *Am. J. Anat.* 1985; **174**:331–346.

6. Drobnis EZ, Katz DF. Videomicroscopy of mammalian fertilization. In: Wassarman PM, ed., *Elements of Mammalian Fertilization*. Boca Raton: CRC Press. 1991; 269–300.

7. Nomikos M, Kashir J, Swann K, Lai FA. Sperm PLCζ: from structure to Ca^{2+} oscillations, egg activation and therapeutic potential. *FEBS Lett.* 2013; **587**:3609–3616.

8. Sutovski P, Moreno RD, Ramalho-Santos J, et al. Ubiquitin tag for sperm mitochondria. *Nature* 1999; **402**:371–372.

9. Navot D, Scott RT, Droesch K, et al. The window of embryo transfer and the efficiency of human conception in vitro. *Fertil. Steril.* 1991; **55**:114–118.

10. Duc-Goiran P, Mignot TM, Bourgeois C, Ferré F. Embryo-maternal interactions at the implantation site: a delicate equilibrium. *Eur. J. Obstet. Gynecol. Reprod. Biol.* 1999; **83**:85–100.

11. Lessey BA. The role of the endometrium during embryo implantation. *Hum. Reprod.* 2000; **15**:39–50.

12. Edwards RG. Implantation, interception and contraception. *Hum. Reprod.* 1994; **9**:985–995.

13. Franasiak JM, Forman EJ, Hong KH, et al. The nature of aneuploidy with increasing age of the female partner: a review of 15 169 consecutive trophectoderm biopsies evaluated with comprehensive chromosomal screening. *Fertil. Steril.* 2014; **101**:656–663.

14. Adams SM, Gayer N, Hosie MJ, Murphy CR. Human uterodomes (pinopods) do not display pinocytotic function. *Hum. Reprod.* 2002; **17**:1980–1986.

15. Nikas G, Drakakis P, Loutradis D, et al. Uterine pinopodes as markers of "nidation window" in cycling women receiving exogenous oestradiol and progesterone. *Hum. Reprod.* 1995; **10**:1208–1213.

16. Licht P, von Volff M, Berkholz A, Wildt L. Evidence for cycle-dependent expression of full-length human chorionic gonadotropin/luteinizing hormone receptor mRNA in human endometrium and decidua. *Fertil. Steril.* 2003; **79**:718–723.

17. Nikas G, Aghajanova L. Endometrial pinopodes: some more understanding on human implantation? *RBM Online* 2002; **4**:18–23.

18. Macklon NS, Brosens JJ. The human endometrium as a sensor of embryo quality. *Biol. Reprod.* 2014; **91**:98.

19. Wilcox AJ, Baird DD, Weinberg CR. Time of implantation of the conceptus and loss of pregnancy. *N. Engl. J. Med.* 1999; **340**:1796–1799.

20. Bentin-Ley U. Relevance of endometrial pinopodes for human blastocyst implantation. *Hum. Reprod.* 2000; **15**:67–73.

21. Aplin JD, Ruane PT. Embryo-epithelium interactions during implantation at a glance. *J. Cell Sci.* 2017; **130**:15–22.

22. Feng Y, Ma X, Deng L, et al. Role of selectins and their ligands in human implantation stage. *Glycobiology* 2017; **27**:385–391.

23. Genbacev OD, Prakobphol A, Foulk RI, et al. Trophoblast L-selectin-mediated adhesion at the maternal-fetal interface. *Science* 2003; **299**:405–408.

24. Soygur B, Moore H. Expression of syncytin 1 (HERV-W), in the preimplantation human blastocyst, embryonic stem cells and trophoblast cells derived in vitro. *Hum. Reprod.* 2016; **31**:1455–1461.

25. Mori M, Bogdan A, Balassa T, Csabai T, Szekeres-Bartho J. The decidua—the maternal bed embracing

the embryo—maintains the pregnancy. *Semin. Immunopathol.* 2016; **38**:635–649.

26. Liu S, Diao L, Huang C, et al. The role of decidual immune cells on human pregnancy. *J. Reprod. Immunol.* 2017; **124**:44–53.

27. Han SW, Lei ZM, Rao CV. Treatment of human endometrial stroma cells with chorionic gonadotropin promotes their morphological and functional differentiation into decidua. *Mol. Cell. Endocrinol.* 1999; **147**:7–16.

28. Yang M, Lei ZM, Rao CV. The central role of human chorionic gonadotropin in the formation of human placental syncytium. *Endocrinology* 2003; **144**:1108–1120.

29. Casper RF. Basic understanding of gonadotropin-releasing hormone-agonist triggering. *Fertil. Steril.* 2015; **103**:867–869.

30. Fournier T, Guibourdenche J, Evain-Brion D. Review: hCGs: different sources of production, different glycoforms and functions. *Placenta* 2015; **36**:S60–S65.

31. Sivalingam VN, Duncan WC, Kirk E, Shephard LA, Horne AW. Diagnosis and management of ectopic pregnancy. *J. Fam. Plann. Reprod. Health Care* 2011; **37**:231–240.

32. Tuckey RC. Progesterone synthesis by the human placenta. *Placenta* 2005; **26**:273–281.

33. Illingworth PJ, Reddi K, Smith K, Baird DT. Pharmacological "rescue" of the corpus luteum results in increased inhibin production. *Clin. Endocrinol. (Oxf).* 1990; **33**:323–332.

34. Duffy DM, Stouffer RL. Gonadotropin versus steroid regulation of the corpus luteum of the rhesus monkey during simulated early pregnancy. *Biol. Reprod.* 1997; **57**:1451–1460.

35. Yoshimi T, Strott CA, Marshall JR, Lipsett MB. Corpus luteum function in early pregnancy. *J. Clin. Endocrinol.* 1969; **29**:225–230.

36. Nakajima ST, Nason FG, Badger GJ, Gibson M. Progesterone production in early pregnancy. *Fertil. Steril.* 1991; **55**:516–521.

37. Gagliardi CL, Goldsmith LT, Saketos M, Weiss G, Schmidt CL. Human chorionic gonadotropin stimulation of relaxin secretion by luteinized human granulosa cells. *Fertil. Steril.* 1992; **58**:314–320.

38. Conrad KP. Maternal vasodilation in pregnancy: the emerging role of relaxin. *Am. J. Physiol. Regul. Integr. Comp. Physiol.* 2011; **301**:R267–R275.

39. Craciunas L, Gallos I, Chu J, et al. Conventional and modern markers of endometrial receptivity: a systematic review and meta-analysis. *Hum. Reprod. Update* 2019; **25**:202–223, doi:10.1093/humupd/dmy044.

40. Balasch J, Fábregues F, Creus M, Vanrell JA. The usefulness of endometrial biopsy for luteal phase evaluation in infertility. *Hum. Reprod.* 1992; **7**:973–977.

41. Pantos K, Nikas G, Makrakis E, et al. Clinical value of endometrial pinopodes detection in artificial donation cycles. *RBM Online* 2004; **9**:86–90.

42. Jin XY, Zhao LJ, Luo DH, et al. Pinopode score around the time of implantation is predictive of successful implantation following frozen embryo transfer in hormone replacement cycles. *Hum. Reprod.* 2017; **32**:2394–2403.

43. Díaz-Gimeno P, Horcajadas JA, Martínez-Conejero JA, et al. A genomic diagnostic tool for human endometrial receptivity based on the transcriptomic signature. *Fertil. Steril.* 2011; **95**:50–60.

44. Hashimoto T, Koizumi M, Doshida M, et al. Efficacy of the endometrial receptivity array for repeated implantation failure in Japan: a retrospective, two-centers study. *Reprod. Med. Biol.* 2017; **16**:290–296.

45. Tan J, Kan A, Hitkari J, et al. The role of the endometrial receptivity array (ERA) in patients who have failed euploid embryo transfers. *J. Assist. Reprod. Genet.* 2018; **35**:683–692.

46. Wang J, Xia F, Zhou Y, et al. Association between endometrial/subendometrial vasculature and embryo transfer outcome: a metaanalysis and subgroup analysis. *J. Ultrasound Med.* 2018; **37**:149–163.

47. Simón C, Martin JC, Pellicer A. Paracrine regulators of implantation. *Baillieres Best Pract. Res. Clin. Obstet. Gynaecol.* 2000; **14**:815–826.

48. Aghajanova L, Stavrèus-Evers A, Nikas Y, Hovatta O, Landgren BM. Coexpression of pinopodes and leukemia inhibitory factor, as well as its receptor, in human endometrium. *Fertil. Steril.* 2003; **79**:808–814.

49. Lindhard A, Bentin-Ley U, Ravn V, et al. Biochemical evaluation of endometrial function at the time of implantation. *Fertil. Steril.* 2002; **78**:221–233.

50. Stavrèus-Evers A, Aghajanova L, Brismar H, et al. Co-existence of heparin-binding epidermal growth factor-like growth factor and pinopodes in human endometrium at the time of implantation. *Mol. Hum. Reprod.* 2002; **8**:765–769.

51. Daiter E, Pampfer S, Yeung YG, et al. Expression of colony stimulating factor-1 in the human uterus and placenta. *J. Clin. Endocrinol. Metab.* 1992; **74**:850–858.

52. Licht P, Russu V, Lehmeyer S, et al. Intrauterine microdialysis reveals cycle-dependent regulation of endometrial insulin-like growth factor binding protein-1 secretion by human chorionic gonadotrophin. *Fertil. Steril.* 2002; **78**:252–258.

53. Slayden OD, Rubin JS, Lacey DL, Brenner RM. Effects of keratinocyte growth factor in the endometrium of rhesus macaques during the luteal-follicular transition. *J. Clin. Endocrinol. Metab.* 2000; **85**:275–285.

54. Tei C, Maruyama T, Kuji N, et al. Reduced expression of alphavbeta3 integrin in the endometrium of unexplained infertility patients with recurrent IVF-ET failures: improvement by danazol treatment. *J. Assist. Reprod. Genet.* 2003; **20**:13–20.

55. Bischof P. Endocrine, paracrine and autocrine regulation of trophoblastic metalloproteinases. *Early Pregnancy* 2001; **5**:30–31.

56. Xu P, Wang YL, Zhu SJ, et al. Expression of matrix metalloproteinase-2, -9, and -14, tissue inhibitors of metalloproteinase-1, and matrix proteins in human placenta during the first trimester. *Biol. Reprod.* 2000; **62**:988–994.

57. Nguyen HPT, Simpson RJ, Salamonsen LA, Greening DW. Extracellular vesicles in the intrauterine environment: challenges and potential functions. *Biol. Reprod.* 2016; **95**:109.

58. Gross N, Kropp J, Khatib H. MicroRNA signaling in embryo development. *Biology (Basel)* 2017; **6**:34.

59. Chegini N, Tang XM, Dou Q. The expression, activity and regulation of granulocyte macrophage-colony stimulating factor in human endometrial epithelial and stromal cells. *Mol. Hum. Reprod.* 1999; **5**:459–466.

60. Paiva P, Hannan NJ, Hincks C, et al. Human chorionic gonadotrophin regulates FGF2 and other cytokines produced by human endometrial epithelial cells, providing a mechanism for enhancing endometrial receptivity. *Hum. Reprod.* 2011; **26**:1153–1162.

61. Sjöblom C, Roberts CT, Wikland M, Robertson SA. Granulocyte-macrophage colony-stimulating factor alleviates adverse consequences of embryo culture on fetal growth trajectory and placental morphogenesis. *Endocrinology* 2005; **146**:2142–2153.

62. Robertson SA, Roberts CT, Farr KL, Dunn AR, Seamark RF. Fertility impairment in granulocyte-macrophage colony-stimulating factor-deficient mice. *Biol. Reprod.* 1999; **60**:251–261.

63. Perez-Garcia, V, Fineberg E, Wilson R, et al. Placentation defects are highly prevalent in embryonic lethal mouse mutants. *Nature* 2018; **555**:463–468.

64. Hemberger M, Hanna CW, Dean W. Mechanisms of early placental development in mouse and humans. *Nat. Rev. Genet.* 2019; **21**:27–43. doi:10.1038/s41576-019-0169-4.

65. Noyes RW, Hertig AT, Rock J. Dating the endometrial biopsy. *Fertil. Steril.* 1950; **1**:3–25.

66. Pijnenborg R, Vercruysse L, Hanssens M. The uterine spiral arteries in human pregnancy: facts and controversies. *Placenta* 2006; **27**:939–958.

67. Malassine A, Frendo J-L, Evain-Brion D. A comparison of placental development and endocrine functions between the human and mouse model. *Hum. Reprod. Update* 2003; **9**:531–539.

68. Jarvela IY, Ruokonen A, Tekay A. Effect of rising hCG levels on the human corpus luteum during early pregnancy. *Hum. Reprod.* 2008; **23**:2775–2781.

69. Gamliel M, Goldman-Wohl D, Isaacson B, et al. Trained memory of human uterine NK cells enhances their function in subsequent pregnancies. *Immunity* 2018; **48**:951–962.

70. Hanna J, Goldman-Wohl D, Hamani Y, et al. Decidual NK cells regulate key developmental processes at the human fetal-maternal interface. *Nat. Med.* 2006; **12**:1065–1074.

71. Kalkunte SS, Mselle TF, Norris WE, et al. Vascular endothelial growth factor C facilitates immune tolerance and endovascular activity of human uterine NK cells at the maternal-fetal interface. *J. Immunol.* 2009; **182**:4085–4092.

72. Klentzeris LD, Bulmer JN, Warren MA, et al. Lymphoid tissue in the endometrium of women with unexplained infertility: morphometric and immunohistochemical aspects. *Hum. Reprod.* 1994; **9**:646–652.

73. Hunt JS, Miller L, Platt JS. Hormonal regulation of uterine macrophages. *Dev. Immunol.* 1998; **6**:105–110.

74. Bulmer JN, Williams PJ, Lash GE. Immune cells in the placental bed. *Int. J. Dev. Biol.* 2010; **54**:281–294.

75. Abrahams VM, Kim YM, Straszewski SL, Romero R, Mor G. Macrophages and apoptotic cell clearance during pregnancy. *Am. J. Reprod. Immunol.* 2004; **51**:275–282.

76. Jiang TT, Chaturvedi V, Ertelt JM, et al. Regulatory T cells: new keys for further unlocking the enigma of fetal tolerance and pregnancy complications. *J. Immunol.* 2014; **192**:4949–4956.

77. Fisher SJ. Why is placentation abnormal in preeclampsia? *Am. J. Obstet. Gynecol.* 2015; **213**:S115–S122.

78. Hunt JS, Petroff MG, McIntire RH, Ober C. HLA-G and immune tolerance in pregnancy. *FASEB J.* 2005; **19**:681–693.

79. Helige C, Ahammer H, Hammer A, et al. Trophoblastic invasion in vitro and in vivo:

similarities and differences. *Hum. Reprod.* 2008; **23**:2282–2291.

80. Maltepe E, Fisher SJ. Placenta: the forgotten organ. *Annu. Rev. Cell Dev. Biol.* 2015; **31**:523–552.

81. Chetty M, Duncan WC. Investigation and management of recurrent miscarriage. *Obstet. Gynecol. Reprod. Med.* 2015; **25**:31–36.

82. Lucas ES, Dyer NP, Murakami K, et al. Loss of endometrial plasticity in recurrent pregnancy loss. *Stem Cells* 2016; **34**:346–356.

83. Sotiriadis A, Makrigiannakis A, Stefos T, Paraskevaidis E, Kalantaridou SN. Fibrinolytic defects and recurrent miscarriage: a systematic review and meta-analysis. *Obstet. Gynecol.* 2007; **109**:1146–1155.

Chapter

6

Hormonal Ovarian Treatment

Raoul Orvieto and Eliezer Girsh

Two-Cell and Two-Gonadotropin Theory

At the beginning of the menstrual cycle, there is an increase in bioactive follicle-stimulating hormone (FSH) levels, a stimulus for the growth and differentiation of follicular granulosa cells (GCs). GC steroidogenic enzymes are also inducible by FSH and are necessary for the production of estradiol (E_2) and progesterone (P_4), as well as expression of luteinizing hormone (LH) receptors on theca cells (TCs). LH then stimulates theca cells to produce androgens, which are metabolized to E_2 by GCs under the influence of FSH. Elevated levels of E_2 then inhibit FSH secretion, providing a negative feedback effect. Growth of the leading follicle continues owing to elevated levels of FSH receptors, whereas secondary follicles with fewer FSH receptors undergo atresia. Taken together, FSH and LH work in concert, as depicted by the classic two-cell (TC and GC), two-gonadotropin (FSH and LH) theory. This theory of natural and artificial hormonal activity exists according to ligand–receptor interactions.

Ligand–Receptor Interaction

Cell surface receptors (membrane receptors, transmembrane receptors) take part in communication between the cell and the outside world. Extracellular signaling molecules attach to the receptor and activate cytoplasmic signals, which are then transferred into the nucleus. Steroid hormones bind to cytosolic receptors and are transferred into the nucleus. Once the receptor is occupied, it activates intracellular second messengers. These messengers convey signals to "switch on" or "switch off" gene expression, which then leads to a cellular response.

Ligands that elicit the same biological effects as natural ligands are called "receptor agonists." Agonists bind to the receptor at the same binding site as the natural ligand, resulting in either full (conventional agonists) or partial (partial agonists) activation. Conversely, "receptor antagonists" mimic ligands that bind to a receptor and prevent receptor activation, thereby inhibiting the biological activity of the receptor. Receptor antagonists can be classified as reversible and irreversible (Figure 6.1). Reversible antagonists readily dissociate from their receptor, while irreversible antagonists form a stable chemical bond with their receptor. Receptor and/or ligand polymorphisms exist between different people and within the same body, which could affect signal and/or cellular responses. In addition, mutations of ligands or their receptors can affect cellular responses.

Ovarian Stimulation

Ovarian stimulation technologies have been designed to resolve infertility problems. The treatments can be categorized into three major groups, and are used in accordance with the clinical conditions: 1. ovulation induction, 2. ovarian superovulation, 3. controlled ovarian hyperstimulation (COH). Ovulation induction and ovarian superovulation are technologies used to prepare the ovary for ovulation, after which fertilization occurs by natural intercourse or by intrauterine insemination (IUI). If pregnancy is not achieved by one of these two methods, COH or assisted reproductive technologies (ART) is the next choice of treatment. Its goal is to influence the recruitment of many antral follicles to produce multiple mature oocytes at the final stage, without releasing them. After that, the oocytes are retrieved by aspiration and then fertilized in the laboratory. Our ability to manipulate the selection of follicles is limited; all efforts have been directed toward recruitment in an attempt to bring multiple follicles to dominance instead of the naturally occurring dominance of one follicle only. The aspirated oocytes consist of both mature and immature oocytes.

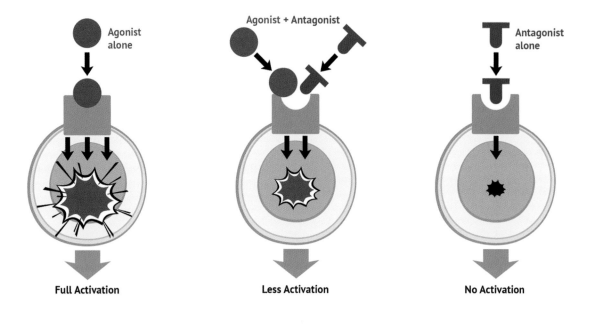

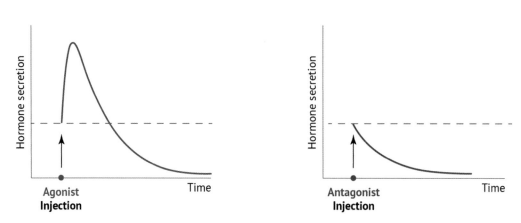

Figure 6.1 Receptor agonist and antagonist binding, and their action scheme.

Before starting the stimulation treatment, a reproductive gynecologist performs transvaginal ultrasounds and blood tests to obtain the baseline hormone levels, and the number of ovarian follicles. The basic hormonal evaluation of women before treatment includes measurement of LH, FSH, prolactin, thyroid-stimulating hormone, E_2, P_4, 17-OH-P_4, testosterone, androstenedione, DHEA, and anti-Müllerian hormone (AMH). Additionally, antral follicle count (AFC), hysteroscopy for women, and semen analysis for men are performed. The results of these tests usually enable clinicians to determine the etiology of infertility and initiate appropriate therapy.

Both AFC and AMH have added value, together with female age and basal FSH, in predicting poor versus high ovarian response to in vitro fertilization (IVF). AMH, recognized as the most accurate biomarker of ovarian reserve, has the advantage of being cycle stage independent. A complete infertility evaluation should be performed before initiating ovarian stimulation to rule out all contributory factors.

Ovulation induction. Traditional indications for ovulation induction include infertility associated with ovulation deficiencies, e.g., amenorrhea, oligomenorrhea, irregular ovulation, hypogonadotropic hypogonadism, and polycystic ovary syndrome (PCOS). All these cases require hormonal induction of ovulation.

Ovarian superovulation. This type of hormonal treatment needs regimens for mild ovarian stimulation to obtain a few dominant follicles (two to three follicles), which are then usually treated by IUI. Indications for superovulation include mild to moderate male factor, unilateral tubal occlusion, and unexplained infertility in both the male and the female partner.

Controlled ovarian hyperstimulation. The purpose of ovarian hyperstimulation is to allow retrieval of multiple mature oocytes during a single IVF cycle. After that, the oocyte is fertilized in vitro, the embryo is cultured, transferred, and implanted. Indications for this approach include mechanical factor and male factor and constitute the second step of treatment after failed ovulation induction and superovulation treatment.

Infertility Due to Defective Ovulation

Ovulation is the result of a delicate, well-synchronized balance between the central nervous system, hypothalamus, hypophysis (pituitary), and ovary. Any disruption of these intricate interactions may lead to defective ovulation and impaired reproduction. Approximately 20% of all female infertility cases can be attributed to ovulatory disorders.

Failure of the hypothalamus to secrete gonadotropin-releasing hormone (GnRH) in the proper pulsatile manner can cause a spectrum of clinical manifestations that range from a normal ovarian cycle to corpus luteum (CL) insufficiency, anovulatory cycle, and oligomenorrhea, to amenorrhea. These disorders are characterized by normal to low serum FSH and LH, and decreased E_2 and P_4 levels. While direct etiology is not always known, most hypothalamic ovulatory disorders are associated with or are due to physical stress, diet, body composition, emotional stress, environment, and other lifestyle-related aspects.

It is well accepted that emotional stress and psychological factors can influence the hypothalamic–pituitary–ovarian axis, resulting in ovarian dysfunction. Furthermore, psychological counseling or a change in lifestyle was shown to be effective in restoring ovulation in affected individuals. Individuals with amenorrhea and significant weight loss may have anorexia nervosa, or bulimia, or both. Other causes of functional hypothalamic defective ovulation may include malnutrition, malabsorption, and malignancies. All affect the hypothalamus via deregulation of the central nervous system – deregulation of hypothalamic neurotransmitters and neuromodulators. The apparent causes of most cases of hypothalamic ovulatory dysfunctions are related to abnormalities in the neuroendocrine factors that regulate pulsatile GnRH secretion. Hence, the majority of patients with hypothalamic ovulatory dysfunction present an unstable GnRH pulse frequency, which results in the absence of regular cyclical changes in serum FSH and LH concentrations, and regular or enhanced pituitary responsiveness to exogenous GnRH.

A classic developmental disorder is Kallmann syndrome or isolated gonadotropin deficiency. The syndrome results from the early degeneration of GnRH-producing neurons due to maldevelopment of the olfactory bulbs and the sulci of the rhinencephalon, leading to insufficient GnRH production and improper pituitary function.

Hypogonadotropism-associated defective ovulation can result from pituitary disorders that damage gonadotropin-secreting cells. Clinical appearance depends on the age of onset, the etiology, and the nutritional status of the patient and can be obvious or very subtle.

Clomiphene Citrate for Ovulation Induction

First synthesized in 1956, clomiphene citrate (CC) has been used clinically for ovulation induction since the 1960s. CC is a mixture of cis- and trans-isomers of a triphenylethylene derivative that acts as an E_2 receptor blocker, with the cis-isomer seemingly constituting the active form [1]. CC is well absorbed orally and is metabolized by the liver to inactive metabolites. CC has an antiestrogenic role at the level of the hypothalamus, which leads to a significant increase in the pulse frequency of LH on cycle day 5 after treatment initiation [2]. CC regimens are initiated at a dose of 50 mg daily and increased until an appropriate E_2 rise is registered, up to a maximum of 250 mg/day. CC is discontinued after an E_2 response is noted, and human chorionic gonadotropin (hCG) is then administered when ultrasound demonstrates a lead follicle of 18 mm to 19 mm in diameter. Approximately 80% of patients will ovulate on CC treatment, while the associated pregnancy rate is only about 40% [3]. The negative effects of CC are ovarian cysts in about 13% of cycles and delayed endometrial development, which subsequently decreases receptivity. CC remains the drug of choice for normoestrogenic anovulation and can be used for mild stimulation.

Letrozole for Ovulation Induction

Letrozole inhibits the aromatase activity in the cytochrome P450 enzyme complex and induces an acute hypoestrogenic state that stimulates the release of FSH. Letrozole also inhibits the spontaneous LH surge. The efficiency of letrozole is dependent on the patient's body mass index (BMI). Letrozole is found to be teratogenic, embryotoxic, and fetotoxic in animal models [4]. However, studies in humans have demonstrated its safety with regards to the health of offspring [4]. Letrozole is administered at a dose of 5 mg daily, for 5 days, from day 3 of the menstrual cycle.

In recent years, oral drugs, such as antiestrogens, aromatase inhibitors, insulin sensitizers, androgens, and others, have been increasingly used in the context of ovarian stimulation, either alone or in combination with exogenous gonadotropin preparations.

Superovulation for Intrauterine Insemination (IUI)

IUI was the first treatment made available for infertility. The major indications for IUI are mild to moderate male factor, mild to moderate endometriosis, unexplained infertility, and cervical factor. The rationale for performing IUI is to increase the number of highly motile spermatozoa (by its concentration in a small volume of medium and injection into the uterine space) proximal to the site of fertilization. In most cases, ovarian stimulation for IUI is achieved using a superovulation protocol with CC, an E_2 antagonist that elevates secretion of endogenous gonadotropins, or with exogenous gonadotropins. Daily doses are adjusted (increased or reduced) every 2–4 days, in accordance with the ovarian

response. When the dominant follicle(s) reaches 18–24 mm, ovulation is induced with hCG (an LH receptor agonist). If two dominant follicles are present, the risk of a multiple pregnancy is about 4%. However, if three or four dominant follicles are present, the risk increases to 18% [3]. If the ovulating dose of hCG is not administered, the follicles will usually become atretic. Since the life span of the fertilizable ovum is estimated to be only 12–24 hours, the timing of the insemination procedure may critically influence success rates. There is controversy as to the optimal number of inseminations per cycle. The majority of published series have documented the efficacy of one IUI performed on the day after the LH surge [5]. The procedures were performed on the day after receiving positive LH test results (one insemination) or on the day of the LH surge and the following day (two inseminations).

Immobilization of the women, by maintaining them in a supine position after IUI, has no positive effect on pregnancy rates. Comparable cumulative ongoing pregnancy rates per couple have been found, with no significant difference between the group of women who lay down for 15 minutes only (32.2%) after IUI versus those that did not (40%) [6]. No difference was found in miscarriage rate, time to pregnancy, or live birth rate between the groups.

Uterine contraction and weak or moderate endometrial movement on the day of IUI are preferable for the success of pregnancy. A cervico-fundal direction of movement, consistent with sperm transport, has also been implicated as beneficial for a successful outcome [7]. For this reason, coitus after IUI could be suggested.

The majority of pregnancies in IUI cycles with gonadotropins occur within three (in younger patients) to six cycles (in older patients) of therapy [8]. Pregnancy rates following one versus two IUIs close to ovulation time have been shown to be similar [9]. As in other ART procedures, catheter choice during IUI also does not seem to be a significant factor affecting pregnancy rates [10], which stands at ~18% and live births at ~8% [11–12].

In the case of unsuccessful IUI, the patient is then prepared for IVF, which, in the past, usually began with a pretreatment, which is less commonly performed today. Pretreatment is defined as administration of steroids (combined oral contraceptive pill, P_4 alone or E_2 alone) before commencing pituitary downregulation in the case of GnRH agonists or before FSH administration in the case of GnRH antagonist protocols. Pretreatment for 5–8 days suppresses natural hormone production and may help synchronize the development of the follicular cohort and aid in IVF cycle planning [13].

The stimulation phase includes the injection of medications for 8–14 days to induce the ovaries to produce follicles. IVF medications often involve self-administration of a combination of injections, patches, and pills. Once the patient is taking medications to stimulate the ovaries, regular blood tests are needed to measure the levels of hormones in the circulation. Because every woman responds to IVF medications differently, hormones must be adjusted on a day-to-day basis to ensure that sufficient follicles are stimulated, and to reduce the risk of ovarian hyperstimulation syndrome (OHSS), which can cause severe morbidity [14]. Other potential side effects include: swelling or rash at the injection site, mood swings and depression, enlarged ovaries, abdominal pain, and bloating.

All treatment regimens used to induce multiple follicular development in IVF programs result in a significant increase in circulating FSH concentrations, either by indirect stimulation of endogenous FSH secretion (e.g., regimens involving CC) or by direct exogenous administration of FSH (e.g., gonadotropin preparations). Although recruitment of a large number of preovulatory follicles (not all the growing follicles develop synchronously) after COH could lead to the retrieval of subpar oocytes [15], several studies have indicated that, for younger patients, the pregnancy rates per cycle after COH are higher than in natural cycles. The cumulative live birth rates are comparable between COH and natural cycles. However, in older patients, COH could lead to retrieval of suboptimal oocytes. Indeed, in older patients (35–42 years of age), COH is associated with lower implantation rates compared with natural cycles.

Human Menopausal Gonadotropins (hMG) for Controlled Ovarian Hyperstimulation

Many stimulation protocols have been introduced for COH of patients undergoing IVF. They include the different stimulation protocols using FSH in combination with GnRH analogs, oral supplementations, and ovarian triggering. Some protocols have shown a better outcome in terms of the live birth rate when extracted highly purified urine human menopausal gonadotropins (hMG), also called menotropins, were used for ovarian stimulation compared with use of recombinant FSH (rFSH) in the GnRH agonist protocol. One of the most efficient stimulation protocols uses a combined protocol of human-derived urinary FSH (uFSH) and rFSH. The combined protocol has brought a significant increase in the proportion of mature metaphase II oocytes and high-quality embryos when compared with either rFSH or uFSH alone. In poor and normal responders, a significantly higher delivery rate was achieved in rFSH + uFSH compared with the other protocols.

Initially, ovarian stimulation was predominantly performed using hMG, showing both FSH and LH bioactivity. However, this bioactivity can vary between different lots of hMG preparation. Differences in biopotency of batches of hMG are consistent with evidence that gonadotropins secreted by the pituitary are released as groups of proteins with some fractions being more bioactive than others. Menotropins are supplied in ampules containing 75 or 150 international units (IU) of FSH and an equal amount of LH per ampule. Purer FSH can be obtained by immunochromatographically isolating LH from urinary preparations of hMG. Variations in the bioactivity of urinary gonadotropins are also reflected by the unpredictable responses of women. hMG treatment is initiated following spontaneous menses or induced withdrawal bleeding, with an initial dose of 150 IU. This same dose is administered daily for 3 days, and then serum E_2 is determined. If the E_2 level has doubled, the same dose of hMG is continued, with serum E_2 monitoring every 1–2 days. Sonograms provide information on follicle number and size. Usually, the first ultrasound is performed when the E_2 level approaches 300 pg/ml. Sonograms are then performed every 1–3 days. Follicular growth is linear and usually proceeds at a rate of 2–3 mm each day. In spontaneous ovulation, the mean follicular diameter before ovulation ranges from 20 mm to 25 mm. In hMG-stimulated cycles, the mean follicular diameter ranges from 18 mm to 21 mm (~5 ml of follicular fluid) before ovulation induction with hCG administration [16].

Stimulation protocol with no desensitization of hypophysis: administration of FSH on days 4–6 of the cycle to induce folliculogenesis (not used in young and good responders). Then, FSH + LH from day 7 up to day 12, and then administration of hCG on day 13 with ovum pickup (OPU) by aspiration on day 15 (Figure 6.2).

Recombinant gonadotropins. rFSH was developed to reduce the inherent variability that resulted from the inconsistent starting materials of uFSH production, and to make FSH production independent of urine collection, thus expanding availability. Since glycosylation is essential to the function of FSH, the recombinant molecules must be produced using mammalian cell lines capable of this post-translational modification.

The glycosylation pattern of gonadotropins varies throughout the menstrual cycle, and the desired glycosylation profile of rFSH also had to be selected. After considering the feasibility of producing three FSH preparations with different glycan profiles, matching the glycosylation at the start, middle, and endpoints of the menstrual cycle, the decision was made to use the midcycle glycosylation pattern, as it was the most bioactive. rFSH is pure (99%) and has a more homogeneous glycosylation pattern than highly purified urinary and pituitary FSH or hMG preparations; the manufacturing process allows for high batch-to-batch consistency in both isoform profile and glycan-species distribution. After the successful production of rFSH, a similar process was used to produce recombinant human versions of LH and recombinant hCG.

Further development of gonadotropins has been a process focused on producing purer products that are safer and more efficacious. Biochemical differences from the original product (strength, purity, and composition of isoforms and/or glycosylation profiles) can cause differences in biological activity (including biopotency, receptor binding, postreceptor biochemistry in the cell, pharmacokinetics, and pharmacodynamics). The currently available products can be injected subcutaneously rather than intramuscularly, and pen injection devices are available, eliminating the need to reconstitute the product before injection and improving ease of use compared with syringe and vial. This has led to the current state of the art, where fertility treatment can be personalized using pure gonadotropin preparations at the start of and during ovarian stimulation, with the aim of maximizing safety and efficacy.

Exogenous gonadotropins may contribute to epigenetic changes in four imprinted genes, *Peg1*, *Kcnq1ot1*, *Zac,* and *H19* [17], and may impair oocyte and embryo development [18]. The imprinting defects involved may lead to clinical implications in ART, such as failure of the embryo to implant, spontaneous abortion, and/or fetal growth retardation attributed to dysfunctional placentas.

When FSH injections are used, multi-follicular development is encouraged. As multi-follicular development is associated with increased serum E_2 concentrations, there are high incidences of a premature LH surge before the follicles have fully matured. To prevent premature LH surge, GnRH analogs (GnRH antagonist) are implemented.

GnRH for Controlled Ovarian Hyperstimulation

The GnRH analogs are synthetic compounds based on amino acid(s) substitution to the originally isolated GnRH (GnRH-I and GnRH-II isoforms) decapeptide. Two types of analog have been synthesized, namely agonists and antagonists. While agonists occupy the GnRH receptors, initially release gonadotropins (flare-up), and downregulate the receptors over a period of time, antagonists block the action of GnRH at its receptors without initial pituitary gonadotropin release. Following an initial stimulation of GnRH receptors by GnRH agonists, the end result, much like with antagonists, is a reversible reduction of endogenous pituitary gonadotropin secretion, leading to a reduction in ovarian steroid production. Dose–response studies indicate that it suppresses both LH and FSH within 10 hours, with the duration of suppression being dose-related.

In the early 1980s, births after IVF were reported after CC-stimulated IVF cycles [19] followed by the

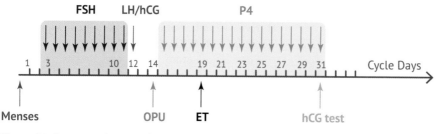

Figure 6.2 Conventional superovulation strategy for IVF. ET, embryo transfer.

use of urinary gonadotropins. In this type of treatment, the ongoing development of multiple follicles coincident with the supraphysiological production of E_2, frequently associated with a premature late follicular phase rise in LH and P_4, resulted in compromised IVF outcomes. For this reason, the downregulation of endogenous gonadotropin synthesis resulting from the co-administration of GnRH agonists was introduced in the late 1980s and rapidly became standard of care. At first, there were only GnRH agonists available. The duration of ovarian stimulation protocols increased significantly due to the initial stimulatory (so-called "flare-up") effect of GnRH agonists on pituitary gonadotropin release, in which both serum LH and FSH are increased. The GnRH agonist-induced surge of gonadotropins can last for 24–36 hours [20]. Unfortunately, agonist suppression increased the incidence of OHSS, most likely due to the synchronization of the follicular cohort. Over the last several years, clinicians have slowly shifted away from GnRH agonist co-treatment towards treatment with GnRH antagonists and, today, there are two main COH protocols: the GnRH antagonist protocol and the long agonist protocol. This shift provided multiple advantages over use of agonists, and also allowed agonist trigger of ovulation with an associated dramatic reduction in OHSS.

GnRH antagonist protocol. GnRH antagonist protocols have been demonstrated to significantly improve the clinical pregnancy rates for expected poor and high responders, and in women at high risk of developing OHSS. Treatment begins on day (D) 2–3 of the menstrual cycle, with daily administration of FSH. On D 5–6, GnRH antagonist is injected (Figure 6.3). The antagonist is designed to prevent premature ovulation

that might hinder treatment success. The combined treatment is continued until mature follicles are obtained. Once mature follicles (generally over 17 mm diameter) appear, an hCG injection is administered to induce final maturation of the follicles and oocytes. Although some practitioners begin the antagonist treatment on a predetermined cycle day of stimulation (known as a fixed start), others rely on feedback from each cycle, including the size of the lead follicle, to individualize timing of antagonist treatment initiation (known as a flexible start) [21–22]. The highest clinical pregnancy rates are achieved when the antagonist is started with a lead follicle of 14–16 mm in size and E_2 levels between 300 pg/ml and 600 pg/ml [23]. If the response of the ovary is low, the agonist short (flare-up) protocol is recommended.

GnRH agonist long protocol. Treatment largely begins with GnRH analog from D 21 of the previous menstrual cycle (~1 week before the scheduled menstruation) (Figure 6.4). The agonist, like the antagonist, is designed to prevent premature ovulation. Unlike treatment with the antagonist, the agonist must be administered for about 2 weeks until the full blockade of FSH and LH secretion. Once FSH and LH suppression is achieved, stimulation of the ovaries with gonadotropins can begin in order to produce follicles. The long protocol yields better implantation rates than the short protocol. The disadvantage of this protocol is the formation of a luteal cyst from the corpus luteum (CL).

If GnRH agonist injections are started during the follicular phase, rather than D 21 of the previous cycle, the surge of gonadotropins might be associated with the development of persistent follicular cysts as follicle growth is transiently stimulated. Starting GnRH agonists in the luteal phase seems to improve the

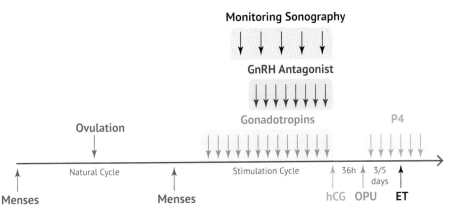

Figure 6.3 Example of GnRH antagonist superovulation strategy for IVF.

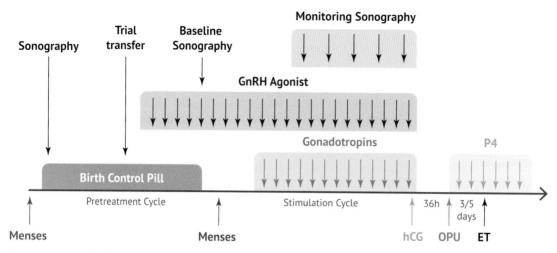

Figure 6.4 Example of GnRH agonist superovulation strategy for IVF.

outcome of the stimulation cycle. Throughout the world, the GnRH agonist long protocol treatment cycles, in which treatment is started in the luteal phase, remain popular, and facilitate standardized treatment protocols.

Additional less frequently used COH protocols include the GnRH agonist short protocol, GnRH agonist ultra-short protocol, spontaneous cycle, natural ovarian cycle, modified natural ovarian cycle, and mild ovarian stimulation.

GnRH agonist short protocol. GnRH agonist is administered from D 1 (or any day between D 1 and D 3) of the menstrual cycle and continued until the full blockade of the pituitary. After that, the administration of gonadotropins is initiated. Today, the short protocol with an agonist is rare, and the term "short protocol" generally refers to a short protocol with an antagonist.

GnRH agonist ultra-short protocol. Gonadotropins are administered from the start of menses until D 10 of the cycle. GnRH agonist is initiated on D 3 and administered up to D 11 of the cycle. On D 11, ovulation is induced using hCG. OPU is performed on D 13 (36 hours post-hCG).

Patients with hypothalamic amenorrhea respond most favorably to pulsatile GnRH agonist administration, with reported ovulation rates of approximately 90%, conception rates of 25–30% per ovulation cycle, and hyperstimulation rates of less than 1% [24].

Spontaneous Cycle IVF

The original IVF procedure developed by Steptoe and Edwards was based on obtaining mature oocytes during spontaneous natural cycles from patients with Fallopian tube defects. Louise Brown, the first ART baby, born on July 25, 1978, was conceived from an ovum that was captured during a spontaneous natural cycle. The initial enthusiasm for this technology waned quickly because the capture technique of the late 1970s and early 1980s yielded only about 60% ovum recovery. On the other hand, natural cycle ART eliminates the drug complications associated with other protocols.

Natural Ovarian Cycle

Natural ovarian cycle – cycle without ovarian stimulation.

Modified Natural Ovarian Cycle

Modified natural ovarian cycle – use of minimal ovarian stimulation for retrieval of a single oocyte. Pharmacological compounds are administered to block the spontaneous LH surge.

Mild Ovarian Stimulation

Mild ovarian stimulation uses a fixed low dose of ovarian stimulation. Advantages include reduced risk of multiple pregnancy, OHSS, and stress [25].

Induction of Final Oocyte Maturation

Follicular rupture is the final part of the ovulation process (final follicle and oocyte maturation that culminates in follicular rupture), occurring ~42 hours after the start of the LH (or human chorionic gonadotropin injection) surge. Thus, in an IVF cycle, oocyte retrieval is carried out 36 ± 2 hours after the artificial LH surge (administration of a single bolus dose of hCG), before follicular rupture [26].

Ovulation induction triggers the final maturation of the oocyte, which can be achieved with an hCG regimen or GnRH agonist, or both [27]. hCG and LH activate the same receptor but differ significantly in their half-life, which is less than 60 minutes for LH and more than 24 hours for hCG.

Following the GnRH antagonist regimen during ovarian stimulation, final oocyte maturation at the end of the follicular phase can also be induced by a bolus dose of a GnRH agonist, inducing a relatively short endogenous LH (and FSH) surge, just like in the normal menstrual cycle [20]. In 1994, a GnRH antagonist was introduced into controlled ovarian stimulation protocols to prevent unwanted LH surges. This resulted in a renewed interest in the GnRH agonist trigger as an alternative to hCG and to prevent OHSS in women who had an excessive response to stimulation. Since GnRH agonists have a greater affinity for GnRH receptors than GnRH antagonists, the agonist can displace the antagonist from the receptor, resulting in LH and FSH release [28].

It quickly became apparent that triggering oocyte maturation with a GnRH agonist in the GnRH antagonist protocol is associated with inadequate luteal phases and lower pregnancy rates with fresh embryo transfer [29]. The reason for early luteolysis or diminished luteal function under GnRH agonist/antagonist management is not clear; however, GnRH receptors are expressed in GCs of preovulatory follicles and CL [30] and may be a target of such treatment.

The physician must select the ovarian induction protocol taking into account previous response to ovulation induction protocols, woman's age, weight, and basal hormonal profile.

The Optimal Number of Oocytes per Stimulatory Cycle

The optimal number of oocytes to be retrieved remains a topic of ongoing debate. Many clinicians believe that retrieval of more oocytes is associated with higher IVF pregnancy rates, also referred to as "the more, the better" approach. However, some ovarian stimulation protocols may affect the quality of acceptable oocytes.

Clustering of ~600 genes and DNA methylation are involved in the process of follicular growth and maturation at any ovarian stimulation protocol, and

they have different involvement from one stimulation protocol to another and from stimulation protocol to a natural cycle. This raises questions as to the identity of the optimal protocol, providing the optimal number and quality of follicles per stimulation, activating a gene profile most similar to the nature profile, and yielding high-quality oocytes and overall IVF success. Studies in mice showed that ovarian hyperstimulation reduces oocyte quality, embryo quality, and implantation rates and causes fetal growth retardation and has negative impacts on oviductal and uterine milieu [31]. In humans, lower doses of gonadotropins are correlated with lower aneuploidy rates [32]. The pregnancy rate was shown to be optimal when 5–13 oocytes were retrieved per cycle [33], and live birth was established as optimal when 6–13 mature oocytes were retrieved per fresh cycle [34]. Other reports show a strong positive association between the number of retrieved oocytes and top/good-quality embryos [35]. The chromosomal error rate of mature oocytes in women less than 35 years old was elevated from 23% in groups of up to 5 oocytes to 35% and 51% in groups of up to 10 oocytes and higher, respectively [36]. Moreover, a mean of 5 mature oocytes are needed to produce 1 euploid blastocyst in women less than 35 years old, while 8 and 13 mature oocytes, respectively, are required in women of ages 39–40 years and women of ages 42–43 years. Thus, to achieve optimal results by IVF, ovarian stimulation should be fine-tuned to the follicle number limit for the relevant age group.

Management of a Patient with Disorders

Ovulation induction is always unsuccessful in women with elevated FSH levels and is contraindicated. PCOS is usually associated with mildly elevated LH levels and normal to low FSH levels. If the patient is markedly underweight, weight-loss amenorrhea should be suspected, and attempts should be made to increase her weight. Most hypoestrogenic women will not respond to CC and are excellent candidates for GnRH therapy.

Polycystic Ovary Syndrome (PCOS)

PCOS affects ~20% of the female population of reproductive age, with 5–10% of these women having symptomatic manifestations, the most common of which being anovulatory infertility [37]. PCOS is characterized by overexpression of androgen and estrogen receptors and ovarian dysfunction. Women with PCOS may have many small cysts around the edges of their ovaries. AMH may play an important part in the pathophysiology of PCOS. Serum AMH concentrations can be used to differentiate between normal versus PCOS ovaries [38]. Patients with classical PCOS also appear to be more likely to have an abnormal intrafollicular environment and impaired oocyte development [39]. Hyperandrogenic follicles of patients with classical PCOS undergoing ovarian stimulation for IVF contain morphologically normal metaphase II oocytes, with abnormal gene expression [40] involving signal transduction, cell metabolism, DNA transcription, and RNA processing. Impaired oocyte quality in PCOS has also been linked to elevated follicular fluid levels of tumor necrosis factor alpha [41] and interleukins [42]. The endometrium of PCOS women also shows altered gene expression of the P_4 receptor. Nearly 50% of women with PCOS are overweight or obese and have reduced insulin sensitivity. PCOS can lead to a wide range of problems, including body hirsutism, menstrual irregularities, infertility, type 2 diabetes, and heart disease. Unfortunately, not all women with the condition are properly diagnosed. They simply do not know that their acne, weight problems, unusual body hair, and/or fertility trouble are related to PCOS.

CC by IUI can be used as a first-line treatment of infertility for women with PCOS. CC is inexpensive and simple to use, leads to ovulation in about 75% of patients, and is associated with only a low risk of multiple gestations. It is administered daily for 5 days after spontaneous or progestogen-induced menstrual bleeding. The treatment can be started on cycle days 2, 3, 4, or 5 [43]. About 15–40% of women with PCOS are CC resistant with no follicular development after a dose of 150 mg of CC per day for an administration period. The recommendation is six CC cycles of IUI, as the cumulative pregnancy rate among anovulatory women with PCOS is around 46% after four cycles versus 65% after six CC cycles [44]. The median threshold rFSH dose advised is 50 IU/day in nonobese (BMI <25 kg/m^2) patients and 75 IU/day in obese (BMI ≥25 kg/m^2) patients [45]. Metformin, an insulin sensitizer used in the treatment of type 2 diabetes, can regulate the menstrual cycle within 1–3 months of treatment in anovulatory women with PCOS [46–47]. Letrozole may be an efficient treatment for ovulation induction in women with PCOS. Letrozole inhibits aromatase activity and induces an acute hypoestrogenic state that stimulates the release of FSH [4].

Dehydroepiandrosterone (DHEA)

DHEA supplementation up to 6 months before IVF has been reported to improve ovarian function, increase pregnancy chances, reduce aneuploidy, and lower miscarriage rates in patients with diminished ovarian reserve (DOR) [48]. However, a meta-analysis that reviewed ~200 IVF cycles concluded that there is insufficient evidence for the efficiency of DHEA supplementation in women with DOR or poor responders [49]. Furthermore, no improvement in ovarian response markers, ovarian response to gonadotropin stimulation, or IVF outcomes was found in poor responders receiving DHEA pretreatment [50]. Because there is minimal evidence for androgen deficiency in DOR patients, the exact effects of exogenous androgens on follicle growth are difficult to investigate in vivo. It is difficult to interpret the mechanisms underlying putative "positive" effects of exogenous DHEA on follicle development in infertile women.

Side Effects of Hormone Treatment

Infertility hormone treatments are designed to induce ovulation either when a woman fails to ovulate or in order to produce a higher number of oocytes, thereby increasing the chances of pregnancy. Side effects and complications of hormone treatment include:

1. Sensitivity to the hormone preparations – rare, but should any unusual effect occur the patient should seek immediate medical care from the attending physician.
2. Ovarian hyperstimulation syndrome (OHSS) – a complication of ovulation induction treatments that is characterized by significant retention of fluid in different cavities of the body. The syndrome includes a wide range of clinical symptoms that are characterized by two main events: significant ovarian enlargement, which is attributed to the multiple developing follicles in the ovary, and increased permeability of membranes and blood vessels, causing fluids to pass into and out of blood vessels and accumulate in third-space compartments (abdominal cavity, chest, heart, and subcutaneous). Severe OHSS also includes an accumulation of fluid, which occasionally requires repeated aspiration to drain the fluid. Fluid accumulating in cavities

might also result in thromboembolic complications or other rare complications, such as heart failure, kidney failure, and other life-threatening events.

3. Miscarriages and ectopic pregnancies – in pregnancies achieved after ovulation induction, the incidence of miscarriages and ectopic pregnancies is slightly higher.

4. Ovarian torsion, rupture, or bleeding – relatively rare but occasionally require surgical intervention. On rare occasions, the ovaries might need to be removed.

5. Other complications – no causal link has been proven to date between ovulation induction and ovarian cancer. Pregnancy is known to provide excellent protection in lowering the incidence of malignant ovarian tumors. Also, hormone treatments administered to treat fertility problems may result in children with physical or mental problems, including genetic defects, or any other abnormality. The rate of these complications does not generally exceed the frequency of their occurrence in natural pregnancies.

Ovarian Hyperstimulation Syndrome (OHSS)

OHSS is a rare but potentially life-threatening complication of ovarian stimulation for fertility treatment. It occurs during the luteal phase (3–7 days after hCG administration) or early pregnancy (12–17 days after hCG administration) and is characterized by a systemic increase in vascular permeability, thought to result from the ovarian secretion of vasoactive peptides such as vascular endothelial growth factor (VEGF) [51]. Its life-threatening effects are primarily caused by extravasation of fluid from the vascular space, leading to dehydration, which increases the viscosity of the blood and predisposes the cerebral vasculature to thrombosis or thromboembolism [52]. The development of ascites causes a tense fluid-filled abdomen, which can impair renal blood flow and function. The development of pleural effusions can cause breathlessness, impaired oxygen concentration, and even mortality.

OHSS does not occur when many follicles develop following ovarian stimulation with gonadotropins, without administration of hCG for ovulation triggering (a GnRH agonist is used instead of hCG). This shows that hCG is the driver of all pathophysiological events in OHSS, linking it to the vascularization of the developing CL. As VEGF is the key molecule involved

in the establishment of the luteal microvasculature, its concentrations are markedly increased when multiple CLs (cycles with multiple follicular development) are developing at the same time and secrete VEGF into the circulation.

During early pregnancy, hCG stimulates further luteal angiogenesis, and VEGF secretion and late-onset OHSS could occur in the presence of increasing hCG.

OHSS risk factors can be divided into primary and secondary. Primary risk factors include young age (less than 35), history of OHSS, and PCOS. Secondary risk factors include a quick rise in estrogen levels during ovulation induction treatment and high follicles/oocytes count. The incidence of mild OHSS is 10–25% per treatment cycle. Moderate or severe OHSS is even less common and generally requires hospitalization. Moderate OHSS also includes nausea, diarrhea, and vomiting. The use of markers for ovarian reserve has improved the risk assessment of OHSS. A cutoff value of 3.36 ng/ml serum AMH levels has been considered a good predictor of OHSS. Levels more than 10 ng/ml are associated with a three-fold increase in OHSS incidence. AFC is also predictive of OHSS, with a risk of OHSS increasing from 2.2% in women with an AFC less than 24 to 8.6% with an AFC greater than 24 [53]. Aspiration of more than 15 oocytes significantly increases the chance of OHSS [20]. For high-risk OHSS patients, a GnRH antagonist ovarian stimulation protocol is strongly advised. It is also worth stressing that the dose of gonadotropins used in at-risk women should not exceed 150 IU/day.

Dopamine agonists, including cabergoline, quinagolide, and bromocriptine, may reduce vascular permeability and help prevent leakage of fluid into the abdominal and pleural cavities. An additional strategy to avoid OHSS is to freeze all embryos and perform embryo transfer during the next cycle.

Social ART

With time, we have been faced with the social questions posed by ART, including its application as a social solution and not solely as a medical solution for infertility. More specifically, single women desiring a child turn to "social egg freezing" to ensure fertility retention and the possibility of having a child with her oocytes later in life, even after having become infertile. In addition, the morality of preimplantation genetic testing for reasons of sex selection versus the morality of abortion of "wrong sex" has been debated.

References

1. Pandya G, Cohen MR. The effect of cis-isomer of clomiphene citrate (cis-clomiphene) on cervical mucus and vaginal cytology. *J. Reprod. Med.* 1972; **8**:133–138.

2. Kerin JF, Liu JH, Phillipou G, Yen SS. Evidence for a hypothalamic site of action of clomiphene citrate in women. *J. Clin. Endocrinol. Metab.* 1985; **61**:265–268.

3. Kelly JL, Adashi EY. Ovulation induction. *Obstet. Gynecol. Clin. North Am.* 1987; **14**:831–864.

4. Palomba S. Aromatase inhibitors for ovulation induction. *J. Clin. Endocrinol. Metab.* 2015; **100**:1742–1747.

5. Deary AJ, Seaton JE, Prentice A, et al. Single versus double insemination: a retrospective audit of pregnancy rates with two treatment protocols in donor insemination. *Hum. Reprod.* 1997; **12**:1494–1496.

6. van Rijswijk J, Caanen MR, Mijatovic V, et al. Immobilization or mobilization after IUI: an RCT. *Hum. Reprod.* 2017; **32**:2218–2224.

7. Kim A, Young Lee J, Il Ji Y, et al. Do endometrial movements affect the achievement of pregnancy during intrauterine insemination? *Int. J. Fertil. Steril.* 2015; **8**:339–408.

8. Akino N, Isono W, Wada-Hiraike O. Predicting suitable timing for artificial reproductive technology treatment in aged infertile women. *Reprod. Med. Biol.* 2016; **15**:253–259.

9. Cantineau AE, Heineman MJ, Cohlen BJ. Single versus double intrauterine insemination in stimulated cycles for subfertile couples: a systematic review based on a Cochrane review. *Hum. Reprod.* 2003; **18**:941–946.

10. Abou-Setta AM, Mansour RT, Al-Inany HG, et al. Intrauterine insemination catheters for assisted reproduction: a systematic review and meta-analysis. *Hum. Reprod.* 2006; **21**:1961–1967.

11. Guzick DS, Carson SA, Coutifaris C, et al. Efficacy of superovulation and intrauterine insemination in the treatment of infertility. National Cooperative Reproductive Medicine Network. *N. Engl. J. Med.* 1999; **340**:177–183.

12. Collins J. Stimulated intra-uterine insemination is not a natural choice for the treatment of unexplained subfertility. Current best evidence for the advanced treatment of unexplained subfertility. *Hum. Reprod.* 2003; **18**:907–912.

13. Cèdrin-Durnerin I, Bständig B, Parneix I, et al. Effects of oral contraceptive, synthetic progestogen or natural estrogen pre-treatments on the hormonal profile and the antral follicle cohort before GnRH antagonist protocol. *Hum. Reprod.* 2007; **22**:109–116.

14. La Marca A, Sunkara SK. Individualization of controlled ovarian stimulation in IVF using ovarian reserve markers: from theory to practice. *Hum. Reprod. Update* 2014; **20**:124–140.

15. Moraloğlu Ö, Tonguc EA, Özel M, et al. The effects of peak and mid-luteal estradiol levels on in vitro fertilization outcome. *Arch. Gynecol. Obstet.* 2012; **285**:857–862.

16. Andersen CY, Westergaard LG, Sinosich MJ, Byskov AG. Human preovulatory follicular fluid: inhibin and free steroids related to optimal follicular maturation in ovarian stimulation regimes and possible function in ovulation. *Hum. Reprod.* 1992; **7**:765–769.

17. Ventura-Juncá P, Irarrázaval I, Rolle AJ, et al. In vitro fertilization (IVF) in mammals: epigenetic and developmental alterations. Scientific and bioethical implications for IVF in humans. *Biol. Res.* 2015; **48**:68.

18. Jiang Z, Wang Y, Lin J, et al. Genetic and epigenetic risks of assisted reproduction. *Best Pract. Res. Clin. Obstet. Gynaecol.* 2017; **44**:90–104.

19. Macklon NS, Stouffer RL, Giudice LC, Fauser BC. The science behind 25 years of ovarian stimulation for in vitro fertilization. *Endocr. Rev.* 2006; **27**:170–207.

20. Gonen Y, Balakier H, Powell W, Casper RF. Use of gonadotropin-releasing hormone agonist to trigger follicular maturation for in vitro fertilization. *J. Clin. Endocrinol. Metab.* 1990; **71**:918–922.

21. Albano C, Smitz J, Camus M, et al. Comparison of different doses of gonadotropin-releasing hormone antagonist cetrorelix during controlled ovarian hyperstimulation. *Fertil. Steril.* 1997; **67**:917–922.

22. Tarlatzis B, Fauser B, Kilibianakis E, Diedrich K, Devroey P. GnRH antagonists in ovarian stimulation for IVF. *Hum. Reprod. Update* 2006; **12**:333–340.

23. Lyttle Schumacher MB, Mersereau JE, Steiner AZ. Cycle day, estrogen level, and lead follicle size: analysis of 27,790 in vitro fertilization cycles to determine optimal start criteria for gonadotropin-releasing hormone antagonist. *Fertil. Steril.* 2018; **109**:633–637.

24. Blunt SM, Butt WR. Pulsatile GnRH therapy for the induction of ovulation in hypogonadotropic hypogonadism. *Acta Endocrinol. Suppl. (Copenh.)* 1988; **288**:58–65.

25. Nargund G, Hutchison L, Scaramuzzi R, Campbell S. Low-dose HCG is useful in preventing OHSS in high-risk women without adversely affecting the outcome of IVF cycles. *RBM Online* 2007; **14**:682–685.

26. Wang W, Zhang X-H, Wang W-H, et al. The time interval between hCG priming and oocyte retrieval in ART program: a meta-analysis. *J. Assist. Reprod. Genet.* 2011; **28**:901–910.

27. Bosch E, Labarta E, Kolibianakis E, Roen M, Meldrum D. Regimen of ovarian stimulation affects oocyte quality and therefore embryo quality. *Fertil. Steril.* 2016; **105**:560–570.

28. Itskovitz-Eldor J, Kol S, Mannaerts B. Use of a single bolus of GnRH agonist triptorelin to trigger ovulation after GnRH antagonist ganirelix treatment in women undergoing ovarian stimulation for assisted reproduction, with special reference to the prevention of ovarian hyperstimulation syndrome: preliminary report: short communication. *Hum. Reprod.* 2000; **15**:1965–1968.

29. Kolibianakis EM, Schultze-Mosgau A, Schroer A, et al. A lower ongoing pregnancy rate can be expected when GnRH agonist is used for triggering final oocyte maturation instead of HCG in patients undergoing IVF with GnRH antagonists. *Hum. Reprod.* 2005; **20**:2887–2892.

30. Choi JH, Gilks CB, Auersperg N, Leung PC. Immunolocalization of gonadotropin-releasing hormone (GnRH)-I, GnRH-II, and type I GnRH receptor during follicular development in the human ovary. *J. Clin. Endocrinol. Metab.* 2006; **91**:4562–4570.

31. Laprise SL. Implications of epigenetics and genomic imprinting in assisted reproductive technologies. *Mol. Reprod. Dev.* 2009; **76**:1006–1018.

32. Rubio C, Mercader A, Alamá P, et al. Prospective cohort study in high responder oocyte donors using two hormonal stimulation protocols: impact on embryo aneuploidy and development. *Hum. Reprod.* 2010; **25**:2290–2297.

33. van der Gaast MH, Eijkemans MJ, van der Net JB, et al. Optimum number of oocytes for a successful first IVF treatment cycle. *RBM Online* 2006; **13**:476–480.

34. Steward RG, Lan L, Shah AA, et al. Oocyte number as a predictor for ovarian hyperstimulation syndrome and live birth: an analysis of 256,381 in vitro fertilization cycles. *Fertil. Steril.* 2014; **101**:967–973.

35. Vermey BG, Chua SJ, Zafarmand MH, et al. Is there an association between oocyte number and embryo quality? A systematic review and meta-analysis. *RBM Online* 2019; **39**:751–763.

36. Haaf T, Lambrecht A, Grossmann B, et al. A high oocyte yield for intracytoplasmic sperm injection treatment is associated with an increased chromosome error rate. *Fertil. Steril.* 2009; **91**:733–738.

37. ESHRE Capri Workshop Group. Health and fertility in World Health Organization group 2 anovulatory women. *Hum. Reprod. Update* 2012; **18**:586–599.

38. Homburg R, Ray A, Bhide P, et al. The relationship of serum anti-Mullerian hormone with polycystic ovarian morphology and polycystic ovary syndrome: a prospective cohort study. *Hum. Reprod.* 2013; **28**:1077–1083.

39. Dumesic DA, Padmanabhan V, Abbott DH. Polycystic ovary syndrome and oocyte developmental competence. *Obstet. Gynecol. Surv.* 2008; **63**:39–48.

40. Wood JR, Dumesic DA, Abbott DH, Strauss JF 3rd. Molecular abnormalities in oocytes from women with polycystic ovary syndrome revealed by microarray analysis. *J. Clin. Endocrinol. Metab.* 2007; **92**:705–713.

41. Amato G, Conte M, Mazziotti G, et al. Serum and follicular fluid cytokines in polycystic ovary syndrome during stimulated cycles. *Obstet. Gynecol.* 2003; **101**:1177–1182.

42. Gallinelli A, Ciaccio I, Giannella L, et al. Correlations between concentrations of interleukin-12 and interleukin-13 and lymphocyte subsets in the follicular fluid of women with and without polycystic ovary syndrome. *Fertil. Steril.* 2003; **79**:1365–1372.

43. Wu CH, Winkel CA. The effect of therapy initiation day on clomiphene citrate therapy. *Fertil. Steril.* 1989; **52**:564–568.

44. Dickey RP, Taylor SN, Lu PY, et al. Effect of diagnosis, age, sperm quality, and number of preovulatory follicles on the outcome of multiple cycles of clomiphene citrate-intrauterine insemination. *Fertil. Steril.* 2002; **78**:1088–1095.

45. Veltman-Verhulst SM, Fauser BC, Eijkemans MJ. High singleton live birth rate confirmed after ovulation induction in women with anovulatory polycystic ovary syndrome: validation of a prediction model for clinical practice. *Fertil. Steril.* 2012; **98**:761–768.

46. Mathur R, Alexander CJ, Yano J, Trivax B, Azziz R. Use of metformin in polycystic ovary syndrome. *Am. J. Obstet. Gynecol.* 2008; **199**:596–609.

47. Sinawat S, Buppasiri P, Lumbiganon P, Pattanittum P. Long versus short course treatment with metformin and clomiphene citrate for ovulation induction in women with PCOS. *Cochrane Database Syst. Rev.* 2012; **10**:CD006226. doi:10.1002/14651858.CD006226.pub3.

48. Gleicher N, Barad DH. Dehydroepiandrosterone (DHEA) supplementation in diminished ovarian reserve (DOR). *Reprod. Biol. Endocrinol.* 2011; **9**:67, doi:10.1186/1477-7827-9-67.

49. Narkwichean A, Maalouf W, Campbell BK, Jayaprakasan K. Efficacy of dehydroepiandrosterone to improve ovarian response in women with diminished ovarian reserve: a meta-analysis. *Reprod. Biol. Endocrinol.* 2013; **11**:44, doi:10.1186/1477-7827-11-44.

83

50. Yeung T, Chai J, Li R, et al. A double-blind randomised trial on the effect of dehydroepiandrosterone on ovarian reserve markers, ovarian response and number of oocyte in anticipated normal ovarian responders. *BJOG* 2016; **123**:1097–1105.

51. Gómez R, Soares SR, Busso C, et al. Physiology and pathology of ovarian hyperstimulation syndrome. *Sem. Reprod. Med.* 2010; **28**:448–457.

52. Kasum M, Danolic D, Oreskovic S, et al. Thrombosis following ovarian hyperstimulation syndrome. *Gynecol. Endocrinol.* 2014; **30**:764–768.

53. Practice Committee of the American Society for Reproductive Medicine. Prevention and treatment of moderate and severe ovarian hyperstimulation syndrome. *Fertil. Steril.* 2016; **106**:1634–1647.

Luteal Support

Eliezer Girsh and Raoul Orvieto

The corpus luteum (CL) is a transitory endocrine gland that develops from the postovulatory ruptured follicle during the luteal phase. Human chorionic gonadotropin (hCG), produced by the embryo, maintains the secretory activity of the CL due to its structural similarity to luteinizing hormone (LH) and subsequent activation of the same receptor. It maintains and stimulates the CL to produce estradiol (E_2) and progesterone (P_4). Luteal P_4 is involved in the transition of the endometrium from a proliferative to a secretory type, with increasing decidualization – an essential facilitator of implantation [1] – and relaxation of the uterine muscle. Preparation of the endometrium lining the uterus for implantation of the embryo begins toward the end of a proliferative phase and extends throughout the luteal phase. This is important for the implantation process and maintenance of pregnancy until the placenta takes over steroid hormone production at approximately 7 weeks.

The Luteal Phase in Stimulated Cycles

The luteal phase is distinctly abnormal following ovarian stimulation. This was already reported by Professor Robert Edwards in the 1970s when he attempted to develop in vitro fertilization (IVF) using clomiphene citrate (CC) stimulation. Changes in the endocrine environment brought on by the gonadotropins used for ovarian stimulation are thought to underlie the CL dysfunction associated with IVF cycles.

The etiology of luteal phase defects in stimulated IVF cycles has been debated for decades. Initially, it was thought that the removal of large quantities of granulosa cells during oocyte retrieval might diminish the most important source of P_4 synthesis, leading to inadequate CL formation and function [2] and subfertility. Others suggested that the prolonged pituitary recovery that follows the gonadotropin-releasing

hormone (GnRH) agonist co-treatment designed to prevent spontaneous LH rise in stimulated cycles results in luteal phase defects. The introduction of GnRH antagonists in IVF raised speculations that the rapid recovery of the pituitary function would obviate the need for luteal phase supplementation. However, studies have confirmed that luteolysis is also initiated prematurely in antagonist-co-treated IVF cycles, compromising the chances for pregnancy. Despite the rapid recovery of pituitary function in GnRH antagonist protocols, luteal phase supplementation remains mandatory [3].

For many years, hCG administration was the standard form of luteal phase support. The disadvantage is the risk of ovarian hyperstimulation syndrome (OHSS), particularly in patients who respond well to stimulation. The pregnancy rate has been found to increase when excess hCG was administered during the luteal phase in which embryo transfer took place [4].

Luteal Progesterone Supplementation

The CL secretes more P_4 than is required for fertility, and there is no definite evidence that P_4 replacement in a natural cycle would improve the chances of conception. As a defective luteal phase has also been reported in hyperstimulated cycles, the optimal dose of P_4 is not known.

The ideal time of an inadequate luteal function is during the resumption of gonadotropins secretion. Women who are breastfeeding, or who have pathological elevations of prolactin, have inhibited LH concentrations and, as such, are less capable of generating a sufficient LH surge. Similarly, women with recovering hypogonadotropic hypogonadism, secondary to low body fat as seen in anorexia, overexercise, or chronic illness, are also less likely to be able to generate an adequate LH surge [5]. In contrast, women with polycystic ovary syndrome tend to have higher baseline LH concentration and pulsatility, with a reduced area under the curve for the LH surge; the same is true in the perimenopausal state, where basal LH concentrations are elevated [5–6]. Also, women taking 5-day courses of antiestrogen fertility drugs, such as CC, tamoxifen, or letrozole, in the early follicular phase, may have reduced estrogen-regulated positive feedback to generate the LH surge, particularly if follicular growth is rapid [6] and the proliferation index in glands and stroma of endometrium during early luteal phase is low. These endometrial alterations may adversely affect implantation.

After ovulation in a stimulated cycle, the patient is advised to take medication to promote implantation. Commonly prescribed medications include P_4, which is delivered in the form of oral, vaginal, rectal, subcutaneous (SC), and intramuscular (IM) preparations. In frozen–thawed embryo transfer cycles, P_4 intake is proposed on the theoretical day of oocyte retrieval [7].

Although P_4 alone can promote implantation and maintain pregnancy, there is evidence that the addition of E_2 may have a synergistic effect [8]. E_2 has been shown to upregulate the P_4 receptor and may play a role in further promoting P_4 action [1]. In clinical practice, it is now routine to replace both P_4 and E_2 for the first 10–12 weeks of gestation in artificial embryo replacement cycles.

Oral P_4. Orally administered natural micronized P_4 undergoes first-pass prehepatic and hepatic metabolism. Thus, oral administration of P_4 leads to variable levels of absorption and poorly sustained plasma P_4 concentrations, and its use as luteal phase support in IVF yields inferior results. Parenteral administration (vaginal, rectal, SC, and IM) of P_4 overcomes the metabolic challenges of oral P_4 administration. The efficacy of oral dydrogesterone 30 mg daily (10 mg, three times daily) was demonstrated in two large randomized control trials and proved non-inferior to micronized vaginal P_4 (MVP) 600 mg daily (200 mg three times daily) and to P_4 gel (Crinone 8%; 90 mg) for luteal support in IVF [9–12]. Due to the more patient-friendly route of administration, and its high tolerability and efficacy, oral dydrogesterone may replace MVP as the standard of care for luteal phase support in IVF [13].

Subcutaneous and intramuscular P_4. P_4 is rapidly absorbed after IM injection, with peak concentrations achieved after approximately 8 hours. However, the IM application of P_4 may be painful and is often not the patient's first choice. SC P_4 is well tolerated and comparable in efficacy to vaginal administration [14].

Rectal and vaginal P_4. Rectal P_4 administration yields improved uterine P_4 levels compared with the oral route. Vaginal administration is associated with high uterine levels of P_4 with low systemic exposure [15]. Following vaginal application (a vaginal gel or vaginal capsules), serum P_4 concentrations reach maximal levels after 3–8 hours and then fall continuously over the next 8 hours. In the majority of cases, 300–600 mg vaginal P_4 is administered daily, divided into two or three doses. Independent of the measured serum P_4 levels, adequate secretory endometrial transformation is achieved following vaginal P_4 use. Also, endometrial P_4 levels are higher after vaginal compared with IM P_4 administration [16]. Vaginally administered P_4 exerts a direct local effect on the endometrium and myometrium before entering the systemic circulation.

hCG or P_4 administration during the luteal phase of assisted reproductive technology (ART) cycles has been suggested to yield higher rates of live birth or ongoing pregnancy than placebo or no treatment, but the evidence is still inconclusive [17]. hCG may increase the risk of OHSS and administration with or without P_4 is associated with higher rates of OHSS than P_4 alone. Neither the addition of E_2 nor the route of P_4 administration appears to be associated with improved pregnancy rates.

Duration of luteal phase support. Administration of hCG or steroids is considered essential to prevent luteolysis. Luteolysis will occur when LH support is withdrawn from the CL for ~3 days, but CL function can be rescued if LH activity is resumed within approximately 72 hours [18]. In early pregnancy, a deficiency of endogenous LH will be compensated for by rapid increases in hCG levels, produced by the developing embryo. Triggering of follicle maturation and ovulation by recombinant hCG elevates endogenous P_4, which peaks on day 3–4 after ovum pickup, earlier than the natural P_4 peak, which occurs on day 6–7 after ovulation. This earlier peak of P_4 may shorten the implantation window and decrease embryo implantation rates.

The use of P_4 supplementation after oocyte retrieval is practically universal, but the optimal concentration (in early- and mid-luteal phase) and duration of P_4 administration remain controversial. It was suggested that P_4 supplementation beyond the first positive hCG test after IVF/intracytoplasmic sperm injection might be unnecessary [19]. The optimal chance of pregnancy was achieved with serum P_4 levels of 60–100 nmol/l in the early luteal phase. During the mid-luteal phase, a P_4 level of 150–250 nmol/l resulted in an optimal chance of live birth: 54% compared with 38% when P_4 levels were higher than 400 nmol/l [20]. High P_4 doses during IVF luteal support may also potentially cause testicular dysgenesis, disrupt the male androgen axis, and disturb normal male genital embryogenesis [21].

The real-life clinical practices regarding luteal phase supplementation in ART have found that most practitioners start luteal phase supplementation on the day of egg collection, with vaginal P_4 as the most frequently used single agent and administered in combination with P_4 IM in 17% of cases. hCG as a single agent for luteal phase supplementation is not being used at all [22]. In 72% of cycles, luteal phase supplementation is administered until 8–10 weeks of gestation or beyond.

References

1. Jabbour HN, Kelly RW, Fraser HM, Critchley HO. Endocrine regulation of menstruation. *Endocr. Rev.* 2006; **27**:17–46.

2. Garcia J, Jones GS, Acosta AA, Wright GL. Corpus luteum fuction after follicle aspiration for oocyte retrieval. *Fertil. Steril.* 1981; **36**:565–572.

3. Fatemi HM, Popovic-Todorovic B, Papanikolaou E, Donoso P, Devroey P. An update of luteal phase support in stimulated IVF cycles. *Hum. Reprod. Update* 2007; **13**:581–590.

4. O'Neill C, Ferrier AJ, Vaughan J, Sinosich MJ, Saunders DM. Causes of implantation failure after in-vitro fertilization and embryo transfer. *Lancet* 1985; **2**:615.

5. The ESHRE Capri Workshop Group. Anovulatory infertility. *Hum. Reprod.* 1995; **10**:1549–1553.

6. Duncan WC. A guide to understanding polycystic ovary syndrome (PCOS). *J. Fam. Plann. Reprod. Health Care* 2014; **40**:217–225.

7. Mackens S, Santos-Ribeiro S, van de Vijver A, et al. Frozen embryo transfer: a review on the optimal endometrial preparation and timing. *Hum. Reprod.* 2017; **32**:2234–2242.

8. Kutlusoy F, Guler I, Erdem M, et al. Luteal phase support with estrogen in addition to progesterone increases pregnancy rates in in-vitro fertilization cycles with poor response to gonadotropins. *Gynecol. Endocrinol.* 2014; **30**:363–366.

9. Ho CH, Chen SU, Peng FS, Chang CY, Yang YS. Luteal support for IVF/ICSI cycles with Crinone 8% (90 mg) twice daily results in higher pregnancy rates than with intramuscular progesterone. *J. Chin. Med. Assoc.* 2008; **71**:386–391.

10. Barbosa MW, Silva LR, Navarro PA, et al. Dydrogesterone vs progesterone for luteal-phase support: systematic review and meta-analysis of randomized controlled trials. *Ultrasound Obstet. Gynecol.* 2016; **48**:161–170.

11. Saccone G, Khalifeh A, Elimian A, et al. Vaginal progesterone vs intramuscular 17α-hydroxyprogesterone caproate for prevention of recurrent spontaneous preterm birth in singleton gestations: systematic review and meta-analysis randomized controlled trials. *Ultrasound Obstet. Gynecol.* 2017; **49**:315–321.

12. Child T, Leonard SA, Evans JS, Lass A. Systematic review of the clinical efficacy of vaginal progesterone for luteal phase support in assisted reproductive technology cycles. *RBM Online* 2018; **36**:630–645.

13. Tournaye H, Sukhikh G, Kuhler E, Griesinger G. A phase III randomized controlled trial comparing the efficacy, safety and tolerability of oral dydrogesterone versus micronized vaginal progesterone for luteal support in in vitro fertilization. *Hum. Reprod.* 2017; **32**:1019–1027.

14. Baker V, Jones C, Doody K, et al. A randomized controlled trial comparing the efficacy and safety of aqueous subcutaneous progesterone with vaginal progesterone for luteal phase support of in vitro fertilization. *Hum. Reprod.* 2014; **29**:2210–2220.

15. Kleinstein J. Efficacy and tolerability of vaginal progesterone capsules (Utrogest 200) compared with progesterone gel (Crinone 8%) for luteal phase support during assisted reproduction. *Fertil. Steril.* 2005; **83**:1641–1649.

16. Penzias A. Luteal phase support. *Fertil. Steril.* 2002; **77**:318–323.

17. van der Linden M, Buckingham K, Farquhar C, Kremer JA, Metwally M. Luteal phase support for assisted reproduction cycles. *Cochrane Database Syst. Rev.* 2015; CD009154. doi:10.1002/14651858. CD009154.

18. Hutchison JS, Zeleznik AJ. The corpus luteum of the primate menstrual cycle is capable of recovering from a transient withdrawal of pituitary gonadotropin support. *Endocrinology* 1985; **117**:1043–1049.

19. Liu X, Mu H, Shi Q, Xiao X, Qi H. The optimal duration of progesterone supplementation in pregnant

women after IVF/ICSI: a meta-analysis. *Reprod. Biol. Endocrinol.* 2012; **10**:107–115.

20. Thomsen LH, Kesmodel US, Erb K, et al. The impact of luteal serum progesterone levels on live birth rates-a prospective study of 602 IVF/ICSI cycles. *Hum. Reprod.* 2018; **33**:1506–1516. doi:10.1093/humrep/dey226.

21. Silver RI. Endocrine abnormalities in boys with hypospadias. *Adv. Exp. Med. Biol.* 2004; **545**:45–72.

22. Vaisbuch E, de Ziegler D, Leong M, Weissman A, Shoham Z. Luteal-phase support in assisted reproduction treatment: real-life practices reported worldwide by an updated website-based survey. *RBM Online* 2014; **28**:330–335.

Ovum Pickup (OPU)

Initially, oocyte retrieval was considered a significant challenge and originally performed by laparotomy and/or by other laparoscopic techniques. However, apart from the complexity of such techniques, the overall success rate was less than 50% [1] due to severe tubal disease, multiple adhesions, or hidden ovaries. Improvement in the success rate of ovum pickup (OPU) to 60–80% per follicle occurred between 1979 and 1980, upon the introduction of a foot-controlled fixed aspiration pressure control [2] and upon an integration of specially designed teflon-lined aspiration needles with beveled points [3]. A transvaginal oocyte retrieval technique was first developed by Pierre Dellenbach and colleagues in Strasbourg, France, and reported in 1984 [4–5].

OPU: Clinician's Role

An ultrasound evaluation should be performed before OPU to determine the optimal ovarian stimulation protocol and to identify any anatomical abnormalities or ovarian malposition [6]. Also, a transvaginal diagnostic ultrasound is critical for visualization of the uterus, and to check for potential difficulties during oocyte retrieval. Before the OPU, written informed patient consent is mandatory.

OPU is generally performed under general anesthesia, with the aid of transvaginal sonography, at 34–38 hours following trigger, i.e., human chorionic gonadotropin (hCG) administration [7–8]. Serum β-hCG levels below 23 mIU/ml suggest inadequate hCG administration [9].

After covering the probe with a sterile latex probe cover, a metallic needle guide is attached over the probe, in a specified groove. A minimal amount of conducting jelly is then placed on the tip of the probe for better conduction.

To eliminate any infection and contamination, vaginal washing is commonly done with regular saline and not with iodine, because povidone-iodine preparations are toxic to oocytes/embryos [10]. The patient is properly draped, and a vaginal ultrasound transducer is introduced to enable baseline scanning of both the ovaries and the uterus. A 16–18 gauge and 35 cm OPU needle with a double lumen and echo tip marking for better tip orientation during OPU should be used. Smaller-diameter needles seem to provoke less patient discomfort. Double-lumen needles, or variations of them, infuse collection medium into the follicle while the follicular fluid (FF) is being aspirated; one end of the tubing is attached to the collection tube, and another end is attached to the ovum aspiration pump (Figure 8.1). Access via the vaginal route for ultrasound-directed follicle aspiration for oocyte recovery has more advantages than the primary transabdominal and periurethral approach, and has completely replaced laparoscopic procedures for oocyte harvesting. The vessels which lie outside the ovary are visible against the contrast of the ovarian capsule to be sure that a puncturing is done at the correct site. The follicle and the vessels can also be differentiated by viewing the cross-section and the longitudinal section of the two; the follicle will remain oval or ovoid, whereas the vessel will look like a long tunnel. Under ultrasound guidance, the clinician inserts a needle through the vaginal wall into an ovarian follicle. The second end of the needle is attached to a suction device. Once the follicle is penetrated, suction is gently applied (routinely velocity of 20–25 ml/min and negative pressure of 120 ± 40 mm Hg), to aspirate FF and with it, hopefully, the cumulus–oocyte complex (COC). The pressure should be maintained stable during the procedure, as changes can induce turbulence. It is generally postulated that increasing the vacuum aspiration pressure might decrease the quality of oocytes retrieved [11]. The collapse of the follicle should be visualized when aspirating, to avoid oocyte loss. If the collapse of the follicle cannot be seen, the oocyte may still be in the follicular cavity. The FF is then delivered to an embryologist to identify and quantify the COC. Some

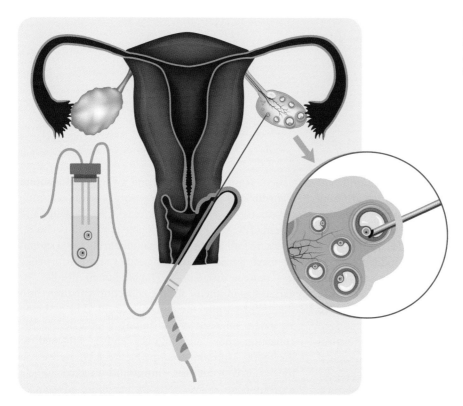

Figure 8.1 Ovum pickup (OPU): vaginal aspiration of follicular fluid with cumulus–oocyte complex (COC) from ovarian follicles.

clinicians suggest first aspirating the larger follicles, while others suggest starting aspiration from the periphery. Most aspirations are based on a "first come, first serve" basis, i.e., after puncturing the ovary, the first follicle to be encountered is aspirated, and aspiration then continues in a sequential fashion. This order of aspiration avoids unnecessary intra-ovarian bleeding and inadvertent rupture of follicles and, most importantly, ensures a precise and continuous view of the needle throughout the procedure. If the aspiration is negative (nothing comes), the aspiration needle should be completely withdrawn, and medium aspirated one or two times to flush the system for any possible blocks. After completing one ovary, the same procedure is repeated in the other ovary. At the end of the procedure, one must look for contours of both the ovaries and pelvis for any blood collection. Vaginal bleeding is generally cause for concern and easily managed by applying pressure with a pad. At the end of the procedure, the ovary should be checked to confirm that all follicles were punctured and to identify any internal bleeding. The OPU procedure takes 10–15 minutes, requires local analgesia and mild sedation, and has a low complication rate. Patients should be kept under observation for about 2 hours until recovery. General status, abdominal distension, blood pressure, and heart rate should be monitored by a nurse.

The main risks are post-procedural pain, infection (0.6%), vaginal hemorrhage (8.6%), and bleeding (more than 100 ml in 0.8% cases) [12], which may be severe or even fatal. Other complications may result from the administration of intravenous sedation or anesthesia. Those include asphyxia, caused by airway obstruction, apnea, hypotension, and pulmonary aspiration of stomach contents.

OPU: Embryologist's Part

The window between administration of hCG to OPU is the period of oocyte maturation in vivo and has a powerful effect on the success of in vitro fertilization (IVF), performed either by in vitro insemination (conventional IVF) or intracytoplasmic sperm injection (ICSI). The performance of OPU, 34–38 hours after ovulation induction (OI), generally ensures the completion of follicular development and oocyte maturation and significantly reduces the risk of spontaneous ovulation (Figure 8.2) [13–14]. Studies have shown that even a slight elongation of this window period led to a higher fertilization rate [15]. In conventional IVF, extending the OI to OPU interval led to a higher fertilization rate and excluded the need to incubate the oocytes before insemination [16]. Late OPU (36 hours + 2 hours) is associated with more available embryos than early OPU (36 hours – 2 hours), and with significantly higher rates of fertilization and pregnancy [17] than after either conventional IVF or ICSI. However, changing the duration of the conventional IVF in vitro culture did not affect the cycle outcome [18]. Prolongation of the OI to OPU interval to the maximum allowable time frame, in selected patients with polycystic ovary syndrome [19] or after repeated cycles with a high rate of aspirated immature oocytes [15], resulted in aspiration of more mature oocytes and higher fertilization rates. The oocyte fertilization rate, number of available embryos, and clinical pregnancy rate were higher at OI to OPU intervals exceeding 36 hours [17].

The final maturation of immature oocytes retrieved after conventional gonadotropin stimulation can be induced by culture in vitro but is associated with lower fertilization and implantation rates [20]. Although completion of the first meiotic division and nuclear maturity are readily achieved in vitro, early removal of the cumulus cells by enzymatic denudation and mechanical stripping reduces the chance of correctly achieving the process to cytoplasmic maturity [21]. The optimal timing of oocyte stripping and ICSI remains undetermined [22–23], and the effect of manipulating these intervals concerning the OI to OPU interval is currently unclear.

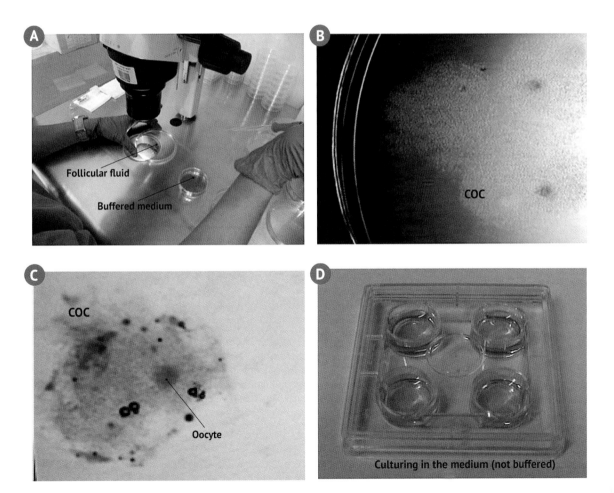

Figure 8.2 Collecting of cumulus–oocyte complexes (COC). (A) COC inspection and transfer from follicular fluid to the buffered medium; (B) collected COC; (C) visualization of oocyte; (D) culturing of COC in the medium.

Empty Follicle Syndrome

Empty follicle syndrome (EFS) is defined as a condition in which no oocytes are obtained after successful ovarian stimulation [24]. It could be frustrating, for the couple and/or for the clinical staff involved. The incidence of EFS has been estimated in a range of 0.6–7% [25]. It is suggested that EFS is occurring due to a technical failure during oocyte aspiration [26], or inappropriate administration of hCG, individual variation in the bioavailability and metabolism of hCG [27], or due to dysfunctional folliculogenesis [28].

Can a follicle be empty of an oocyte? In the growing follicle, the presence of an oocyte is obligatory, and a situation of genuine EFS cannot exist. Tight support between different cell types in the follicle exists. Cooperation between the oocyte and follicular cells in the growing follicle is extremely important. The oocyte regulates cumulus cell functions by growth differentiation factor 9, bone morphogenetic protein 15, and others [29]. However, cumulus cells coordinate oocyte development and maturation, provide energy substrate for oocyte meiosis resumption, regulate oocyte transcription, and promote nuclear and cytoplasmic maturation of the oocyte [30–33]. Different ovarian factors originating from the oocyte and/or follicular cells are involved in firm oocyte–follicle interaction and development. Communication between the oocyte and neighboring follicular cells could be reached by gap junction protein, connexin 43 (Cx43) [34], expression of which is under the control of luteinizing hormone (LH). Interruption in this communication could prevent the maturation of the oocyte. This function of Cx43 could play an important role in female fertility and recurrent EFS [35]. An additional possible factor for EFS could be a mutation in the LH receptor. It was observed that the substitution of aspargine by serine in the LH receptor impaired follicular function and explained the EFS to the repeated administration of hCG [36]. Findings suggest that most cases of EFS are observed in patients with a diminished ovarian reserve and older than 35 years [37]. Another possible reason for EFS is zona pellucida (ZP) mutations [38], resulting in the assembly of a thinner ZP, probably lead to oocyte degeneration or, possibly, an increase in the fragility of oocytes during follicular puncture or stripping of oocytes. For this reason, unsuccessful oocyte aspiration is not evidence for the real empty follicle.

Preparation of Media for OPU

The use of follicle flushing during OPU varies dramatically between clinics. If flushing is used, protocols vary in the many alternative solutions that can be applied. The media for OPU collection is recommended to be prepared up to 24 hours before the procedure. Generally, two types of media are prepared: buffered flushing medium, which can be used for follicular flushing during the aspiration, and buffered flushing medium with heparin (10 IU/ml), a naturally occurring anticoagulant, which can be used for washing of needle (8–10 ml/tube/patient). These media can be stored overnight at 4°C and should be warmed to 37°C just before the OPU procedure.

COC Collection

COCs are collected in a biological laminar flow box (Class II) to maintain the maximal biological safety of the embryologist using human fluids that have infection potential. FF is poured out from the collecting tube to a Petri dish and is examined for COCs under a binocular. Temperature of 37°C and pH of 7.2–7.4 of the flushing medium must be carefully controlled for the collection of COCs. Detected COCs under a binocular are transferred to buffered medium at a temperature and pH identical to those of the flushing medium. The COCs are divided by quotas of four to five COCs per well or dish, so as not to "put all the eggs in one basket." After collection, COCs are counted, transferred to the culture medium (with no buffer and with an osmolarity of 285 mOsm/kg) in the same groups of four to five COCs, and placed in an incubator until the next step of treatment (stripping, fertilization).

References

1. Lopata A, Johnston WIH, Leeton J, et al. Collection of human oocytes by laparotomy and laparoscopy. *Fertil. Steril.* 1974; **25**:1030–1038.

2. Wood C, Leeton J, Talbot M, Trounson AO. Technique for collecting mature human oocytes for in-vitro fertilization. *Br. J. Obstet. Gynaecol.* 1981; **88**:756–760.

3. Renou P, Trounson A, Wood C, Leeton JF. The collection of human oocytes for in-vitro fertilization. An instrument for maximizing oocyte recovery rate. *Fertil. Steril.* 1981; **35**:409–412.

4. Dellenbach P, Nisand I, Moreau L, et al. Transvaginal, sonographically controlled ovarian follicle puncture for egg retrieval. *Lancet* 1984; **1**:1467.

5. Dellenbach P, Nisand I, Moreau L, et al. Transvaginal sonographically controlled ovarian follicle puncture for egg retrieval. *Fertil. Steril.* 1985; **44**:656–662.

6. Grimbizis GF, Di Spiezio Sardo A, Saravelos SH, et al. The Thessaloniki ESHRE/ESGE consensus on diagnosis of female genital anomalies. *Hum. Reprod.* 2016; **31**:2–7.

7. Stelling JR, Chapman ET, Frankfurter D, et al. Subcutaneous versus intramuscular administration of human chorionic gonadotropin during an in vitro fertilization cycle. *Fertil. Steril.* 2003; **79**:881–885.

8. Weiss A, Neril R, Geslevich J, et al. Lag time from ovulation trigger to oocyte aspiration and oocyte maturity in assisted reproductive technology cycles: a retrospective study. *Fertil. Steril.* 2014; **102**:419–423.

9. Matorras R, Aparicio V, Corcostegui B, et al. Failure of intrauterine insemination as rescue treatment in low responders with adequate HCG timing with no oocytes retrieved. *RBM Online* 2014; **29**:634–639.

10. Hershlag A, Feng HL, Scholl GS. Betadine (povidone-iodine) is toxic to murine embryogenesis. *Fertil. Steril.* 2003; **79**:1249–1250.

11. Jeffcoate N. Infertility and assisted reproductive technologies. In: Kumar P, Malhotra N, eds., *Jeffcoate's Principles of Gynaecology*. New Delhi: Jaypee. 2008; 721–723.

12. Bennett SJ, Waterstone JJ, Cheng WC, Parsons J. Complications of transvaginal ultrasound-directed follicle aspiration: a review of 2670 consecutive procedures. *J. Assist. Reprod. Genet.* 1993; **10**:72–77.

13. Mansour RT, Aboulghar MA, Serour GI. Study of the optimum time for human chorionic gonadotropin-ovum pickup interval in in vitro fertilization. *J. Assist. Reprod. Genet.* 1994; **11**:478–481.

14. Nargund G, Reid F, Parsons J. Human chorionic gonadotropin-to-oocyte collection interval in a superovulation IVF program. A prospective study. *J. Assist. Reprod. Genet.* 2001; **18**:87–90.

15. Raziel A, Schachter M, Strassburger D, et al. In vivo maturation of oocytes by extending the interval between human chorionic gonadotropin administration and oocyte retrieval. *Fertil. Steril.* 2006; **86**:583–587.

16. Jamieson ME, Fleming R, Kader S, et al. In vivo and in vitro maturation of human oocytes: effects on embryo development and polyspermic fertilization. *Fertil. Steril.* 1991; **56**:93–97.

17. Garor R, Shufaro Y, Kotler N, et al. Prolonging oocyte in vitro culture and handling time does not compensate for a shorter interval from human chorionic gonadotropin administration to oocyte pickup. *Fertil. Steril.* 2015; **103**:72–75.

18. Fisch B, Kaplan-Kraicer R, Amit S, Ovadia J, Tadir Y. The effect of preinsemination interval upon fertilization of human oocytes in vitro. *Hum. Reprod.* 1989; **4**:495–496.

19. Bokal EV, Vrtovec HM, Virant Klun I, Verdenik I. Prolonged HCG action affects angiogenic substances and improves follicular maturation, oocyte quality and fertilization competence in patients with polycystic ovarian syndrome. *Hum. Reprod.* 2005; **20**:1562–1568.

20. Fauque P, Guibert J, Jouannet P, Patrat C. Successful delivery after the transfer of embryos obtained from a cohort of incompletely in vivo matured oocytes at retrieval time. *Fertil. Steril.* 2008; **89**:991.e1–991.e4.

21. Van de Velde H, De Vos A, Joris H, Nagy ZP, Van Steirteghem AC. Effect of timing of oocyte denudation and micro-injection on survival, fertilization and embryo quality after intracytoplasmic sperm injection. *Hum. Reprod.* 1998; **13**:3160–3164.

22. Dozortsev D, Nagy P, Abdelmassih S, et al. The optimal time for intracytoplasmic sperm injection in the human is from 37 to 41 hours after administration of human chorionic gonadotropin. *Fertil. Steril.* 2004; **82**:1492–1496.

23. Isiklar A, Mercan R, Balaban B, et al. Impact of oocyte pre-incubation time on fertilization, embryo quality and pregnancy rate after intracytoplasmic sperm injection. *RBM Online* 2004; **8**:682–686.

24. Stevenson T, Lashen H. Empty follicle syndrome: the reality of a controversial syndrome, a systematic review. *Fertil. Steril.* 2008; **90**:691–698.

25. Awonuga A, Govindbhai J, Zierke S, Schnauffer K. Continuing the debate on empty follicle syndrome: can it be associated with normal bioavailability of β-human chorionic gonadotrophin on the day of oocyte recovery? *Hum. Reprod.* 1998; **13**:1281–1284.

26. van Heusden AM, van Santbrink EJ, de Jong D. The empty follicle syndrome is dead. *Fertil. Steril.* 2008; **89**:746.

27. Bustillo M. Unsuccessful oocyte retrieval: technical artifact or genuine empty follicle syndrome? *RBM Online* 2004; **8**:59–67.

28. Tsuiki A, Rose BI, Hung TT. Steroid profiles of follicular fluids from a patient with the empty follicle syndrome. *Fertil. Steril.* 1988; **49**:104–107.

29. Eppig JJ. Oocyte control of ovarian follicular development and function in mammals. *Reproduction* 2001; **122**:829–838.

30. Feuerstein P, Cadoret V, Dalbies-Tran R, et al. Gene expression in human cumulus cells: one approach to oocyte competence. *Hum. Reprod.* 2007; **22**:3069–3077.

31. Hamel M, Dufort I, Robert C, et al. Identification of differentially expressed markers in human follicular

cells associated with competent oocytes. *Hum. Reprod.* 2008; **23**:1118–1127.

32. Adriaenssens T, Wathlet S, Segers I, et al. Cumulus cell gene expression is associated with oocyte developmental quality and influenced by patient and treatment characteristics. *Hum. Reprod.* 2010; **25**:1259–1270.

33. Assidi M, Montag M, van der Ven K, Sirard MA. Biomarkers of human oocyte developmental competence expressed in cumulus cells before ICSI: a preliminary study. *J. Assist. Reprod. Genet.* 2011; **28**:173–188.

34. Granot I, Dekel N. Cell-to-cell communication in the ovarian follicle: developmental and hormonal regulation of the expression of connexin-43. *Hum. Reprod.* 1998; **13**:85–97.

35. Onalan G, Pabuccu R, Onalan R, Ceylaner S, Selam B. Empty follicle syndrome in two sisters with three cycles: case report. *Hum. Reprod.* 2003; **18**:1864–1867.

36. Yariz KO, Walsh T, Uzak A, et al. Inherited mutation of the luteinizing hormone/choriogonadotropin receptor (LHCGR) in empty follicle syndrome. *Fertil. Steril.* 2011; **96**:E125–E130.

37. Girsh E, Makovski Lev-Tov E, Umansky N, et al. Empty follicle syndrome-oocyte could be retrieved in consecutive cycle. *JFIV Reprod. Med. Genet.* 2016; **4**:4. doi:10.4172/2375-4508.1000193.

38. Dai C, Chen Y, Hu L, et al. ZP1 mutations are associated with empty follicle syndrome: evidence for the existence of an intact oocyte and a zona pellucida in follicles up to the early antral stage. A case report. *Hum. Reprod.* 2019; **34**:2201–2207. doi:10.1093/humrep/dez 174.

Chapter 9

In Vitro Fertilization (IVF)

Preparation for Fertilization

In vitro fertilization (IVF) is a complex series of techniques used to help with fertility or prevent genetic problems and assist with the conception. During IVF, oocytes are collected from ovaries and fertilized by spermatozoa in a laboratory. The fertilization can be done using the patient's oocytes and the partner's sperm or donor oocytes and partner's/donor sperm. All gametes (spermatozoa and oocytes) should be correctly prepared and selected before the initiation of the fertilization process.

Sperm Preparation (for IUI, IVF, ICSI)

For assisted reproductive technology (ART), semen samples must first be processed in a procedure that imitates the natural conditions, where the best viable spermatozoa are separated from other elements of the ejaculate and actively migrate through the cervical mucus. To maintain fertilization capacity of sperm, viable sperm cells must be separated from other elements of the ejaculate within 30–60 minutes of ejaculation [1]. It is also recommended by the World Health Organization (WHO) and suggested to limit damage from cells (leukocytes, dead and dying sperm cells) present in the semen. All sperm preparation procedures should be conducted under aseptic conditions, i.e., in a biological class II laminar flow biosafety cabinet.

Sperm must be personally delivered to the IVF laboratory by the ovum pickup (OPU) patient's male partner presenting a photo ID card as proof of the specimen ownership. The sperm specimen should be collected into a sterile container (tissue grade and sperm-toxicity tested) by masturbation following a 24–72-hour period of abstinence [2–3], or by 1–3 hours of abstinence according to other references [4], and delivered to the laboratory within 1 hour of ejaculation (Figure 9.1). After liquefaction (sperm liquefies typically within 5–20 minutes of ejaculation [5]),

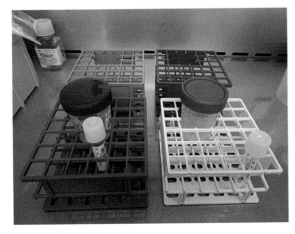

Figure 9.1 The sperm specimen should be collected into a sterile container (tissue grade and sperm-toxicity tested) following a 24–72-hour period of abstinence and delivered to the laboratory within 1 hour of ejaculation. Each sperm specimen should be treated in separate stands.

the ejaculate volume is measured, and sperm cells are counted and tested for motility, all this visually observed under a light microscope (Figure 9.2). Following complete liquefaction, sperm wash medium is added to the ejaculate to remove the seminal plasma containing prostaglandins (to prevent uterine contractions in case of intrauterine insemination [IUI]), seminal particulate debris, crystals of spermin phosphate, proteins, and microbial contamination, and to minimize reactive oxygen species (ROS) and keep spermatozoa at neutral pH. Also, the presence of large numbers of nonviable spermatozoa in the sample can inhibit the capacitation of viable spermatozoa [6]. Prolonged sperm cell exposure to seminal plasma is not recommended.

A number of methods for spermatozoa separation and isolation from the seminal plasma have been developed, including swim-up, swim-down, two-layer discontinuous gradient centrifugation, sedimentation

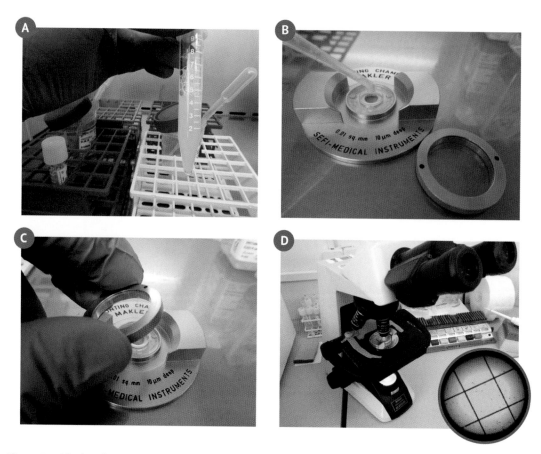

Figure 9.2 After liquefaction the ejaculate volume is measured, and sperm cells are counted. (A) Sperm volume measurement; (B) and (C) sperm preparation in counting chamber; (D) sperm cells visually observed under a light microscope for motility.

methods, polyvinylpyrrolidone (PVP) droplet swim-out, magnetic-activated cell sorting (MACS), fluorescence cell sorting methods, glass wool filtration, and electrophoresis. The ideal sperm preparation method should be cost-effective and allow for the processing of a large ejaculate volume, maximizing the number of spermatozoa available. Examination of spermatozoa in the ejaculate cannot evaluate the spermatozoa capacitation capacities, the acquisition of sperm cell surface proteins required for zona pellucida (ZP) binding and penetration, and the ability to fertilize the oocyte.

Swim-up technique. Swim-up is one of the most universally used sperm preparation techniques and can be used on a cell pellet or a liquefied semen sample covered with culture medium (sperm wash). Tubes are incubated at a 45° angle for 1 hour at a temperature ranging between 4 and 30°C (do not go above 34–35°C), which allows active, motile sperm to naturally swim up and come out of the sample into the clear medium, where they are aspirated. The main disadvantage of this method is the relatively low yield of motile spermatozoa retrieved. Only 5–10% of the sperm cells subjected to swim-up are retrieved; when a concentrated cell pellet is used, some motile spermatozoa may be trapped in the middle of the pellet and cannot move up as far as those that are located at the edges of the pellet.

Migration–sedimentation technique. The migration–sedimentation method is usually used for samples with low motility, as it relies on the natural movement of spermatozoa due to gravity. Specially developed tubes, called Tea-Jondet tubes, are used for migration–sedimentation. Sperm cells swim from a ring-shaped well into the culture medium above and then settle through the central hole of the ring. The advantage of this method is that it is a gentle method, and thus the amount of ROS produced is negligible. However, the special tubes that are used are relatively expensive.

Swim-down technique. The swim-down technique relies on the natural movement of spermatozoa. The semen sample is placed above a discontinuous serum albumin medium, which becomes progressively less concentrated toward the bottom of the tube; the tube is then incubated for 1 hour. During migration, the most motile sperm move downward into the gradient.

Density gradient centrifugation. Density gradient centrifugation separates sperm cells by their density, which differs between morphologically normal and abnormal spermatozoa (Figure 9.3). A mature morphologically normal spermatozoon has a density of 1.10 g/ml or more, whereas an immature and morphologically abnormal spermatozoon has a density of 1.06–1.09 g/ml [7]. Density gradient sperm separation fraction includes a colloidal suspension of silica

particles stabilized with covalently bonded hydrophilic silane supplied in HEPES. The two gradients used are a lower phase (90%) and an upper phase (45%). Semen is gently layered on top of the upper phase. After centrifugation, the interphases between seminal plasma and 45% density gradient, and 45% and 90% gradient containing the leukocytes, cell debris, and morphologically abnormal sperm with poor motility are discarded. The highly motile, morphologically normal, viable spermatozoa form a pellet at the bottom of the tube. Centrifugal force and time are kept at the lowest possible values (~300 × g) in order to minimize the production of ROS by leukocytes and nonviable sperm cells [8]. Sperm washing medium (with 5.0 mg/ml human albumin) is used to wash and resuspend the final pellet.

Magnetic-activated cell sorting (MACS). MACS separates apoptotic spermatozoa from non-apoptotic spermatozoa. During apoptosis (programmed cell death), phosphatidylserine residues are translocated from the inner membrane of the spermatozoa to the

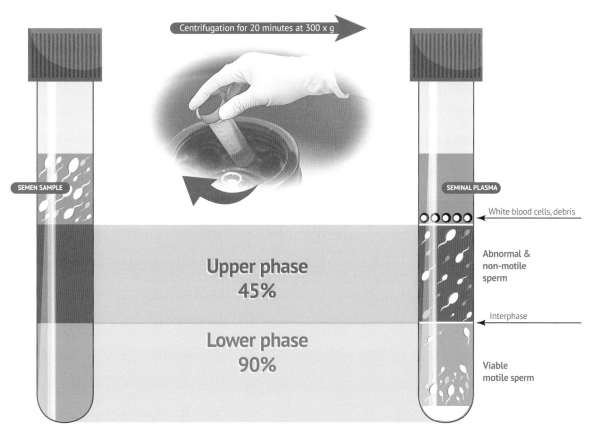

Figure 9.3 Sperm density gradient centrifugation.

outside. Annexin V has a strong affinity for phosphatidylserine but cannot pass through the intact sperm membrane. Thus, annexin V binding to spermatozoa indicates compromised sperm membrane integrity. Colloidal magnetic beads (~50 nm in diameter) are conjugated to specific anti-annexin V antibodies and used on a column to separate dead and apoptotic spermatozoa by MACS. All the unlabeled, annexin V-negative, non-apoptotic spermatozoa pass through the column, while the annexin V-positive (apoptotic) fraction is retained on the column.

For the isolation of functionally normal spermatozoa, sperm migration techniques and gradient centrifugation remain the most popular methods [9]. Sperm preparation using density gradient centrifugation has become a standard technique for sperm preparation for use in ART. Semen quality is better preserved in a two-layer density gradient compared with the swim-up isolation process [10]. Thus, the most commonly used method for sperm recovery is a combined method of density gradient, followed by swim-up.

Density gradient combined with swim-up. After initial semen specimen washing and centrifugation (900 × g for 5–7 minutes), the formed pellet is resuspended and gently dispensed onto the top of a two-layer density gradient (90% lower phase and gently dispensed 45% upper phase, or 80% and 40% respectively) tube. The gradient must be used within a short time of preparation as the two phases eventually blend into one another, blurring the initially sharp interface between the two. An accepted three-layered column at a ratio of 1:3 v/v (90%, 45% gradient, and upper phase of washed resuspended sperm fraction) provides for good separation of the cells. The three-layered tube is centrifuged at 300 × g for 20 minutes. After centrifugation, all layers are carefully aspirated, without disturbing the pellet, and discarded. The formed pellet, containing suitable motile spermatozoa, is extensively washed with sperm washing medium and centrifuged at 900 × g for 5–7 minutes. The supernatant is discarded, and the pellet with motile spermatozoa is covered with a small volume of fresh sperm washing medium and then incubated at room temperature at an angle of ~45° to ensure increase in surface area. Active, motile sperm cells swim out from the pellet into the clear medium, which is then aspirated and stored until the fertilization process (IUI, classic IVF, or intracytoplasmic sperm injection [ICSI]). This method of sperm preparation results in a high percentage of motile spermatozoa with nuclear integrity

[10–12]. To protect spermatozoa from "cold shock," it is essential to ensure that all components of the gradient and sperm wash medium are at room temperature before use. Sperm cells incubated at 37°C have a shorter life span than sperm cells incubated at room temperature.

Spermatozoa retrieved from the uterine cavity or vicinity of oocytes, with the potential to bind oocytes, were found to be more uniform in appearance than those from a native semen sample. This in vivo observation helped define the appearance of potentially fertilizing, morphologically normal spermatozoa [13]. Human sperm morphology has been defined as an essential parameter for the diagnosis of male infertility and a prognostic indicator of natural [14] or assisted [15] pregnancies.

Oocyte Preparation

Oocytes for IVF. In stimulated cycles, 36 ± 2 hours after triggering of ovulation, a typical mature preovulatory cumulus–oocyte complex (COC) displays radiating corona cells surrounded by an expanded, loose mass of cumulus cells (CCs). The COCs intended for classical IVF post-OPU are incubated in an equilibrated medium under 5% CO_2, 5% O_2, 90% N_2 at 37°C, until insemination.

Oocyte denudation for ICSI. The optimal timing for oocyte denudation (or stripping) and ICSI remains under debate [16–18], and the effect of manipulating these intervals concerning the human chorionic gonadotropin (hCG)/agonist–OPU interval is currently unclear. Late OPU is associated with more available embryos than early OPU and significantly higher rates of fertilization and pregnancy. Some studies showed that the length of incubation before or after denudation did not affect fertilization and pregnancy rates, regardless of OPU timing [19]. Immediate (up to 30 minutes) and early (0.5–2 hours) denudation showed no statistically significant differences in fertilization and pregnancy rates between these groups [20].

Oocytes are denuded using enzymatic (hyaluronidase) and then mechanical (stripper tips of ~300–140 μm) techniques. Commercial denudation solution typically consists of 80 IU/ml hyaluronidase in a HEPES buffered medium supplemented with human serum albumin (5 mg/ml) and gentamicin (10 μg/ml). A lower concentration of hyaluronidase (8 IU/ml) has been suggested to improve the fertilization rate and embryo quality [21].

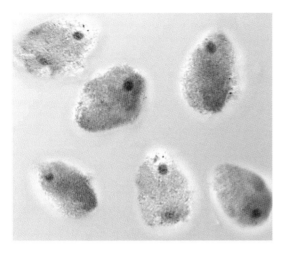
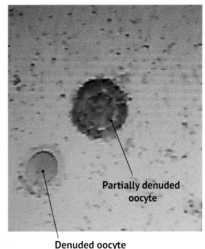

Partially denuded oocyte

Denuded oocyte

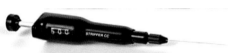

Figure 9.4 Denudation of oocytes.

CCs are partially removed from retrieved oocytes within 1–2 minutes of pipetting in hyaluronidase, which is followed by further mechanical stripping of oocytes in buffered washing medium by gradually reducing the diameter of the stripper tips from ~300 μm to ~140 μm to complete denudation (Figure 9.4). The oocyte size must be appropriately defined visually as incorrect use of a narrow tip for a large oocyte may damage the oocyte. After stripping, oocytes should be thoroughly washed to remove traces of hyaluronidase. Removal of the CC mass provides the unique opportunity of evaluating oocyte morphology before the fertilization process, and in particular, the nuclear maturation status. Oocyte nuclear maturity status, as assessed by light microscopy, is assumed to be at the metaphase II (MII) stage when the first polar body (PB) is visible in the perivitelline space. Generally, 85% of the oocytes retrieved following ovarian hyperstimulation display the first PB and are classified as MII, whereas 10% present show an intracytoplasmic nucleus called the germinal vesicle (GV). Approximately 5% of the oocytes have neither a visible GV nor a first PB, and these oocytes are generally classified as metaphase I (MI) oocytes [22]. Following a morphological assessment of the stripped oocyte, all oocytes are separated by maturity level and cultured until fertilization.

The current literature remains contradictory with regards to the value of oocyte morphology as a predictor of IVF outcome (Figure 9.5) [23–24].

Nuclear maturity alone is insufficient for the determination of oocyte quality. Nuclear and cytoplasmic maturation should be completed in a coordinated manner to ensure optimal conditions for subsequent fertilization. In the fully matured oocyte (MII), the meiotic spindle aligns with the first PB position. The appearance of the spindle is time dependent, with maximal appearance occurring between 39 and 40.5 hours post-hCG [25]. Mature oocytes have a short fertile life span and are highly sensitive to external conditions, e.g., pH, temperature, light, accuracy of stripping, and others (Figure 9.6).

Spontaneous maturation of immature oocytes, generally at the MI stage, retrieved after conventional gonadotropin stimulation, can be induced by in vitro culture, but are associated with lower fertilization and implantation rates compared with in vivo-matured oocytes [26–27]. Human oocytes matured in vitro require at least 1 hour to complete nuclear maturation after first PB extrusion [28].

Incomplete denudation (oocytes with attached CCs) was shown to increase the quality of subsequent cleavage embryo and blastocyst development by improving the cytoplasmic and nuclear maturation of retrieved oocytes and preimplantation development [29]. The oocyte would be cultured also with other autologous CCs and then transferred to the uterus. This process is called cumulus-assisted embryo transfer and has been shown to increase pregnancy rates [30].

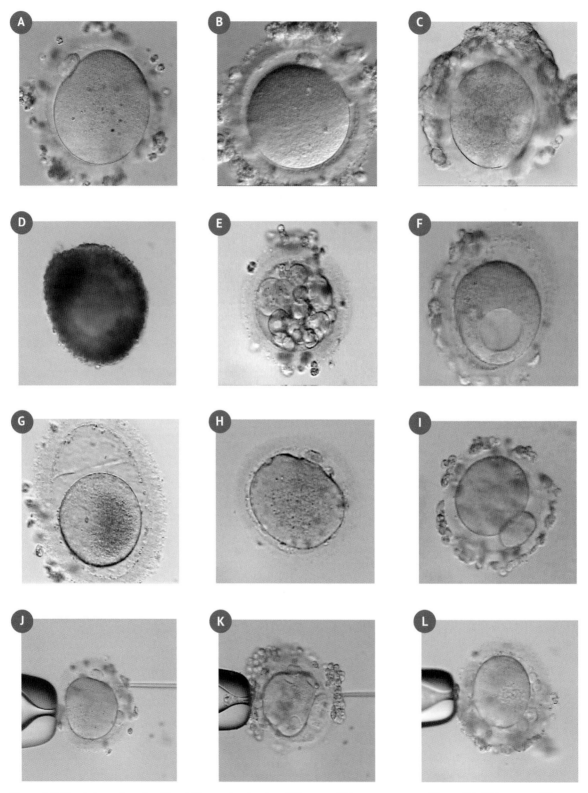

Figure 9.5 Morphology of oocytes: (A) and (B) normal and mature (MII) oocyte; (C) immature oocyte with two GVs; (D) immature (MI) oocyte with compact CC; (E) fragmented oocyte, (F) vacuolated oocyte; (G) dark ooplasm and septum in perivitelline space; (H) non-regular edges; (I) huge PB; (J) two (or fragmented) PBs; (K) formless oocyte; (L) granulated ooplasm and a few PBs; (M) absence of perivitelline space; (N) big perivitelline space; (O) oval oocyte; (P) pear-shaped oocyte; (Q) two oocytes with common ZP; (R) connected oocytes.

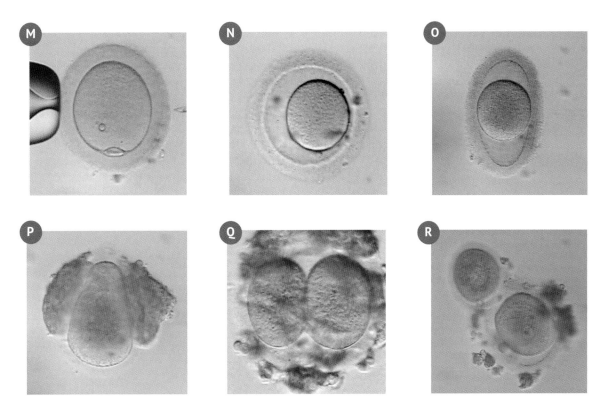

Figure 9.5 (cont.)

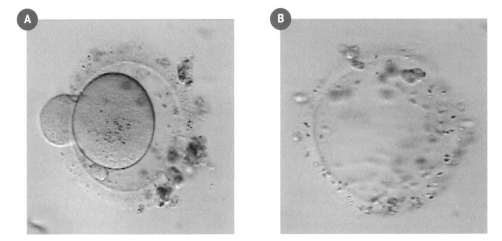

Figure 9.6 Damaged oocyte after stripping process. (A) Partial extrusion of the ooplasm from damaged oolemma; (B) leaked ooplasm from damaged oolema.

Fertilization

Human life is created with the fertilization of an oocyte. This procedure in the laboratory is highly sensitive ethically; therefore, a double check of the identity of gametes before starting fertilization is mandatory. Once the oocyte and the sperm fuse, the oocyte and sperm chromosomes are first packaged into two separate male and female membrane-enclosed nuclei. Both nuclei then slowly move toward each other to the center of the fertilized egg, called the zygote. There, they continue occupying distinct territories in the zygote throughout the first cellular division. How the autonomy of parental genomes is retained after fertilization remains unclear, but involves male and female chromosome separation machinery, which increases the probability that chromosomes are separated into multiple, unequal groups, which may compromise embryo development and give rise to spontaneous miscarriage.

Fertilization by Intrauterine Insemination (IUI)

IUI is considered the simplest and least invasive insemination procedure, with reasonable live birth rates and costs. Inseminations have been performed in domestic and farm animals since the 1900s, while artificial inseminations in humans began only in the 1940s. Human IUIs were first reported in 1962 [31].

While sperm motility seems to be the most valuable predictor of IUI success [32], total motile sperm cell count (TMC) used for insemination has been cited as the most predictive index of conception after IUI cycles [33]. A minimal TMC of 1 million for insemination was initially reported to be required to achieve pregnancy [34], but later it was found that the native sperm TMC in the range of 5–10 million is the best correlate with IUI success [35–36].

We suggest an ejaculatory abstinence period of 1–2 days before IUI, despite a lower TMC inseminated compared with more prolonged ejaculatory abstinence, which is generally associated with increased sperm count, but decreased motility and no impact on sperm morphology [37]. An extended period of abstinence (more than 5–7 days) may be related to a higher exposure of sperm cells to ROS and, consequently, to greater sperm DNA damage.

Age is the most important factor in the success rate of IUI. The chances of achieving a live birth are negatively correlated with advanced maternal age [38]. The age-related drop in female fecundity has been well documented in women undergoing IUI with donor spermatozoa [39]. In women older than 40 years, IVF treatment is more preferred as the most successful strategy [40].

IUI performed in natural cycles has roughly half the pregnancy rate of that of cycles stimulated with either clomiphene citrate or gonadotropins [41–42]. In stimulated cycles two preovulatory follicles are suitable. Three preovulatory follicles, especially in older women, are acceptable [35], while most centers cancel the procedure if more than three mature follicles are observed. The hCG–IUI interval showed no impact on clinical pregnancy (any conception that is detected by ultrasound or serum hCG levels developed to pregnancy): 24 versus 36 hours of an interval [43] or 24 versus 48 hours of an interval [44]. Either one or two inseminations are valid for this procedure, and should ideally be performed within the window of 12–38 hours after ovulation induction. Follicle rupture and uterine contractions visualized by ultrasound following IUI are favorable prognostic factors.

In Vitro Insemination (classic IVF)

In vitro insemination (or classic IVF) provides a higher probability for sperm–oocyte collision through the availability of high concentrations of spermatozoa, which include numbers of motile and morphologically normal spermatozoa adequate to achieve fertilization [45]. Desirable sperm counts should provide for a ratio of 2000–10 000 sperm cells per oocyte, depending on semen parameters [46]. Insemination is carried out by placing one oocyte with sperm cells in each ~20 µl microdroplet of carbon dioxide pre-equilibrated culture medium overlaid with light paraffin oil and incubated in a 5% CO_2, 5% O_2, 90% N_2 humidified atmosphere, at 37°C. Up to five oocytes can be cultured with 50 000 sperm cells in a volume of 300 µl. For standard IVF procedures, oocytes are incubated with spermatozoa for 16 hours, mainly for practical reasons because it corresponds to the timing for the observation of pronuclei. According to several studies, prolonged oocyte exposure to high concentrations of spermatozoa may be detrimental, especially in male factor infertility cases, because of ROS formation [47].

In humans, sperm entry into the COC occurs within 15 minutes of in vitro insemination [48]. Following 1 hour of oocyte exposure to spermatozoa, a large part of the cumulus oophorus is disassociated, verifying an immediate interaction between the gametes. However, it is interesting to note that in some male factor cases, although the CCs are still intact after 1 hour of in vitro insemination, fertilization still occurs. Consequently, this could mean that the cumulus plays an essential role in the entrapment

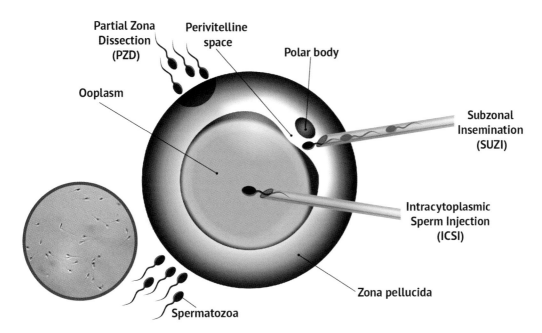

Figure 9.7 Types of fertilization.

of spermatozoa within the vicinity of the oocyte [49]. The higher fertilization rates and enhanced embryo development and viability achieved after a short (1 hour) insemination indicate that prolonged exposure of oocytes to high concentrations of spermatozoa is detrimental [50].

Initial micromanipulation techniques. The first micromanipulation techniques, e.g., partial zona dissection (PZD) and subzonal insemination (SUZI), were developed in the 1980s, to enhance the success of IVF in couples with male factor infertility.

PZD facilitates sperm entry into the oocyte by creating one or more holes in the ZP. The hole is mechanically created with a needle or chemically induced using acidic Tyrode's solution [51]. Results of PZD in cases of male factor infertility were promising with fertilization rates of 68% compared with 33% with conventional insemination [51]. However, PZD results in up to 57% polyspermy, as the number of sperm entering the perivitelline space cannot be controlled.

SUZI is a more direct method of fertilization, involving the insertion of one or more spermatozoa directly into the perivitelline space, under the ZP [52]. This method effectively addresses severe male factor infertility and decreases rates of polyspermy due to control over the number of spermatozoa injected [53]. It has been demonstrated that up to four spermatozoa can be

injected without increasing the rate of polyspermy, while injection of 5–10 sperm is associated with a 50% rate of polyspermy [54]. Initial studies reported fertilization rates of 25–71% with this technique [52]; however, overall clinical pregnancy rates remain low, at a rate of only 2.9% of the embryos transferred [54].

Intracytoplasmic Sperm Injection (ICSI)

ICSI involves the direct injection of a single immobilized sperm cell into the oolema of a mature oocyte and is superior to PZD or SUZI, methods which have been used before 1992 (Figure 9.7). ICSI is used for the cases when sperm cells may not penetrate the oocyte (male/female factors) during natural conception and classical IVF. A randomized comparison found that ICSI doubled the fertilization rate compared with SUZI and generated embryos in 83% compared with 50% of SUZI cycles [55].

The first births after the use of ICSI technology were reported by Palermo and colleagues in 1992 [56]. The direct injection of a single sperm cell into a mature oocyte bypasses the natural processes of sperm selection; oocyte survival rate after this mechanical intervention was 94%. The use of ICSI in IVF cycles has increased from 36.4% in 1996 to 93.3% in 2012 among cycles with male factor infertility [57]. ICSI has become a well-established universal method

103

as an effective form of treatment for couples with infertility and has become the standard of care for patients with male factor infertility, with fertilization rates of 60–70%, similar to rates of conventional insemination in men with normal semen parameters [58].

Sperm suspensions after preparation are combined with medium containing PVP or hyaluronate to increase viscosity and to facilitate spermatozoa handling, though the efficacy and safety of these substances have been questioned [59]. Micromanipulation for ICSI involves a standard holding pipette for the oocyte and a sharpened injection pipette for the sperm cell. For injection, a single, motile, and overtly morphologically normal sperm cell is selected from the PVP drop and immobilized using the injection pipette. The tail of the sperm cell is positioned at a 90° angle to the injection pipette, which is lowered and drawn across the tail, resulting in membrane permeability as in nature (initiation of capacitation) and loss of motility; both of these factors enhance fertilization [60]. The immobilized sperm cell is aspirated tail first, into the injection pipette. The oocyte is held with the holding pipette and positioned such that the PB is adjacent to 6 or 12 o'clock, a position which prevents spindle destruction by the injection pipette (3 o'clock entry point of the injection pipette). The injection pipette is gently inserted through the ZP and into the plasma membrane of the oocyte. The membrane must be ruptured by gentle manipulation of the injection pipette. The sign of broken membrane is the ooplasm backflow into the injection pipette. The sperm cell is then carefully released into the ooplasm and the pipette is withdrawn, completing the procedure.

The spindle view (PolScope) system has been developed to identify a location of the spindle, useful information to prevent oocyte damage at the time of ICSI, thereby increasing the likelihood of successful, normal fertilization [61].

The survival rate of oocytes following the ICSI procedure is 94%, and the fertilization rate with ejaculated spermatozoa and surgically obtained spermatozoa is 75% and 69.8%, respectively [62]. Complete fertilization failure following ICSI has been linked to oocyte activation failure or incomplete sperm decondensation [63–65]. DNA fragmentation in female or male gametes is believed to be the primary cause of fertilization failure [66].

The timing of the ICSI procedure may be critical. The time between OPU and ICSI ranges from 1 to 10 hours. No effect of the OPU–ICSI interval on fertilization rate or embryo quality was found on day 2 or day 3 of embryo development [67]; no statistically significant differences were found between early (1–2 hours post-denudation) and late (5 hours post-denudation) injection on ICSI outcomes, embryo implantation, clinical pregnancy or live birth rates [68]. However, the aging of oocytes after OPU has been described and late fertilization (more than 5 hours) remains a controversial topic.

In contrast to in vivo fertilization, ICSI introduces a whole sperm cell into the ovum cytoplasm (Figure 9.8). In such a way, paternal mitochondria from sperm neck is introduced into the ovum. There is a theory that the paternal mitochondria are tagged with ubiquitin shortly after fertilization, successfully eliminating them from the cytoplasm [69].

Selection of Spermatozoa for Fertilization

Sperm selection for ICSI is based on the visual morphological assessment by an embryologist. Therefore, exploring the relationship between sperm morphology and fertilization capacity is of critical importance to the success of ICSI [70]. Since structurally abnormal human sperm cells do not necessarily contain an abnormal chromosome constitution [71], it is not surprising that many normal babies have been born after ICSI using a low morphology sperm cell, including round-headed sperm cell without acrosomal caps [72], stump-tail sperm cell [73], and immotile sperm cell of men with axonemal defects [74]. It has even been possible to produce pregnancy and birth from oocytes fertilized by ICSI with immature spermatozoa as round spermatids [75].

Sperm cells from some men may be immotile due to low intracellular concentrations of cAMP. "Awakening" such spermatozoa using a phosphodiesterase inhibitor, e.g., pentoxifylline or theophylline, that elevates cAMP levels and enhances motility before performing ICSI has resulted in healthy children [76]. Some immotile spermatozoa are acceptable for ICSI use, as indicated by functional sperm tail membrane integrity, measured by a pulse of diode laser at the tail; a viable spermatozoon curls its tail in response to the laser. ICSI results are significantly improved when spermatozoa are selected through diode laser, as opposed to the hypo-osmotic swelling sperm selection technique [77].

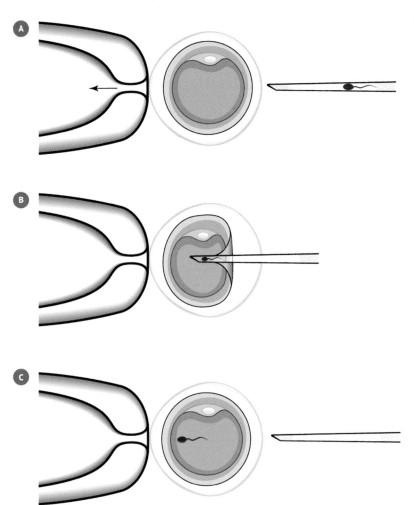

Figure 9.8 Intracytoplasmic sperm cell injection (ICSI).

MACS adapted to separate apoptotic spermatozoa from non-apoptotic spermatozoa was found to improve sperm specimen quality. Spermatozoa isolated by density gradient centrifugation followed by MACS have a higher percentage of motile and viable sperm cells and lower expression of apoptotic markers than samples prepared by density gradient centrifugation only [78].

It was also found that impaired morphology of the sperm cell head, which can be observed by embryologists in the routine sperm selection process, correlates with poorer ICSI outcomes. Motile sperm organellar morphology examinations demonstrated a positive correlation between the morphological normalcy of the sperm cell nucleus and the potential to achieve fertilization and pregnancy after ICSI [79].

Hyaluronic acid (HA) is naturally present in the extracellular matrix of the cumulus oophorus surrounding the oocyte during the natural human fertilization process. The extracellular matrix is a barrier that can only be overcome by mature spermatozoa that have extruded their specific receptors to HA and digest the matrix by hyaluronidase. After that, they penetrate the ZP and fertilize the oocyte [80]. Spermatozoa which are unable to bind HA exhibit many aspects of immaturity; they retain cytoplasm on the sperm neck and excess histones in the nucleus, show greater aberrant sperm head morphology, and have lower genomic integrity [81–82]. To improve fertilization results the noninvasive method, based on selective binding of the mature sperm cells to HA, was suggested. This method has been associated with a higher quality of embryo scores with significant decrease in aneuploidies and higher pregnancy rates [83]. HA-based spermatozoa selection is useful to improve the results of fertilization in some IVF cycles. Nevertheless, sperm cell morphology in conjunction with its motility is considered to be the best predictor of successful fertilization during natural conception, IUI conception, conventional IVF method, and ICSI. Selection of sperm cells for ICSI by a combination of different methods is highly recommended.

During the ICSI procedure, the whole spermatozoon is injected, including its outer plasma membrane and acrosome cap. Then enzymes within the ooplasm break down the sperm cell plasma membrane before sperm-derived oocyte-activating factor can activate the oocyte [84]. This delay of oocyte activation often results in an extension of the normal sperm head remodeling progression. Consequently, an asymmetry in sperm chromatin decondensation develops due to the persistence of perinuclear theca at the base of the acrosome. This delay in chromatin decondensation leads to a delay in the subsequent nuclear remodeling process, including the recruitment of nuclear pore constituents, and also leads to a delay in DNA replication and the first cell cycle following fertilization [85].

A sperm cell may not be able to induce Ca^{2+} oscillations if it undergoes premature chromatin condensation, or fails to undergo decondensation at the appropriate time [86]. Application of a Ca^{2+} ionophore to rescue an oocyte, which failed to activate, resulted in a healthy child delivery [87]. Implantation rates after ICSI with testicular spermatozoa improved when artificial oocyte activation using a Ca^{2+} ionophore was performed but were not improved when ejaculated or epididymal spermatozoa were used [88]. Sperm-specific cytosolic phospholipase C zeta (PLCζ) induces Ca^{2+} oscillations within the oocyte. Globozoospermic sperm cells can have deficient production or release of PLCζ, which is associated with oocyte activation failure. Injection of PLCζ with such sperm cell to oocyte could greatly improve the rate of oocyte activation and fertilization [89].

It has been noted that the rates of fertilization by cryopreserved sperm cells were consistently higher than with fresh sperm cells. This phenomenon can be explained due to the plasma membrane damaging of freeze–thaw cycles. During the cryopreservation process, the sperm cell plasma membrane weakens and ruptures under the stress of osmotic pressure and the formation of ice crystals. This membrane condition may accelerate sperm chromatin release from the sperm cell upon entry into the ovum by ICSI, resulting in higher fertilization rates [90].

Semen Viscosity

To reduce semen viscosity, specimens can be diluted with a sperm wash medium. Liquefaction achieved due to this procedure is not suitable for highly viscous samples. Alternatively, the viscous semen can be forced through a needle with a narrow gauge but it is associated with sperm cell damage [5]. A commonly used treatment to reduce viscosity involves enzymatic liquefaction using trypsin. If the semen fails to liquefy after a 20-minute incubation at 37°C, trypsin is added directly to the semen specimen. The specimen is then swirled and incubated for an additional 10 minutes, resulting in complete liquefaction of the sample. However, no data regarding the effect of trypsin treatment on integrity and health status of sperm cells are available.

Sperm Preparation after Retrograde Ejaculation

Retrograde ejaculation occurs when semen is redirected into the urinary bladder during ejaculation. The acidity of the urine, toxicity of urea, and hypotonic osmotic conditions in urine quickly affect the viability of sperm cells. In cases of low sperm volume and a low number of spermatozoa in the ejaculate, the urine needs to be analyzed for sperm cells. Upon arrival at the laboratory, the patient should empty his bladder, and drink a cup or two of water. As soon as the patient feels an urge to urinate, he should masturbate and collect the ejaculated specimen. Immediately after the semen collection, the patient should empty his bladder into a large container. The total volume and pH of the urine are measured and recorded, and the urine is poured into 50 ml conical centrifuge tubes. Following centrifugation for 10 minutes at 800–1000 × g, the supernatant is discarded and pellets are resuspended in a small volume of sperm wash medium. The treated retrograde and antegrade specimens are tested for sperm cells.

For clinical application of retrograde sperm for fertilization, the patient is asked to drink one tablespoon of bicarbonate with a glass of water 2 to 3 hours before masturbation. If urine pH is still too low, increase the amount of bicarbonate to two tablespoons at the next evaluation. The concentrated retrograde specimen and the antegrade specimen are usually prepared using density gradient centrifugation [91].

Sperm Preparation after Assisted Ejaculation

Direct penile vibratory stimulation (PVS) [92] or indirect rectal electro-stimulation [93] are used to retrieve semen from men who have disturbed ejaculation or who cannot ejaculate due to health conditions, such as spinal cord injury (SCI), or young boys (before oncology treatments). Infertility is a significant complication of SCI in men, 90% of whom cannot create children via sexual intercourse. Patients with SCI often have ejaculates with a high sperm concentration, low sperm motility, and contaminations of red blood cells and white blood cells. It has been reported that semen obtained by PVS has better quality than semen obtained by rectal electro-ejaculation for men with SCI [94]. Obtained ejaculates are most effectively prepared with density gradient centrifugation [91].

Variation in sperm preparation methods is available to process sperm for ART use. A suitable sperm preparation method should be carefully examined and chosen for each infertile couple.

Abnormalities after Fertilization

Concerns about fertilization and genetic abnormalities arising after classic IVF and ICSI have been voiced. Following ICSI, decondensation and remodeling of the sperm chromatin are delayed and structurally distinct, resulting in a delay in the onset of DNA synthesis in the first cell cycle [85; 95]. The ICSI method bypasses and mimics the natural events of sperm–ovum interaction and fusion. One of the critical events during this interaction is membrane fusion and exocytosis of the sperm acrosome. These events result in an extension of the normal sperm head remodeling process as well as the creation of asymmetry in chromatin decondensation. The apical portion of the sperm cell chromatin is disturbed, leading to decondensation of the posterior portion of the sperm chromatin, while the apical portion remains intact. This delay in chromatin decondensation leads to a delay in subsequent nuclear remodeling processes, including the recruitment of nuclear pore constituents, and a delay in DNA replication (by both maternal and paternal pronuclei) and the first cell cycle following fertilization [96].

During ICSI, the oocyte membrane is ruptured by the ICSI pipette, and ooplasm aspiration into the injection pipette damages the cytoskeleton structure of the oocyte. Additionally, the sperm cell is injected with PVP/hyaluronate into the oocyte. These structural alterations and injection of chemical compounds may have epigenetic effects on the fertilized oocyte and gene expression in the newly formed embryo.

It was suggested that men with nonobstructive azoospermia and extreme oligozoospermia are at increased risk of hiding genetic lesions related to infertility, including Y chromosome deletions [97]. As such, men can successfully father children by the ICSI method, but the genetic trait relating to their infertility may be transmitted to their male offspring [98].

It was shown that use of semen with impaired quality significantly reduces the fertilization rate [99]. The ICSI procedure has proven to be successful in achieving fertilization in cases of a broad spectrum of male factor issues, including the most severe oligozoospermia, and ejaculates completely lacking normal sperm cells [100]. Apparent sperm cell motility deficiencies can result from a variety of conditions, such as infection and obstructive azoospermia. However, genetic reasons, such as immotile cilia syndrome, can also result in spermatozoa with inherently nonfunctional flagella [101]. ICSI outcomes with this patient population are particularly poor [102]. It has been estimated that there are various levels of spermatogenesis present in at least 60% of azoospermic men, and surgical sperm cell isolation followed by ICSI has been successful even in cases classified as Sertoli cell-only syndrome [103]. The well-characterized correlation between cystic fibrosis (CF) mutations and congenital bilateral absence of the vas deferens is another distinct infertility risk factor requiring surgical retrieval [104]. Men with idiopathic obstructive azoospermia are also at increased risk of harboring CF mutations [105].

It was shown that immature male germ cells can be used to reach fertilization by ICSI. A few pregnancies have been reported following the oocyte injection with round spermatids; however, the success rate of obtaining a viable embryo is extremely low [106]. Theoretically, it was assumed that if round spermatids exist in a biopsy or ejaculate, then later stages, such as elongated spermatids and mature spermatozoa, should also be present. Normal children births have been reported following elongated spermatid injection; however, the overall success of these techniques is also much lower than ICSI with mature spermatozoa [107].

107

Safety of ICSI

The direct injection of a single sperm cell into a mature oocyte bypasses the natural physiological processes of typical sperm selection. This method raises questions regarding the potential risk of congenital malformations and genetic defects in children born after ICSI [108]. ICSI with testicular sperm cells raised even more questions with regard to the safety of the ICSI technique itself. The chromosomal or genetic constitution of testicular sperm cells increases the risk of possibility of genomic imprinting at the time of fertilization [109–110].

Prenatal Diagnosis in ICSI Pregnancies

Prenatal evaluations have shown a statistically significant increase in sex chromosome aberrations and *de novo* structural aberrations after ICSI procedures compared with the control neonatal population [111].

Genetic consultation for patients with infertility is strongly recommended due to general and specific risk factors present in this population and the risk of chromosomal aberrations in IVF-treated fetuses. All of these patients are advised for prenatal diagnosis (invasive or noninvasive). A strong preference is for noninvasive prenatal screening such as ultrasound and serum markers. Invasive prenatal screening has additional risks and should be discussed with patients.

Congenital Malformations in ICSI Children

The current literature does not provide a full picture of the outcome of ICSI pregnancies. In the first 30 years of IVF, ~40% of children originated from multiple pregnancies, mostly twin pregnancies. It is evident that this excessive number of multiple pregnancies results in complications appearing either immediately or later in life. In the last decade, multiple pregnancy rates have reduced substantially. The major and minor congenital malformation rate is challenging to compare between the different surveys because of the differences in methodology used. The major and minor congenital malformation rate in ICSI children is estimated as ~3–9%, versus 1–3% in the general population, and is non-statistically different from that in classic IVF children [108; 111–112]. Controversial data are claiming the increased risk of inhibition of mental development among ICSI children compared with the general population [113–116].

Children conceived through IVF or ICSI are six times more likely to have Beckwith–Wiedemann syndrome, a disease where there is a loss of imprinting of the *H19* gene on chromosome 11 (locus 11p15.5). Beckwith–Wiedemann syndrome patients with loss of imprinting tend to display hypermethylation of *H19*, resulting in an under-expression of *H19* and, therefore, hyperactivation of insulin-like growth factor-II, leading to tumor growth [117]. Also, children conceived through ART have a greater tendency to develop Angelman syndrome, a neurogenetic disorder characterized by severe intellectual and developmental disability caused by the loss or inactivation of genes located at q11-q13 on chromosome 15.

References

1. Bjorndahl L, Mortimer D, Barratt CLR, et al. Sperm preparation. In: *A Practical Guide to Basic Laboratory Andrology*, 1st ed. New York: Cambridge University Press. 2010; 167–187.

2. Levitas E, Lunenfeld E, Weiss N, et al. Relationship between the duration of sexual abstinence and semen quality: analysis of 9,489 semen samples. *Fertil. Steril.* 2005; **83**:1680–1683.

3. Pons I, Cercas R, Villas C, Braña C, Fernández-Shaw S. One abstinence day decreases sperm DNA fragmentation in 90 % of selected patients *J. Assist. Reprod. Genet.* 2013; **30**:1211–1218.

4. Bahadur G, Almossawia O, Zeirideen Zaid R, et al. Semen characteristics in consecutive ejaculates with short abstinence in subfertile males. *RBM Online* 2016; **32**:323–328.

5. Henkel RR, Schill WB. Sperm preparation for ART. *Reprod. Biol. Endocrinol.* 2003; **108**:1–22.

6. Makker K, Agarwal A, Sharma R. Oxidative stress and male infertility. *Indian J. Med. Res.* 2009; **129**:357–367.

7. Oshio S, Kaneko S, Iizuka R, Mohri H. Effects of gradient centrifugation on human sperm. *Arch. Androl.* 1987; **19**:85–93.

8. Bourne H, Edgar DH, Baker HWG. Sperm preparation techniques. In: Gardner DK, Weissman A, Howles CM, Shoham Z, eds., *Textbook of Assisted Reproductive Techniques: Laboratory and Clinical Perspectives*, 2nd ed. USA: Informa Healthcare. 2004; 79–91.

9. Sakkas D, Manicardi GC, Tomlinson M, et al. The use of two density gradient centrifugation techniques and the swim-up method to separate spermatozoa with chromatin and nuclear DNA anomalies. *Hum. Reprod.* 2000; **15**:1112–1116.

10. Allamaneni SS, Agarwal A, Rama S, Ranganathan P, Sharma RK. Comparative study on density gradients and swim-up preparation techniques utilizing neat and cryopreserved spermatozoa. *Asian J. Androl.* 2005; **7**:86–92.

11. May-Panloup P, Chrétien MF, Savagner F, et al. Increased sperm mitochondrial DNA content in male infertility. *Hum. Reprod.* 2003; **18**:550–556.

12. Jackson RE, Bormann CL, Hassun PA, et al. Effects of semen storage and separation techniques on sperm DNA fragmentation. *Fertil. Steril.* 2010; **94**:2626–2630.

13. Menkveld R, Stander FS, Kotze TJ, Kruger TF, van Zyl JA. The evaluation of morphological characteristics of human spermatozoa according to stricter criteria. *Hum. Reprod.* 1990; **5**:586–592.

14. Bonde JP, Ernst E, Jensen TK, et al. Relation between semen quality and fertility: a population-based study of 430 first-pregnancy planners. *Lancet* 1998; **352**:1172–1177.

15. Kruger TF, Menkveld R, Stander FS, et al. Sperm morphologic features as a prognostic factor in in vitro fertilization. *Fertil. Steril.* 1986; **46**:1118–1123.

16. Jacobs M, Stolwijk AM, Wetzels AM. The effect of insemination/injection time on the results of IVF and ICSI. *Hum. Reprod.* 2001; **16**:1708–1713.

17. Dozortsev D, Nagy P, Abdelmassih S, et al. The optimal time for intracytoplasmic sperm injection in the human is from 37 to 41 hours after administration of human chorionic gonadotropin. *Fertil. Steril.* 2004; **82**:1492–1496.

18. Isiklar A, Mercan R, Balaban B, et al. Impact of oocyte pre-incubation time on fertilization, embryo quality and pregnancy rate after intracytoplasmic sperm injection. *RBM Online* 2004; **8**:682–686.

19. Garor R, Shufaro Y, Kotler N, et al. Prolonging oocyte in vitro culture and handling time does not compensate for a shorter interval from human chorionic gonadotropin administration to oocyte pickup. *Fertil. Steril.* 2015; **103**:72–75.

20. Naji O, Moska N, Dajani Y, et al. Early oocyte denudation does not compromise ICSI cycle outcome: a large retrospective cohort study. *RBM Online* 2018; **37**:18–24.

21. de Moura BR, Gurgel MC, Machado SP, et al. Low concentration of hyaluronidase for oocyte denudation can improve fertilization rates and embryo quality. *JBRA Assist. Reprod.* 2017; **21**: 27–30.

22. Rienzi L, Ubaldi F. Oocyte retrieval and selection. In: Gardner DK, Weissman A, Howles CM, Shoham Z, eds., *Textbook of Assisted Reproductive Technologies: Laboratory and Clinical Perspectives*, 3rd ed. London: Informa Healthcare, 2009; 5–101.

23. Rienzi L, Vajta G, Ubaldi F. Predictive value of oocyte morphology in human IVF: a systematic review of the literature. *Hum. Reprod. Update* 2011; **17**:34–45.

24. Lazzaroni-Tealdi E, Barad DH, Yu Y, et al. Oocyte scoring system with better predictability of clinical IVF pregnancies than currently practiced embryo quality assessment. *PLoS One* 2015; **10**: e0143632.

25. Kilani S, Cooke S, Chapman M. Time course of meiotic spindle development in MII oocytes. *Zygote* 2011; **19**:55–62.

26. Alvarez C, García-Garrido C, Taronger R, González de Merlo G. In vitro maturation, fertilization, embryo development & clinical outcome of human metaphase-I oocytes retrieved from stimulated intracytoplasmic sperm injection cycles. *Indian J. Med. Res.* 2013; **137**:331–338.

27. Fauque P, Guibert J, Jouannet P, Patrat C. Successful delivery after the transfer of embryos obtained from a cohort of incompletely in vivo matured oocytes at retrieval time. *Fertil. Steril.* 2008; **89**:991.e1–991.e4.

28. Hyun C-S, Cha J-H, Son W-Y, et al. Optimal ICSI timing after the first polar body extrusion in *in vitro* matured human oocytes. *Hum. Reprod.* 2007; **22**:1991–1995.

29. Ebner T, Moser M, Sommergruber M, Shebl O, Tews G. Incomplete denudation of oocytes prior to ICSI enhances embryo quality and blastocyst development. *Hum. Reprod.* 2006; **21**:2972–2977.

30. Parikh FR, Nadkarni SG, Naik NJ, Naik DJ, Uttamchandani SA. Cumulus coculture and cumulus-aided embryo transfer increases pregnancy rates in patients undergoing *in vitro* fertilization. *Fertil. Steril.* 2006; **86**:839–847.

31. Cohen MR. Intrauterine insemination. *Int. J. Fertil.* 1962; 7:235–240.

32. Sakhel K, Schwarck S, Ashraf M, Abuzeid M. Semen parameters as determinants of success in 1662 cycles of intrauterine insemination after controlled ovarian hyperstimulation. *Fertil. Steril.* 2005; **84**:248–249.

33. Papillon-Smith J, Baker SE, Agbo C, Dahan MH. Pregnancy rates with intrauterine insemination: comparing 1999 and 2010 World Health Organization semen analysis norms. *RBM Online* 2015; **30**:392–400.

34. Marshburn PB, Alanis M, Matthews ML, et al. A short period of ejaculatory abstinence before intrauterine insemination is associated with higher pregnancy rates. *Fertil. Steril.* 2010; **93**:286–288.

35. Merviel P, Heraud MH, Grenier N, et al. Predictive factors for pregnancy after intrauterine insemination (IUI): an analysis of 1038 cycles and a review of the literature. *Fertil. Steril.* 2010; **93**:79–88.

36. Zhang E, Tao X, Xing W, Cai L, Zhang B. Effect of sperm count on success of intrauterine insemination in couples diagnosed with male factor infertility. *Mater Sociomed* 2014; **26**:321–323.

37. Jurema MW, Vieira AD, Bankowski B, et al. Effect of ejaculatory abstinence period on the pregnancy rate after intrauterine insemination. *Fertil. Steril.* 2005; **84**:678–681.

38. Speyer BE, Abramov B, Saab W, et al. Factors influencing the outcome of intrauterine insemination (IUI): age, clinical variables and significant thresholds. *J. Obstet. Gynaecol.* 2013; **33**:697–700.

39. van Noord-Zaadstra BM, Looman CW, Alsbach H, et al. Delaying childbearing: effect of age on fecundity and outcome of pregnancy. *BMJ* 1991; **302**:1361–1365.

40. Goldman MB, Thornton KL, Ryley D, et al. A randomized clinical trial to determine optimal infertility treatment in older couples: the Forty and Over Treatment Trial (FORT-T). *Fertil. Steril.* 2014; **101**:1574–1581.

41. Tomlinson MJ, Amissah-Arthur JB, Thompson KA, Kasraie JL, Bentick B. Prognostic indicators for intrauterine insemination (IUI): statistical model for IUI success. *Hum. Reprod.* 1996; **11**:1892–1896.

42. Honda T, Tsutsumi M, Komoda F, Tatsumi K. Acceptable pregnancy rate of unstimulated intrauterine insemination: a retrospective analysis of 17,830 cycles. *Reprod. Med. Biol.* 2015; **14**: 27–32.

43. Tonguc E, Var T, Onalan G, et al. Comparison of the effectiveness of single versus double intrauterine insemination with three different timing regimens. *Fertil. Steril.* 2010; **94**:1267–1270.

44. Khalifa Y, Redgment CJ, Tsirigotis M, Grudzinskas JG, Craft IL. The value of single versus repeated insemination in intra-uterine donor insemination cycles. *Hum. Reprod.* 1995; **10**:153–154.

45. Trounson AO. The choice of the most appropriate fertilization technique for human male factor infertility. *Reprod. Fertil. Dev.* 1994; **6**:37–43.

46. Fiorentino A, Magli MC, Fortini D, et al. Sperm:oocyte ratios in an in vitro fertilization (IVF) program. *J. Assist. Reprod. Genet.* 1994; **2**:97–103.

47. Ron-el R, Nachum H, Herman A, et al. Delayed fertilization and poor embryonic development associated with impaired semen quality. *Fertil. Steril.* 1991; **55**:338–344.

48. Gianaroli L, Tosti E, Magli MC, et al. Fertilization current in the human oocyte. *Mol. Reprod. Dev.* 1994; **3**:209–214.

49. Bedford JM, Kim HH. Cumulus oophorus as a sperm sequestering device in vivo. *J. Exp. Zool.* 1993; **265**:321–328.

50. Gianaroli L, Fiorentino A, Magli MC, Ferraretti AP, Montanaro N. Prolonged sperm-oocyte exposure and high sperm concentration affect human embryo viability and pregnancy rate. *Hum. Reprod.* 1996; **11**:2507–2511.

51. Malter HE, Cohen J. Partial zona dissection of the human oocyte: a nontraumatic method using micromanipulation to assist zona pellucida penetration. *Fertil. Steril.* 1989; **51**:139–148.

52. Laws-King A, Trounson A, Sathananthan AH, Kola I. Fertilisation of human oocytes by micro-injection of a single spermatozoon under the zona pellucida. *Fertil. Steril.* 1987; **48**:637–642.

53. Ng SC, Bongso A, Ratnam SS. Microinjection of human oocytes: a technique for severe oligoasthenoteratozoospermia. *Fertil. Steril.* 1991; **56**:1117–1123.

54. Sakkas D, Gianaroli L, Diotallevi L, et al. IVF treatment of moderate male factor infertility: a comparison of mini-Percoll, partial zona dissection and sub-zonal sperm insertion techniques. *Hum. Reprod.* 1993; **8**:587–591.

55. Levran D, Bider D, Yonesh M, et al. A randomized study of intracytoplasmic sperm injection (ICSI) versus subzonal insemination (SUZI) for the management of severe male factor infertility. *J. Assist. Reprod. Genet.* 1995; **12**:319–321.

56. Palermo G, Joris H, Devroey P, Van Steirteghem AC. Pregnancies after intra-cytoplasmic injection of single spermatozoon into an oocyte. *Lancet* 1992; **340**:17–18.

57. Boulet SL, Mehta A, Kissin DM, et al. Trends in use of and reproductive outcomes associated with intracytoplasmic sperm injection. *JAMA* 2015; **313**:255–263.

58. Wang J, Sauer MV. In vitro fertilization (IVF): a review of 3 decades of clinical innovation and technological advancement. *Ther. Clin. Risk Manag.* 2006; **2**:355–364.

59. Tsai MY, Huang FJ, Kung FT, et al. Influence of polyvinylpyrrolidone on the outcome of intracytoplasmic sperm injection. *J. Reprod. Med.* 2000; **45**:115–120.

60. Dozortsev D, Rybouchkin A, De Sutter P, Dhont M. Sperm plasma membrane damage prior to intracytoplasmic sperm injection: a necessary condition for sperm nucleus decondensation. *Hum. Reprod.* 1995; **10**:2960–2964.

61. Rienzi L, Ubaldi F, Martinez F, et al. Relationship between meiotic spindle location with regard to the polar body position and oocyte developmental potential after ICSI. *Hum. Reprod.* 2003; **18**:1289–1293.

62. Palermo GD. ICSI: technical aspects. In: Gardner DK, Weissman A, Howles CM, Shoham Z, eds., *Textbook of Assisted Reproductive Techniques: Laboratory and*

Clinical Perspectives. Boca Raton: CRC Press. 2001; 147–157.

63. Sousa M, Tesarik J. Ultrastructural analysis of fertilization failure after intracytoplasmic sperm injection. *Hum. Reprod.* 1994; **9**:2374–2380.

64. Flaherty SP, Payne D, Swann NJ, Mattews CD. Aetiology of failed and abnormal fertilization after intracytoplasmic sperm injection. *Hum. Reprod.* 1995; **10**:2623–2629.

65. Ebner T, Moser M, Sommergruber M. Jesacher K, Tews G. Complete oocyte activation failure after ICSI can be overcome by a modified injection technique. *Hum. Reprod.* 2004; **19**:1837–1841.

66. Bosco L, Ruvolo G, Morici G, et al. Apoptosis in human unfertilized oocytes after intracytoplasmic sperm injection. *Fertil. Steril.* 2005; **84**:1417–1423.

67. Bárcena P, Obradors A, Vernaeve V, Vassena R. Should we worry about the clock? Relationship between time to ICSI and reproductive outcomes in cycles with fresh and vitrified oocytes. *Hum. Reprod.* 2016; **31**:1182–1191.

68. Van de Velde H, De Vos A, Joris H, Nagy ZP, Van Steirteghem AC. Effect of timing of oocyte denudation and micro-injection on survival, fertilization and embryo quality after intracytoplasmic sperm injection. *Hum. Reprod.* 1998; **13**:3160–3164.

69. Reynier P, May-Panloup P, Chretien MF, et al. Mitochondrial DNA content affects the fertilizability of human oocytes. *Mol. Hum. Reprod.* 2001; **7**:425–429.

70. Celik-Ozenci C, Jakab A, Kovacs T, et al. Sperm selection for ICSI: shape properties do not predict the absence or presence of numerical chromosomal aberrations. *Hum. Reprod.* 2004; **19**:2052–2059.

71. Viville S, Mollard R, Bach ML, et al. Do morphological anomalies reflect chromosomal aneuploidies?: case report. *Hum. Reprod.* 2000; **15**:2563–2566.

72. Zeyneloglu HB, Baltaci V, Duran HE, Erdemli E, Batioglu S. Achievement of pregnancy in globozoospermia with Y chromosome microdeletion after ICSI. *Hum. Reprod.* 2002; **17**:1833–1836.

73. Stalf T, Sánchez R, Köhn FM, et al. Pregnancy and birth after intracytoplasmic sperm injection with spermatozoa from a patient with tail stump syndrome. *Hum. Reprod.* 1995; **10**:2112–2114.

74. Okada H, Fujioka H, Tatsumi N, et al. Assisted reproduction for infertile patients with 9 + 0 immotile spermatozoa associated with autosomal dominant polycystic kidney disease. *Hum. Reprod.* 1999; **14**:110–113.

75. Tesarik J, Rolet F, Brami C, et al. Spermatid injection into human oocytes. II. Clinical application in the treatment of infertility due to non-obstructive azoospermia. *Hum. Reprod.* 1996; **11**:780–783.

76. Terriou P, Hans E, Giorgetti C, et al. Pentoxifylline initiates motility in spontaneously immotile epididymal and testicular spermatozoa and allows normal fertilization, pregnancy, and birth after intracytoplasmic sperm injection. *J. Assist. Reprod. Genet.* 2000; **17**:194–199.

77. Aktan TM, Montag M, Duman S, et al. Use of a laser to detect viable but immotile spermatozoa. *Andrologia* 2004; **36**:366–369.

78. Said TM, Agarwal A, Grunewald S, et al. Evaluation of sperm recovery following annexin V magnetic-activated cell sorting separation. *RBM Online* 2006;**13**:336–339.

79. Bartoov B, Berkovitz A, Eltes F, et al. Real-time fine morphology of motile human sperm cells is associated with IVF–ICSI outcome. *J. Androl.* 2002; **23**:1–8.

80. Parmegiani L, Cognigni GE, Bernardi S, et al. "Physiologic ICSI": hyaluronic acid (HA) favors selection of spermatozoa without DNA fragmentation and with normal nucleus, resulting in improvement of embryo quality. *Fertil. Steril.* 2010; **93**:598–604.

81. Huszar G, Ozkavukcu S, Jakab A, et al. Hyaluronic acid binding ability of human sperm reflects cellular maturity and fertilizing potential: selection of sperm for intracytoplasmic sperm injection. *Curr. Opin. Obstet. Gynecol.* 2003; **18**:260–267.

82. Yagci A, Murk W, Stronk J, Huszar G. Spermatozoa bound to solid state hyaluronic acid show chromatin structure with high DNA chain integrity: an acridine orange fluorescence study. *J. Androl.* 2010; **31**:566–572.

83. Chiou Fen C, Ni Lee S, Nee Lim M, Ling Yu S. Relationship between sperm hyaluronan-binding assay (HBA) scores on embryo development, fertilisation, and pregnancy rate in patients undergoing intra-cytoplasmic sperm injection (ICSI). *Proc. Singapore Healthc.* 2013; **22**:120–124.

84. Morozumi K, Shikano T, Miyazaki S, Yanagimachi R. Simultaneous removal of sperm plasma membrane and acrosome before intracytoplasmic sperm injection improves oocyte activation/embryonic development. *Proc. Natl. Acad. Sci. U. S. A.* 2006; **103**:17661–17666.

85. Ramalho-Santos J, Sutovsky P, Simerly C, et al. ICSI choreography: fate of sperm structures after monospermic rhesus ICSI and first cell cycle implications. *Hum. Reprod.* 2000; **15**:2610–2620.

86. Rawe VY, Olmedo SB, Nodar FN, et al. Cytoskeletal organization defects and abortive activation in human oocytes after IVF and ICSI failure. *Mol. Hum. Reprod.* 2000; **6**:510–516.

87. Murase Y, Araki Y, Mizuno S, et al. Pregnancy following chemical activation of oocytes in a couple with repeated failure of fertilization using

ICSI: case report. *Hum. Reprod.* 2004; **19**:1604–1607.

88. Borges E Jr, de Almeida Ferreira Braga DP, de Sousa Bonetti TC, Iaconelli A Jr, Franco JG Jr. Artificial oocyte activation using calcium ionophore in ICSI cycles with spermatozoa from different sources. *RBM Online* 2009; **18**:45–52.

89. Schmiady H, Schulze W, Scheiber I, Pfüller B. High rate of premature chromosome condensation in human oocytes following microinjection with round-headed sperm: case report. *Hum. Reprod.* 2005; **20**:1319–1323.

90. Wald M, Ross LS, Prins GS, et al. Analysis of outcomes of cryopreserved surgically retrieved sperm for IVF/ICSI. *J. Androl.* 2006; **27**:60–65.

91. Chapter 5: Sperm Preparation Techniques. In: Cooper TG, Aitken J, Auger J, et al., eds., *World Health Organization Laboratory Manual for the Examination and Processing of Human Semen*, 5th ed. Switzerland: WHO Press. 2010; 161–168.

92. Brackett NL, Kafetsoulis A, Ibrahim E, Aballa TC, Lynne CM. Application of 2 vibrators salvages ejaculatory failures to 1 vibrator during penile vibratory stimulation in men with spinal cord injuries. *J. Urol.* 2007; **177**:660–663.

93. Saito K, Kinoshita Y, Hosaka M. Direct and indirect effects of electrical stimulation on the motility of human sperm. *Int. J. Urol.* 1999; **6**:196–199.

94. Brackett NL, Padron OF, Lynne CM. Semen quality of spinal cord injured men is better when obtained by vibratory stimulation versus electroejaculation. *J. Urol.* 1997; **157**:151–157.

95. Hewitson L, Simerly C, Schatten G. Cytoskeletal aspects of assisted fertilization. *Semin. Reprod. Med.* 2000;**18**:151–159.

96. Hewitson L, Dominko T, Takahashi D, et al. Unique checkpoints during the first cell cycle of fertilization after intracytoplasmic sperm injection in rhesus monkeys. *Nat. Med.* 1999; **5**:431–433.

97. Silber SJ, Alagappan R, Brown LG, Page DC. Y chromosome deletions in azoospermic and severely oligozoospermic men undergoing intracytoplasmic sperm injection after testicular sperm extraction. *Hum. Reprod.* 1998; **13**:3332–3337.

98. Page DC, Silber S, Brown LG. Men with infertility caused by AZFc deletion can produce sons by intracytoplasmic sperm injection, but are likely to transmit the deletion and infertility. *Hum. Reprod.* 1999; **14**:1722–1726.

99. Tournaye H, Devroey P, Camus M, et al. Comparison of in-vitro fertilization in male and tubal infertility: a 3 year survey. *Hum. Reprod.* 1992; **7**:218–222.

100. Devroey P. Clinical application of new micromanipulative technologies to treat the male. *Hum. Reprod.* 1998; **13**:112–122.

101. Afzelius BA, Eliasson R. Male and female infertility problems in the immotile-cilia syndrome. *Eur. J. Respir. Dis. Suppl.* 1983; **127**:144–147.

102. Liu J, Nagy Z, Joris H, et al. Analysis of 76 total fertilization failure cycles out of 2732 intracytoplasmic sperm injection cycles. *Hum. Reprod.* 1995; **10**:2630–2636.

103. Gul U, Turunc T, Haydardedeoglu B, et al. Sperm retrieval and live birth rates in presumed Sertoli-cell-only syndrome in testis biopsy: a single centre experience. *Andrology* 2013; **1**:47–51.

104. Oates RD, Amos JA. The genetic basis of congenital bilateral absence of the vas deferens and cystic fibrosis. *J. Androl.* 1994; **15**:1–8.

105. Jarvi K, Zielenski J, Wilschanski M, et al. Cystic fibrosis transmembrane conductance regulator and obstructive azoospermia. *Lancet* 1995; **345**:1578.

106. Antinori S, Versaci C, Dani G, et al. Fertilization with human testicular spermatids: four successful pregnancies. *Hum. Reprod.* 1997; **12**:286–291.

107. Araki Y, Motoyama M, Yoshida A, et al. Intracytoplasmic injection with late spermatids: a successful procedure in achieving childbirth for couples in which the male partner suffers from azoospermia due to deficient spermatogenesis. *Fertil. Steril.* 1997; **67**:559–561.

108. Hansen M, Kurinczuk JJ, Bower C, Webb S. The risk of major birth defects after intracytoplasmic sperm injection and in vitro fertilization. *N. Engl. J. Med.* 2002; **10**:725–730.

109. Silber S, Escudero T, Lenahan K, et al. Chromosomal abnormalities in embryos derived from testicular sperm extraction. *Fertil. Steril.* 2003; **79**:30–38.

110. Doornbos ME, Maas SM, McDonnell J, Vermeiden JP, Hennekam RC. Infertility, assisted reproduction technologies and imprinting disturbances. *Hum. Reprod.* 2007; **22**:2476–2480.

111. Van Steirteghem A, Bonduelle M, Devroey P, Liebaers I. Follow-up of children born after ICSI. *Hum. Reprod. Update* 2002; **8**:111–116.

112. Palermo GD, Colombero LT, Schattman GL, Davis OK, Rosenwaks Z. Evolution of pregnancies and initial follow-up of newborns delivered after intracytoplasmic sperm injection. *JAMA* 1996; **276**:1983–1987.

113. Bowen JR, Gibson FL, Leslie GI, Saunders DM. Medical and developmental outcome at 1 year for

children conceived by intracytoplasmic sperm injection. *Lancet* 1998; **351**:1529–1534.

114. Bondulle M, Joris H, Hofmans K, Liebaers I, Van Steirteghem A. Mental development of 201 ICSI children at 2 years of age. *Lancet* 1998; **351**:1553.

115. Sutcliffe AG, Taylor B, Li J, et al. Children born after intracytoplasmic sperm injection: population control study. *BMJ* 1999; **318**:704–705.

116. Winter C, Van Acker F, Bonduelle M, Desmyttere S, Nekkebroeck J. Psychosocial development of full term singletons, born after preimplantation genetic diagnosis (PGD) at preschool age and family functioning: a prospective case-controlled study and multi-informant approach. *Hum. Reprod.* 2015; **3**:1122–1136.

117. DeBaun MR, Niemitz EL, Feinberg AP. Association of in vitro fertilization with Beckwith–Wiedemann syndrome and epigenetic alterations of LIT1 and H19. *Am. J. Hum. Genet.* 2003; **72**:156–160.

Chapter 10

Embryo Culture

Media Preparation for the Embryo Culture

Global tissue culture media were first developed by Ludwig and Ringer, nearly 150 years ago. These were simple salt solutions, simulating the properties of serum. The second generation of culture media, developed in the 1970s, mimics the female reproductive tract environment. A new, third generation of media was more improved and provided optimal growth conditions in vitro. The shift from home-brewed culture media to commercially manufactured media has contributed to improvements in laboratory and clinical outcomes, eliminating inconsistencies, manufacturing errors, and batch-to-batch variability. In 1963, Ralph Brinster designed the method of culture for oocytes and embryos in small droplets of culture medium covered by a layer of paraffin oil [1]. Later on, this "micro-drop" method had become the most widely used for the culture of mammalian embryos in vitro. By the mid-1990s, most IVF laboratories adopted the "closed" under-oil culture system, which has provided a more stable and more suitable culture environment for embryonic growth. Variations of the second-generation media called sequential and third-generation simplex optimized derived media are still in use at present and seem effective in supporting the development of human embryos through 6 days of culture in vitro. Culture for human embryos improved over the past decade by adding of essential amino acids.

After the compaction stage (day 4 of embryo culture), embryos have different requirements of amino acids and energy molecules compared with the cleavage stages (days 1–3). For example, the main energy source provided in an early-stage medium is lactate and pyruvate, as opposed to glucose for embryo culture from late day 3 with the onset of embryo compaction [2]. In addition, essential amino acids and metabolites, such as citrate and malate, are almost completely omitted from media used for early embryo culture, but are included in media used for embryos that have undergone compaction. Also, the chelating agent EDTA is included in early embryo culture media, but omitted from media used for extended culture, based on the assumption that this compound is toxic to blastocyst-stage embryos [3–4]. Solubilized ions, similar to those detected in the oviduct and uterine fluids, are the most abundant chemical constituents of culture media, to support human embryo cleavage and blastocyst formation in vitro. Together with purified water, ionic constituents contribute mainly to the osmolality of a medium. Media at a range of 250–290 mOsm can acceptably support mammalian embryo development [5]. Osmolality higher than 300 mOsm can induce deleterious changes in cell volume. Based on the knowledge of specific media requirements for the optimal embryonic development conditions, companies developed universal one-step media suitable for all embryo stages (Figure 10.1). Media from different manufacturers vary little in their composition of conventional ionic, protein supplements, and the main energy substrates: pyruvate, glucose, and lactate, which regulate mammalian embryo metabolism [6].

Amino acids are found in human reproductive tract fluids [7] and are essential regulators of embryo development. Glutamine was found to support the development of human embryos to the morula and blastocyst stages and increase energy metabolism. Taurine and glycine have been shown to act as osmolytes and, therefore, may help minimize the stress induced by osmotic fluctuations. Protein sources in culture medium play a role in preventing embryo adhesion to the culture plate and also may act as organic osmolytes and pH buffers. However, protein and amino acid metabolites in culture medium may negatively affect embryo development. Supplementation of culture media with protein showed ammonium accumulation (ranging from 8.4 mM to 138.6 mM), primarily from the

Characteristics	Single medium (one step)	Sequential medium (two steps)
Leaves embryos undisturbed	Yes	No
Accumulation of growth factors	Yes	Low
Replacment of essential nutrients	No	Yes
Accumulation of toxins	Yes	Low
Relative stress to embryos	Low	High
Requires control	One medium	Two media
Essential amino acids for blastocyst development	Contains	Cleavage medium does not contain
pH	pH is similar during culture	Cleavage (pH=7.2-7.25) Blast (pH=7.3-7.35)
Relative cost	Low	High

Figure 10.1 Comparison between one-step and two-step culture medium.

amino acid glutamine metabolism by the embryo with the highest level at day 4 of incubation, the level that might inhibit embryo development and have a possible risk for fetal defects [8]. For this reason, embryo culture media have reduced amount of the amino acids and contain the more stable dipeptide forms of glutamine.

The addition of growth factors such as leukemia inhibitory factor, epidermal growth factor, insulin-like growth factor-I (IGF-I), and the cytokine granulocyte-macrophage colony-stimulating factor (GM-CSF) has been shown to support the development of human embryos to the blastocyst stage [9–12]. Furthermore, IGF-I and GM-CSF stimulated the development of the inner cell mass (ICM).

The majority of human embryo culture systems use a bicarbonate/carbon dioxide-buffered medium to maintain a physiological pH of 7.2–7.4. The combination of 25 mM sodium bicarbonate with 5% CO_2 gas atmosphere results in a pH of 7.45 at sea level. An increase of carbon dioxide concentration up to 6% leads to decrease of pH till 7.37. These conditions are optimal for embryo growth and are highly recommended. Extracellular pH (pHe) in the culture medium is recognized to be a critical factor in establishing intracellular pH (pHi). pHi regulates protein conformation, glycolysis, and many of the other critical metabolic and transport processes in the embryo. The embryo can regulate its pHi, specifically acidosis, via the HCO_3^-/Cl^- exchanger; however, even slightly fluctuations of pHi during 3 hours lead to the disorganization of mitochondria and actin cytoskeletal elements [13]. Therefore, appropriate and stable pHe is a crucial factor of the embryo culture system.

The temperature of media varies throughout the lab, and can be affected by the dish manufacture or media volume used. For example, a decrease in the temperature of media culture from 37°C to 36.5°C was associated with a significantly higher cleavage rate, but a lower blastocyst formation rate on day 5. For this reason it is recommended to use media warmed to 37°C [14].

Oxygen concentration is also a crucial factor in embryo culture. Atmospheric oxygen concentration of 20% is highly detrimental to the embryos of all mammalian species studied, negatively affecting metabolism, and the proteome and gene expression. In contrast, the oxygen concentrations in the reproductive tract of mammalian species have been reported to range between 1.5% and 8%. The culture of mammalian embryos at low concentrations of oxygen (5–7%) is thought to minimize the formation of embryotoxic reactive oxygen species. Reduction of oxygen concentrations to 5% did not affect blastocyst development, but increased total cell number compared with the culture at 20% O_2 [15].

Media for fertilized oocyte and/or embryo culturing should be prepared and carbon dioxide/oxygen-saturated in an incubator for approximately 6 hours before use. A dish with prepared culture medium is covered with mineral oil to prevent medium evaporation under carbon dioxide/oxygen-saturated conditions at 37°C. The carbon dioxide/oxygen molecules pass through the oil–medium interface until the oil becomes saturated with carbon dioxide/oxygen. The thermodynamic transition of gas molecules through oil and its saturation takes approximately 4 hours, or more, depending on the type and volume of oil in the dish/plate. Usually, after 6 hours of incubation, the plate with medium covered by oil is ready for use. However, mineral oil may have a negative effect on the cultured embryo. It was shown that lipid-soluble materials are absorbed by mineral oil from the medium, and toxic compounds are released into the medium from the oil, which may lead to adverse effects [16]. For example, mineral oil peroxidation negatively affects media and embryo development. Conditions such as incubation time and high temperature can increase the peroxidation of mineral oil.

The embryo is sensitive to both chemical and physical signals within its microenvironment, which can play a significant role in its development and post-transfer events. These chemical and physical factors include oxygen, ammonium, volatile organics, temperature, pH, volume of oil overlay, medium volume/embryo density, exposure to atmospheric (20%) oxygen, and the accumulation of toxins in the media due to the static and undynamic nature of culture.

Some IVF laboratories culture embryos separately, one embryo per drop of medium, while others culture in groups of three to five embryos per drop. Increasing the fertilized oocyte density to two or four oocytes/culture drop does not affect the fertilization rate and embryo formation [17]. Culture of embryos in groups may have an advantage due to the secretion of growth-promoting factors, which act in an autocrine–paracrine fashion. The benefits of group embryo culture are in debate [18–19]. Embryo-to-embryo communication may not always be positive. The poor-quality embryos possibly exert a negative influence on the development of good-quality embryos in the same culture group [20].

The co-culture of embryos with somatic cells (granulosa cells, cumulus cells) has been reported to improve embryo and blastocyst development, decrease fragmentation, and improve pregnancy and implantation rates [21–22]. Somatic cells may enhance embryo development by providing trophic factors [23]. In summary, the gain in knowledge of both the physiology of the embryo and the environment of the oviduct and uterus leads to improvements in culture media and culture conditions.

Day 1 of Culture (Zygote)

Preparation for division begins when two haploid pronuclei (pN) disappear and syngamy occurs within 20–34 hours after fertilization (Figure 10.2). Mitotic division occurs approximately 35–36 hours after fertilization and results in the formation of two diploid blastomeres.

During the first hours of development after fertilization, the differentiated germ cells, i.e., the oocyte and the sperm cell, must be reprogrammed into a totipotent state. This process ensures that the newly formed zygotic genome can subsequently drive the differentiation of all the diverse cell types of the adult. The reprogramming relies on maternally supplied RNAs and proteins stockpiled in the oocyte. The zygotic genome remains

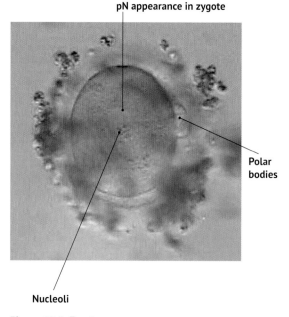

Figure 10.2 Zygote.

transcriptionally silent while reprogramming takes place. As the paternal centrioles pull the chromatids apart, a channel appears between the two poles, and the zygote formed one-cell embryo cleaves into a two-cell embryo at approximately 35–36 hours postfertilization. Early entrance into the first cell division has been used as an indicator of embryo viability. Embryos that had undergone early cleavage within 25 hours of fertilization were associated with higher pregnancy rates [24]. However, for the embryo to continue developing after this initial reprogramming phase, the zygotic genome must be expressed. After the sperm has fertilized the oocyte, the centriole and microtubules arising from the sperm cell bring the female and male pN into juxtaposition [25]. Normally fertilized oocytes are spherical and have two polar bodies (PBs) and two pN. Male and female pNs appear virtually simultaneously at ~6.2 hours postfertilization. However, while the female pN always forms cortically and near the site of emission of the second PB, the initial position of the male pN is cortical, intermediate, or central (15.2%, 31.2%, and 53.6%, respectively) [26]. Pronuclear alignment occurs 16–18 hours postfertilization and failure of this process is indicative of lack of one or more fertilization events. The pN and nucleoli show various presentations [27], named "Z-score" (Z1–Z4, where Z1 is a higher score and Z4 is a lower score), which reflect the chromosomal status and developmental inferiority of the embryo (Figure 10.3). "Z-scoring" is determined by size, number, and distribution of nucleoli. Zygotes with three to seven even-sized

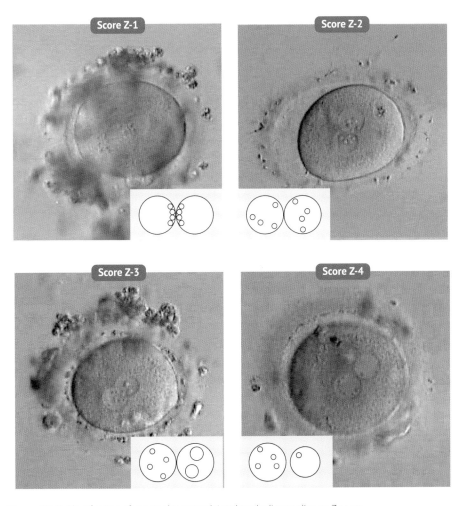

Figure 10.3 Classification of zygotes by pronuclei and nucleoli according to Z-score.

nucleoli per nucleus have a high chance to grow to embryos with greater developmental potential. There have been several attempts to determine embryo viability based on the location and alignment of the nucleolar precursor bodies in the nuclei [27–28]. Appearance of "touching" pN 16–18 hours after fertilization is associated with a higher viability score. The sperm-derived centriole and microtubules arising from fertilization are responsible for the alignment of pN. Pronuclear alignment relative to the PB axis, which positions the nucleoli, has also been assessed as an indicator of embryo viability. Also, it has been suggested that the size variation between the two pN may indicate chromosomal anomalies and limited developmental potential [29]. Before syngamy, pN can rotate within the ooplasm, directing their axes towards the second PB [30]. Embryos failing to achieve an optimal pronuclear orientation may exhibit cleavage anomalies that can manifest as poor morphology, uneven cleavage, or fragmentation. Chromatin from the sperm and the egg is unified to create an entirely new genome. It remains unclear whether activation of the zygotic genome is instructive to the changes in the underlying chromatin or the changes in chromatin are required for genome activation. However, these processes are intimately linked. Two distinct genomes (paternal and maternal) undergo different processes as they are brought together in the zygote. In many species, the paternal genome is repackaged through the exchange of histones for protamines. In the transcriptional silence that follows fertilization, the genome is repackaged back to histones and reprogrammed to prepare the embryo to give rise to a new individuum. The transition from silence to widespread gene expression requires precise regulation. This regulation is accomplished through several coordinated processes, in which transcription factors play a central role. After fertilization, translational upregulation promotes the accumulation of genome-activating transcription factors, which direct chromatin remodeling in reprogramming contexts, helping to erase the previous cell identity (oocyte) while creating a new one (embryo).

It is unknown when and how molecular and morphological symmetry breaking emerges and how these two elements integrate spatially and temporally to control the genetic and epigenetic networks that direct lineage fate and pattern formation in the embryo. The molecular and physical circumstances under which distinct stem cell types can self-organize to form tissues, organs, or even artificial embryos in vitro are also unknown and it is vital that these be defined.

Tripronuclear or tetrapronuclear (or multipronuclear) zygotes form triploid (or multiploid) embryos and some regain a diploid karyotype by the expulsion of a set of chromosomes in a nucleated fragment [31]. Nondisjunction in meiosis I or meiosis II of oogenesis results in an extra set of maternal chromosomes, a state termed digyny. Nondisjunction in meiosis I or meiosis II of spermatogenesis results in an extra set of paternal chromosomes, a state known as diandry. Digyny is a triploid zygote in which the extra haploid set is of maternal origin (like retention of the second PB or binucleate oocyte), while diandry is a triploid zygote in which the extra haploid set is of paternal origin. Giant oocytes might be a possible source of digynic triploidy. It is not recommended to transfer or cryopreserve the embryos developed from giant oocytes or tripronuclear zygotes [31–32]. A monopronuclear zygote may be diploid; some of them may develop to a blastocyst and term after transfer [33–34]. It is suggested that monopronuclear zygotes be rechecked for multiple pN within a few hours and cultured to the blastocyst stage for possible transfer. However, the use of one pN zygotes, and zygotes showing no pN or more than two pN are not recommended by the European Society of Human Reproduction and Embryology (ESHRE).

Day 2 of Culture (Embryo Two to Four Cells)

Embryo score can be evaluated at high magnification (at least 200×, preferably 400×) using an inverted microscope with Hoffman or equivalent optics. Embryos are optimally at the four-cell stage of development by 45–46 hours postfertilization (day 2) [35]. Slowly developing embryos may still be at the two-cell stage at this time point. Some individual cells of the embryo may be asynchronous in their cell division, resulting in embryos with uneven cell numbers. It is accepted that transition from maternal to embryonic gene expression occurs between the four-cell and the eight-cell stage, i.e., during the first 48 hours after fertilization, the embryo primarily relies on maternal transcripts rather than its activated genome [36].

Number and size of blastomeres and embryonic fragmentation score are morphological features used to assess embryo quality [37–38] and which stand as the basis of the embryo classification system (grade 1A to grade 4C), in which the numbers and letters represent fragmentation (<10%; 10–30%; 30–50%; >50%) and blastomeres (size and shape), respectively. In addition to these criteria, blastomeres can exhibit normal nucleation (one per blastomere, no nucleus, or multinucleation. Multinucleated embryos are associated with lower clinical pregnancy and live birth rates than single-nucleated embryos [39]; they are not associated with increased occurrence of congenital anomalies and chromosomal defects. It was suggested that blastomere multinucleation is a consequence rather than a cause of aneuploidy [40]. Fragmentation is the extrusion of the plasma membrane, including the cytoplasm of an embryo, into the extracellular region and appears to be a natural occurrence in human embryos [41]. Mitochondria are the most abundant structures found in the fragments [42]. The mechanisms causing fragmentation are not fully understood, although it has been speculated that developmentally lethal defects or apoptotic events may cause the process. Fragmentation of less than 10% is associated with a 23% live birth rate, 10–25% fragmentation with an 11% live birth rate, and more than 25% fragmentation with an only 1% live birth rate [43]. Fragment removal from the embryos does not improve embryo quality [42].

Day 3 of Culture (Embryo Six to Eight Cells)

By 54–56 hours postfertilization (day 3), embryos are optimally at the eight-cell stage of development (Figure 10.4) [35]. Embryos dividing either too slowly or too quickly may have metabolic and/or chromosomal defects (Figure 10.5). It was reported that more than 60% of the embryos that arrest between the pronuclear and the eight-cell stage are chromosomally abnormal [44]. Similarly, embryos exhibiting irregularly shaped blastomeres and severe fragmentation are considered poor-quality embryos and show a higher incidence of chromosomal abnormalities [45] on day

3 as well as on day 2 (Figure 10.6). Abnormal slow cleaving (two to six cells on day 3) and rapidly cleaving embryos show a higher incidence of chromosomal aneuploidy than embryos showing normal cleavage kinetics [46]. On day 3, embryos may contain blastomeres with more than one nucleus and are chromosomally abnormal compared with nonmultinucleated embryos [47].

On day 3, embryo cells begin to become heterogeneous (first decision for differentiation to be trophectoderm cells or ICM later) [48–50]. Also, on day 3 postfertilization, there is an increase in cell–cell adhesion and partial loss of definition between single blastomeres of embryos that have initiated compaction. During compaction and with the establishment of cell–cell adhesions, blastomeres undergo a rearrangement process leading to communication between blastomeres signaling procession to the next stage – morula.

Day 4 of Culture (Morula)

Approximately 4 days after fertilization, when 16–32 embryo cells have undergone compaction, the embryo is termed a morula (Figure 10.7) [51]. Compaction involves the formation of tight junctions and gap junctions between blastomeres, the formation of philopodia (adhesive contacts that include actin and myosin), and blastomere polarization, resulting in tight communication between blastomeres and segregation of two cellular populations of inside and outside cells [52]. Differentiation of cells to trophectoderm or ICM is continuous from day 3 [53]. These cells' fate decisions are dependent on cell heterogeneity, polarity, position, and origin.

Day 5 of Culture (Blastocyst)

When a cavity forms within the morula, it is termed a blastocyst. Cavitation involves the formation of the blastocoele, the fluid-filled cavity necessary for blastocyst formation. The Na^+/K^+-ATPase pump located on the basolateral membrane expels Na^+ from the cell and into the intercellular spaces, forming an osmotic gradient, which leads to passive following of the water, thereby forming the blastocoele cavity [54]. Today, the function of the blastocyst lumen is unknown. As cavitation proceeds, two populations of cells form by blastomere polarization during compaction and cavitation: the trophectoderm population that forms extraembryonic tissue – trophoblast – and

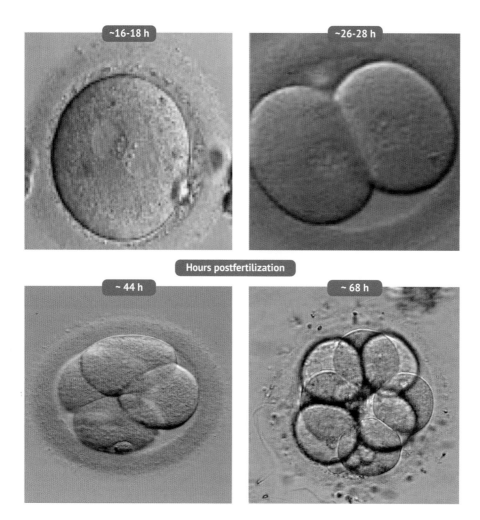

Figure 10.4 Development stages of cultured embryo.

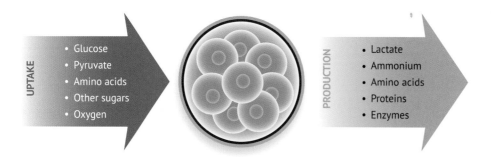

Figure 10.5 The uptake and excretion products of cultured embryo.

the population of ICM that forms the embryo lineages: epiblast and hypoblast [55].

The blastocyst has several different grades, depending on its stage of development (Figure

10.8). When a cavity is apparent, the ICM and trophectoderm are distinct; the embryo is termed an early blastocyst. The blastocyst begins to increase in size, and is then termed an expanding

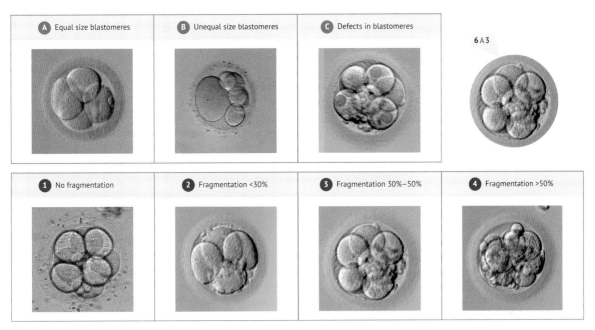

Figure 10.6 Classification of embryo by blastomere count, blastomere size, and fragmentation rate.

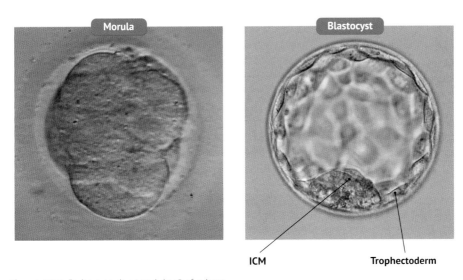

Figure 10.7 Embryo on day 4 and day 5 of culture.

blastocyst until it has fully expanded. During expansion, the blastocyst causes thinning of the ZP, culminating in its rupture, after which, the blastocyst begins to herniate through the ZP in a process called hatching. This hatching process occurs on approximately day 6 or 7. When the blastocyst entirely escapes from the ZP, it is termed a hatched blastocyst.

Blastocysts can appear morphologically similar but contain significantly different cell numbers (range: 24–322 [56]) and bear different hatching abilities [57]. On days 5, 6, and 7, expanded blastocysts have an average of 38, 40, and 80 trophectoderm cells and 20, 42, and 46 ICM cells, respectively [58]. The total number of mitochondrial DNA (mtDNA) copies in the developing embryo does not change from

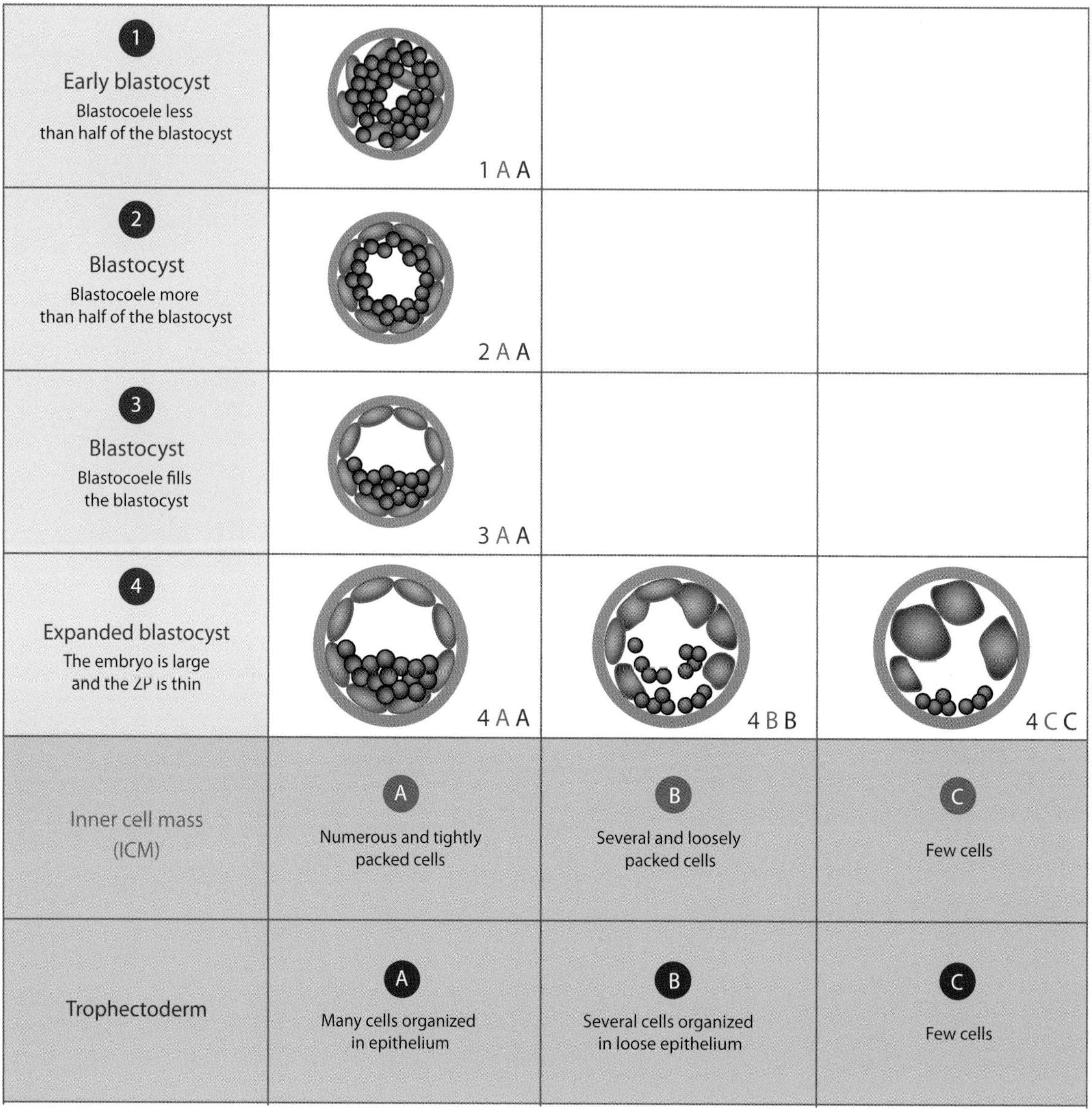

	A	B	C
1 Early blastocyst Blastocoele less than half of the blastocyst	1 A A		
2 Blastocyst Blastocoele more than half of the blastocyst	2 A A		
3 Blastocyst Blastocoele fills the blastocyst	3 A A		
4 Expanded blastocyst The embryo is large and the ZP is thin	4 A A	4 B B	4 C C
Inner cell mass (ICM)	**A** Numerous and tightly packed cells	**B** Several and loosely packed cells	**C** Few cells
Trophectoderm	**A** Many cells organized in epithelium	**B** Several cells organized in loose epithelium	**C** Few cells

Figure 10.8 Gardner's classification of blastocyst according to embryo size, blastocoele size, inner cell mass, and trophectoderm compositions.

fertilization until the blastocyst stage, despite numerous cell divisions, resulting in progressively diluted mtDNA content in each of the blastomeres. At this stage of development (day 5), the blastocyst begins to secrete human chorionic gonadotropin (hCG) at the level of ~5 IU/L/day, with maximal production on ~day 10 [59], necessary for initial stages of embryonic recognition in vivo. hCG production does not appear to begin until the expanded stage [60].

Embryo growth rate and morphology are determinants of embryo quality (Figure 10.9). There is a decrease in embryo quality in embryos generated from oocytes of aging women. This phenomenon may be explained by increased chromosomal abnormalities, time of genomic activation, and the temporal pattern of gene expression during the initial stages of embryo development. Embryos that appear normal morphologically may still contain chromosomal

Embryo testing (Istanbul consensus - 2011, Alfa, ESHRE)	
Day 1	16 ± 1 h for 2pN
Day 2	44 ± 1 h for 4 blastomeres
Day 3	68 ± 1 h for 8 blastomeres
Day 4	92 ± 2 h for compacted or compacting
Day 5	116 ± 2 h for fully expanded

Figure 10.9 Timing for optimal embryonic development stages.

abnormalities and the frequency of these abnormalities increases with maternal age [61]. In general, there is no correlation between morphological and genetic embryo profiles [62].

References

1. Brinster RL. A method for in vitro cultivation of mouse ova from two-cell to blastocyst. *Exp. Cell Res.* 1963; **32**:205–208.

2. Gott AL, Hardy K, Winston RM, Leese HJ. Non-invasive measurement of pyruvate and glucose uptake and lactate production by single human preimplantation embryos. *Hum. Reprod.* 1990; **5**:104–108.

3. Hardarson T, Bungum M, Conaghan J, et al. Noninferiority, randomized, controlled trial comparing embryo development using media developed for sequential or undisturbed culture in a time-lapse setup. *Fertil. Steril.* 2015; **104**:1452–1459.

4. Machtinger R, Racowsky C. Culture systems: single step. *Methods Mol. Biol.* 2012; **912**:199–209.

5. McKiernan SH, Bavister BD. Environmental variables influencing in vitro development of hamster 2-cell embryos to the blastocyst stage. *Biol. Reprod.* 1990; **43**:404–413.

6. Gardner DK, Lane M. Culture and selection of viable blastocysts: a feasible proposition for human IVF? *Hum. Reprod. Update* 1997; **3**:367–382.

7. Borland RM, Biggers JD, Lechene CP, Taymor ML. Elemental composition of fluid in the human Fallopian tube. *J. Reprod. Fertil.* 1980; **58**:479–482.

8. Kleijkers SH, van Montfoort AP, Bekers O, et al. Ammonium accumulation in commercially available embryo culture media and protein supplements during storage at 2–8°C and during incubation at 37°C. *Hum. Reprod.* 2016; **31**:1192–1199.

9. Dunglison GF, Barlow DH, Sargent IL. Leukaemia inhibitory factor significantly enhances the blastocyst formation rates of human embryos cultured in serum-free medium. *Hum. Reprod.* 1996; **11**:191–196.

10. Martin KL, Barlow DH, Sargent IL. Heparin-binding epidermal growth factor significantly improves human blastocyst development and hatching in serum-free medium. *Hum. Reprod.* 1998; **13**:1645–1652.

11. Lighten AD, Moore GE, Winston RM, Hardy K. Routine addition of human insulin-like growth factor-I ligand could benefit clinical in-vitro fertilization culture. *Hum. Reprod.* 1998; **13**:3144–3150.

12. Sjöblom C, Wikland M, Robertson SA. Granulocyte-macrophage colony-stimulating factor promotes human blastocyst development in vitro. *Hum. Reprod.* 1999; **14**:3069–3076.

13. Squirrell JM, Lane M, Bavister BD. Altering intracellular pH disrupts development and cellular organization in preimplantation hamster embryos. *Biol. Reprod.* 2001; **64**:1845–1854.

14. Fawzy M, Emad M, Gad MA, et al. Comparing 36.5°C with 37°C for human embryo culture: a prospective randomized controlled trial. *RBM Online* 2018; **36**:620–626.

15. Gardner DK. Reduced oxygen tension increases blastocyst development, differentiation and viability. *Fertil. Steril.* 1999; **72**:S30–S31.

16. Shimada M, Kawano N, Terada T. Delay of nuclear maturation and reduction in developmental competence of pig oocytes after mineral oil overlay of in vitro maturation media. *Reproduction* 2002; **124**:557–564.

17. Khamsi F, Roberge S, Lacanna IC, Wong J, Yavas Y. Effects of granulosa cells, cumulus cells, and oocyte density on in vitro fertilization in women. *Endocrine* 1999; **10**:161–166.

18. Almagor M, Bejar C, Kafka I, Yaffe H. Pregnancy rates after communal growth of preimplantation human embryos in vitro. *Fertil. Steril.* 1996; **66**:394–397.

19. Rijnders PM, Jansen CA. Influence of group culture and culture volume on the formation of human blastocysts: a prospective randomized study. *Hum. Reprod.* 1999; **14**:2333–2337.

20. Tao T, Robichaud A, Mercier J, Ouellette R. Influence of group embryo culture strategies on the blastocyst development and pregnancy outcome. *J. Assist. Reprod. Genet.* 2013; **30**:63–68.

21. Menezo Y, Hazout A, Dumont M, Herbaut N, Nicollet B. Coculture of embryos on Vero cells and transfer of blastocysts in humans. *Hum. Reprod.* 1992; **7**:101–106.

22. Freeman MR, Whitworth CM, Hill GA. Granulosa cell co-culture enhances human embryo development and pregnancy rate following in-vitro fertilization. *Hum. Reprod.* 1995; **10**:408–414.

23. Liu LP, Chan ST, Ho PC, Yeung WS. Partial purification of embryotrophic factors from human oviductal cells. *Hum. Reprod.* 1998; **13**:1613–1619.

24. Sakkas D, Shoukir Y, Chardonnens D, Bianchi PG, Campana A. Early cleavage of human embryos to the two-cell stage after intracytoplasmic sperm injection as an indicator of embryo viability. *Hum. Reprod.* 1998; **13**:182–187.

25. Sathananthan AH, Kola I, Osborne J, et al. Centrioles in the beginning of human development. *Proc. Natl. Acad. Sci. U. S. A.* 1991; **88**:4806–4810.

26. Papale L, Fiorentino A, Montag M, Tomasi G. The zygote. *Hum. Reprod.* 2012; **27**(Suppl. 1):i22–i49.

27. Gámiz P, Rubio C, de los Santos MJ, et al. The effect of pronuclear morphology on early development and chromosomal abnormalities in cleavage-stage embryos. *Hum. Reprod.* 2003; **18**:2413–2419.

28. Tesarik J, Greco E. The probability of abnormal preimplantation development can be predicted by a single static observation on pronuclear stage morphology. *Hum. Reprod.* 1999; **14**:1318–1323.

29. Sadowy S, Tomkin G, Munné S, Ferrara-Congedo T, Cohen J. Impaired development of zygotes with uneven pronuclear size. *Zygote* 1998; **6**:137–141.

30. Payne D, Flaherty SP, Barry MF, Matthews CD. Preliminary observations on polar body extrusion and pronuclear formation in human oocytes using time-lapse video cinematography. *Hum. Reprod.* 1997; **12**:532–541.

31. Kola I, Trounson A, Dawson G, Rogers P. Tripronuclear human oocytes: altered cleavage patterns and subsequent karyotypic analysis of embryos. *Biol. Reprod.* 1987; **37**:395–401.

32. Balakier H, Bouman D, Sojetcki A, Librach C, Squire JA. Morphological and cytogenetic analysis of human giant oocytes and giant embryos. *Hum. Reprod.* 2002; **17**:2394–2401.

33. Staessen C, Van Steirteghem AC. The chromosomal constitution of embryos developing from abnormally fertilized oocytes after intracytoplasmic sperm injection and conventional in-vitro fertilization. *Hum. Reprod.* 1997; **12**:321–327.

34. Gras L, Trounson AO. Pregnancy and birth resulting from transfer of a blastocyst observed to have one pronucleus at the time of examination for fertilization. *Hum. Reprod.* 1999; **14**:1869–1871.

35. Cummins JM, Breen TM, Harrison KL, et al. A formula for scoring human embryo growth rates in in vitro fertilization: its value in predicting pregnancy and in comparison with visual estimates of embryo quality. *J. In Vitro Fert. Embryo Transf.* 1986; **3**:284–295.

36. Braude P, Bolton V, Moore S. Human gene expression first occurs between the four- and eight-cell stages of preimplantation development. *Nature* 1988; **332**:459–461.

37. Baczkowski T, Kurzawa R, Głabowski W. Methods of embryo scoring in in vitro fertilization. *Reprod. Biol.* 2004; **4**(1):5–22.

38. Moriwaki T, Suganuma N, Hayakawa M, et al. Embryo evaluation by analysing blastomere nuclei. *Hum. Reprod.* 2004; **19**:152–156.

39. Seikkula J, Oksjoki S, Hurme S, et al. Pregnancy and perinatal outcomes after transfer of binucleated or multinucleated frozen-thawed embryos: a case-control study. *RBM Online* 2018; **36**:607–613.

40. Tesarik J. Is blastomere multinucleation a safeguard against embryo aneuploidy? Back to the future. *RBM Online* 2018; **37**:506–507.

41. Buster JE, Bustillo M, Rodi IA, et al. Biologic and morphologic development of donated human ova recovered by nonsurgical uterine lavage. *Am. J. Obstet. Gynecol.* 1985; **153**:211–217.

42. Halvaei I, Khalili MA, Esfandiari N, et al. Ultrastructure of cytoplasmic fragments in human cleavage stage embryos. *J. Assist. Reprod. Genet.* 2016; **33**:1677–1684.

43. Racowsky C, Combelles CM, Nureddin A, et al. Day 3 and day 5 morphological predictors of embryo viability. *RBM Online* 2003; **6**:323–331.

44. Almeida PA, Bolton VN. Cytogenetic analysis of human preimplantation embryos following developmental arrest in vitro. *Reprod. Fertil. Dev.* 1998; **10**:505–513.

45. Almeida PA, Bolton VN. The relationship between chromosomal abnormality in the human preimplantation embryos following developmental in vitro. *Reprod. Fertil. Dev.* 1996; **8**:235–241.

46. Magli MC, Gianaroli L, Munné S, Ferraretti AP. Incidence of chromosomal abnormalities from a morphologically normal cohort of embryos in poor-prognosis patients. *J. Assist. Reprod. Genet.* 1998; **15**:297–301.

47. Kligman I, Benadiva C, Alikani M, Munne S. The presence of multinucleated blastomeres in human embryos is correlated with chromosomal abnormalities. *Hum. Reprod.* 1996; **11**:1492–1498.

48. Piotrowska-Nitsche K, Perea-Gomez A, Haraguchi S, Zernicka-Goetz M. Four-cell stage mouse blastomeres have different developmental properties. *Development* 2005; **132**:479–490.

49. Torres-Padilla ME, Parfitt DE, Kouzarides T, Zernicka-Goetz M. Histone arginine methylation regulates pluripotency in the early mouse embryo. *Nature* 2007; **445**:214–218.

50. Bischoff M, Parfitt DE, Zernicka-Goetz M. Formation of the embryonic-abembryonic axis of the mouse blastocyst: relationships between orientation of early cleavage divisions and pattern of symmetric/asymmetric divisions. *Development* 2008; **135**:953–962.

51. Iwata K, Yumoto K, Sugishima M, et al. Analysis of compaction initiation in human embryos by using time-lapse cinematography. *J. Assist. Reprod. Genet.* 2014; **31**:421–426.

52. Fierro-Gonzalez JC, White MD, Silva JC, Plachta N. Cadherin-dependent filopodia control preimplantation embryo compaction. *Nat. Cell. Biol.* 2013; **15**:1424–1433.

53. Morris SA, Teo RT, Li H, et al. Origin and formation of the first two distinct cell types of the inner cell mass in the mouse embryo. *Proc. Natl. Acad. Sci. U. S. A.* 2010; **107**:6364–6369.

54. Watson AJ, Natale DR, Barcroft LC. Molecular regulation of blastocyst formation. *Anim. Reprod. Sci.* 2004; **82–83**:583–592.

55. White MD, Zenker J, Bissiere S, Plachta N. Instructions for assembling the early mammalian embryo. *Dev. Cell* 2018; **45**:667–679.

56. Hardarson T, Caisander G, Sjögren A, et al. A morphological and chromosomal study of blastocysts developing from morphologically suboptimal human pre-embryos compared with control blastocysts. *Hum. Reprod.* 2003; **18**:399–407.

57. Van Blerkom J. Development of human embryos to the hatched blastocyst stage in the presence or absence of a monolayer of Vero cells. *Hum. Reprod.* 1993; **8**:1525–1539.

58. Hardy K, Handyside AH, Winston RM. The human blastocyst: cell number, death and allocation during late preimplantation development. *Development* 1989; **107**:597–604.

59. Woodward BJ, Lenton EA, Turner K. Human chorionic gonadotrophin: embryonic secretion is a time-dependent phenomenon. *Hum. Reprod.* 1993; **8**:1463–1468.

60. Woodward BJ, Lenton EA, Turner K, Grace WF. Embryonic human chorionic gonadotropin secretion and hatching: poor correlation with cleavage rate and morphological assessment during preimplantation development in vitro. *Hum. Reprod.* 1994; **9**:1909–1914.

61. Munné S, Alikani M, Tomkin G, Grifo J, Cohen J. Embryo morphology developmental rates, and maternal age are correlated with chromosome abnormalities. *Fertil. Steril.* 1995; **64**:382–391.

62. Rienzi L, Capalbo A, Stoppa M, et al. No evidence of association between blastocyst aneuploidy and morphokinetic assessment in a selected population of poor-prognosis patients: a longitudinal cohort study. *RBM Online* 2015; **30**:57–66.

Embryo Transfer

Eliezer Girsh and Irina Ayzikovich

Conditions for an Embryo at Oviduct and Uterus

In vitro fertilization (IVF) strives to ensure an in vitro environment that closely mimics the physiological environment of gametes. However, the providing of such conditions is limited by the lack of our knowledge on the actual natural levels of oxygen concentration, pH, and temperature within the reproductive tract.

The environments within the oviduct and uterus differ significantly in terms of nutrient availability, and the presence of a complex mixture of cytokines and growth factors in the uterus [1]. The oviduct is characterized by relatively high levels of pyruvate (0.14–0.32 mM) and lactate (5.4–10.5 mM), with relatively low levels of glucose (0.5–1.1 mM). In contrast, the uterus contains a relatively high level of glucose (3.15 mM) [2–3]. The relative availability of nutrients within the female reproductive tract precisely reflects the changing requirements of the preimplantation embryo at each stage of development.

The degree of tissue oxygenation is defined by partial pressure (pO_2). In contrast to pO_2, which represents partial pressure in mm Hg, dissolved oxygen (DO) is a measure of oxygen concentration, i.e., the number of DO molecules in the liquid (mg/l). Comparison of pO_2 in tissue with DO in a liquid is not equal; therefore, the environment of the embryo in culture differs from the environment in Fallopian tubes and uterus. DO is reliant on various key physical factors, such as temperature, pH, and salinity, in addition to external pressures. Historically, atmospheric oxygen tension (~21% or 750 mm Hg) has been used in the medium of tissue culture and then in IVF embryo culture. Nevertheless, the physiological oxygen concentration in the female reproductive tract has been found to be lower, ranging between 2% and 8% [4]. This pO_2 in the Fallopian tubes is dependent on the blood circulation in the subepithelial capillary network. Moreover, pO_2 within the uterus during the reproductive cycle, as found in humans, monkeys, rabbits, and hamsters, is less than ambient air pO_2 at sea level. In addition, the intrauterine pO_2 also depends on hormonal activity during estradiol (E_2) and progesterone (P_4) fluctuations [5]. The intrauterine pO_2 has been shown to vary considerably between individuals, with a range of 6.4–32 mm Hg [6]. The fluctuations in intrauterine pO_2 within the estrous/menstrual cycle are not consistent, and there are no clear data about uterine pO_2 around implantation and the early pregnancy states. The physiological significance of reduced pO_2 in the female reproductive tract is mostly unknown. However, it seems that this is a functional phenomenon as a means to protect the developing blastocyst from oxygen toxicity.

Various levels of pH are found in different parts of the female reproductive tract. Lower pH levels are measured within the cervix and vagina compared with the Fallopian tubes and uterus. During ovulation, pH in the uterus and endocervical mucus was shown to be increased [7]. Biological buffers have been introduced into embryo culture media to help stabilize pH [8]; however, the in vivo pH regulation mechanism within the reproductive tract is likely to be more comprehensive than these culture media.

The potential involvement of temperature in embryo development is studied within the IVF procedure. The temperature for embryo culture is accepted to be close to the natural body temperature. Basal body temperature is diurnal, with minimum body temperatures measured in the early morning. Female body temperature also tends to show a biphasic pattern with a phase of the cycle, increasing in the luteal phase by 0.31–0.46°C compared with the follicular phase [9], with the latter attributed to the thermogenic action of P_4 [10]. The regulation of temperature within the reproductive tract is multifarious.

The region of isthmus of the Fallopian tube (sperm storage site) is 1–2°C cooler than the portion of ampulla (fertilization site) [11], and variation in temperature may affect fertilization or embryo development. Extreme changes in body temperature may trigger an immune response, orchestrated by molecular networks of cytokines and miRNAs [12], which may injure the embryo. The temperature of 37°C is accepted as a standard and practically used in embryo culture incubators.

The preimplantation embryo is known to be highly sensitive to the environment as it undergoes a process of dynamic changes and reprogramming in preparation for implantation. Conditions within the uterus and Fallopian tubes fluctuate throughout the estrous and menstrual cycles. They tend to show an oscillatory biorhythm, which may be important for the survival of the preimplantation embryo and may be influenced by hormones, blood supply, tissue integrity, and other external factors. The "natural" environment of the preimplantation embryo remains to be fully characterized. There is no simple single solution which can translate the dynamic physiological conditions to an IVF laboratory setting. Although the transfer of zygotes and cleavage-stage human embryos to the uterus can result in pregnancies, in all mammalian species studied to date, the transfer of cleavage-stage embryos resulted in significantly compromised transfer outcomes compared with transfer at the blastocyst stage. Therefore, the transfer of a cleavage-stage embryo to the uterus places it into an environment that is not ideal.

The relative conditions, such as the pH of commercially available culture media, the temperature, and concentration of oxygen in IVF incubators are based on results extracted from animal studies.

Gamete intrafallopian transfer (GIFT). GIFT is a fertility technique in which both oocytes and sperm are placed directly into the Fallopian tube, allowing for fertilization to occur.

The Fallopian tube is a susceptible and gentle structure, particularly vulnerable to many disease processes and iatrogenic insults. Its lumen is small, ciliated, delicate, and easily damaged by surgical intervention. Patients treated using GIFT underwent routine ovarian stimulation, and oocyte retrieval was performed by laparoscopy or mini-laparotomy. Postretrieval, up to four mature oocytes were drawn into a catheter followed by sperm. The catheter was then laparoscopically passed through the fimbriae and advanced to the ampullary portion of the Fallopian tube where the gametes were injected. The first successful pregnancy conceived through GIFT occurred in 1984. The benefits of GIFT included a more physiological environment for fertilization; however, this technique results in poor fertilization rate and is no longer used.

Zygote intrafallopian transfer (ZIFT). To address concerns of poor fertilization rate with GIFT, a procedure known as ZIFT was introduced in the late 1980s. Oocytes were retrieved laparoscopically or transvaginally, fertilized, and laparoscopically transferred directly into the Fallopian tube. This technique allowed for confirmation of fertilization while also allowing for early development in vitro and zygote/embryonic transport via the Fallopian tube. One of the disadvantages of ZIFT was the inability to select the most viable zygotes from a large cohort for transfer. This procedure also is no longer used.

Intrauterine embryo transfer (ET). ET is a technique involving the intrauterine transfer of embryos. There are a few procedures that allow transfer of embryos to the uterus by noninvasive methods: ultrasound-guided transvaginal ET [13], transmyometrial ET [14], and transcervical ET. The first two methods have been used for patients with anatomical abnormalities of the uterus or severe cervical stenosis that predict difficulty or inability to cannulate the cervical canal. Transcervical ET is a rapid and straightforward technique and does not require analgesics or anesthetics. Disadvantages of the methods described above include the technical difficulty encountered in patients with cervical stenosis and the risk of infection from microorganisms introduced into the endometrial cavity.

Selection of Embryo for Transfer

One of the most lottery aspects of assisted reproductive technology (ART) is the selection of embryos that will be able to yield a healthy pregnancy. A number of selection criteria for rationalization of the process have been suggested, including the zygote appearance score (pronuclei and nucleoli orientation), the rate of embryo development (cleavage rate), morphological assessments (equality of blastomeres, fragmentation), blastocyst development, and preimplantation genetic testing (PGT). Embryo scoring techniques have been developed to help assess fetal implantation potential.

Morphological embryo assessment has been employed for many years as a tool for determining pregnancy potential. Embryos are scored based on cell count, fragmentation pattern, cytoplasmic pitting, blastomere regularity, and vacuole presence [15–18].

Fragmentation is one of the typical morphological features used in assessing embryo quality. Grading systems evaluate embryo quality based on the cell (blastomeres) count and the percentage of fragmentation observed in the embryo. Low implantation rates were reported from embryos with higher than 15% fragmentation on day 2 of development [19]. While not all fragmentation appears to be detrimental to embryo development, its pattern has a profound effect on the embryo's developmental potential. Large fragments appear to be more detrimental than small fragments. The correlation between fragmentation and apoptosis is not clear; however, fragmentation may be a sign of apoptosis if regulatory proteins are altered [20].

Embryo scoring based on cleavage rate and morphology is one of the major predicting factors in maximizing pregnancy rates [19; 21]. Embryos with eight cells (blastomeres) on day 3 have a lower percent of chromosomal abnormalities than embryos with altered (more than eight or less than eight) numbers of blastomeres at this stage of development [22]. Blastomere volume also has an essential impact on embryo quality. A positive correlation exists between blastomere volume and the number of mitochondrial DNA copies [23]. The cell stage at the time of transfer has become a significant factor in identifying the embryos with the greatest implantation potential. Embryonic genome activation occurs between the four-cell and eight-cell stages of preimplantation development [24]. ET on day 3 or day 5 of development allows for the selection of embryos undergoing embryonic activation. In fact, the embryo selection criterion should be based on the dynamics of all embryo development stages from zygote "Z"-scoring of pronuclei to embryo parameters scoring on day 3 or day 5 of development.

Extended embryo culture to the blastocyst stage was suggested as a possible selection criterion of the most vital embryo for transfer (only half of all zygotes have the potential to develop to the blastocyst stage) as a means of reducing the risks of aneuploidy. Nevertheless, extended culture to the blastocyst stage does not eliminate embryos displaying chromosome abnormalities; ~40% of embryos exhibiting normal morphological development to blastocyst are aneuploid. Selection of blastocyst-stage embryos at this time may allow for the transfer of a single blastocyst (day 5). At this stage, the transfer is associated with a significant increase in implantation rate compared with cleavage-stage transfer (day 3) [25]. A scoring system for blastocyst development, based on cavity formation, inner cell mass (ICM) definition, and trophectoderm (TE) distinction, was first described by Dokras et al. [26] and later extended by Gardner et al. [27]. The two grading systems, compared by a randomized study, illustrated the superiority of the Gardner system over the Dokras system in predicting blastocysts with a higher chance of implantation and clinical pregnancy. Although the advantages of blastocyst transfer have been presented, efficacy of this time-point procedure is still in dispute. A subsequent analysis of the various studies involving blastocyst transfer revealed that there were striking differences in culture conditions. In particular, studies that did not find a benefit in blastocyst transfer had used atmospheric oxygen for embryo culture, whereas the studies reporting significant benefits from day 5 transfer had used 5% O_2 for embryo culture. This latter point highlights the difficulties of comparing studies assumed to have performed IVF in the same way. There is proof that blastocyst transfer increased implantation rates, decreased pregnancy losses, and slightly reduced the time to pregnancy.

Both meiotic and mitotic types of chromosome errors have been observed during preimplantation development. Meiotic errors primarily arise during oogenesis and become more frequent with advancing female age. Mitotic errors arise after fertilization and most commonly occur during the first three cleavage divisions. Mitotic errors lead to a phenomenon known as mosaicism (chromosomally distinct cells within the same embryo). PGT is a more reliable and useful technique to eliminate chromosomally abnormal embryos. Regardless of the many criteria proposed to assist in the selection process of the normal embryo, no single criterion offers a significant advantage over the others. Most embryo selection systems are based on a combination of criteria, including morphology, cleavage rate, and embryonic genomic activation.

Older patients (more than 35 years old) are more likely to have "slow" blastocysts, and this asynchrony, which increases with maternal age, should be taken into account when synchronizing the embryo to endometrium receptivity [28].

Despite the intensive research performed on the various aspects of human reproduction (genomics, proteomics, and metabolomics), most embryologists still daily use routine assessments using standard variables, which include developmental rate, based on cell counts on day 2 and day 3 and development of a blastocyst on day 5, and morphological features such as fragmentation, degree of symmetry in cleavage-stage embryos, and ICM or TE quality in blastocysts (Figures 11.1 and 11.2).

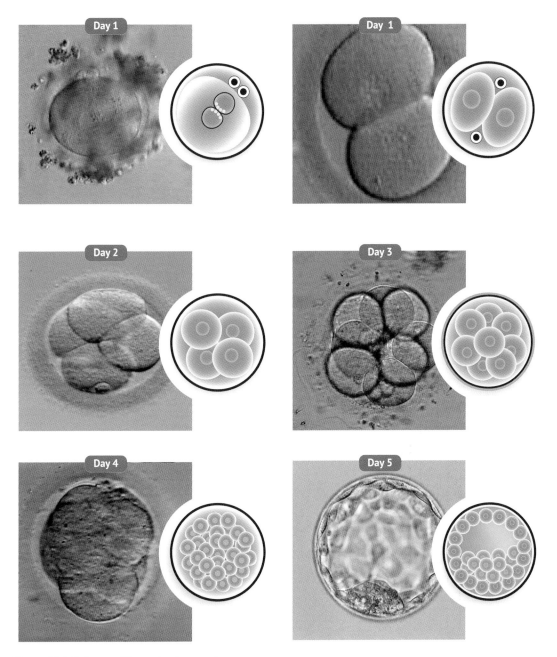

Figure 11.1 Embryo at different developmental stages.

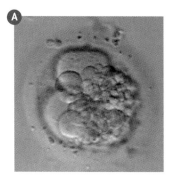 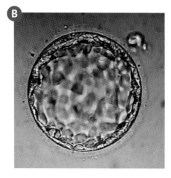

Figure 11.2 Low embryo quality. (A) Cleavage-stage embryo; (B) blastocyst.

Assisted Hatching

Manipulation of the zona pellucida (ZP), termed "assisted hatching" (AH), has been introduced to favor embryo hatching and ultimately improve ART outcomes. Assisted zona hatching is a part of ART in which a small hole is made in the ZP, using a micromanipulation or laser, thereby facilitating ZP hatching. The AH procedure was first described by Jacques Cohen, who, in 1988, reported the first pregnancy after AH [29]. Various AH procedures have been developed to help embryos escape from their ZP during blastocyst expansion. These include mechanical incision of the ZP, chemical ZP drilling with acidic Tyrode's solution (pH = 2.5), enzymatic zona removal with pronase treatment, laser-assisted AH, and piezo (Figure 11.3) [30].

During mechanical incision, the embryo is held firmly in position by the holding pipette, and an opening is made by introducing a dissecting pipette through the ZP, followed by rubbing the embryo gently against the holding pipette until the embryo is released [31].

When drilling with Tyrode's solution, the solution is expelled with a micropipette until one-third of the ZP is dissolved to perform the thinning. A disadvantage of this procedure is the possibility of an embryo damaged by acidic pH.

Bathing embryos in pronase solution and thinning of the ZP by enzyme treatment before transfer yields similar effects to other AH procedures.

The introduction of laser has substituted acidic and enzymatic removal of ZP. Lasers represent an ideal tool for microsurgical procedures, as the energy is easily focused on the targeted area, producing a controlled and precisely positioned hole, with high interoperator consistency. Two methods of laser-assisted AH can be used. In the first method, the contact mode, the laser is guided through optical fibers touching the embryo and ultraviolet light is delivered by a glass pipette, or infrared light is delivered with a quartz fiber. In the second method, the noncontact mode, the laser beam is directed through the ZP using an optical lens tangential to the embryo. The noncontact mode using various laser wavelengths is preferred for gamete micromanipulation. The 1.48 μm laser can be focused through the conventional optics of an inverted microscope, to illuminate a polystyrene culture dish filled with culture medium, providing for easy non-touch and objective-driven targeting of the laser light to specific cellular subcomponents, such as the embryo ZP. The location, duration, and increment of the delivered energy can be precisely defined with the aid of computer programs. A laser can be used to thin or to make actual holes in the ZP. ZP thinning can be performed on the outer or inner side of the ZP. Both light electron microscopy and scanning electron microscopy have revealed no degenerative ultrastructural alterations of oocyte and embryo ZP following laser-mediated zona drilling [32]. In various protocols the time of AH varies, from immediately to 24 hours before ET, as well as irradiation time and size of the hole (10–40 μm). It should be emphasized that the live birth rate is not affected.

The clinical relevance of AH on fresh or frozen embryos within an ART program remains controversial [33–34]. There is no significant evidence that ZP drilling in selective embryos helps in poor-prognosis cases [35] or in cases of older patients [36]. The implantation rate of ZP-drilled embryos and control embryos was 25% and 18%, respectively [37], and selective AH appeared most effective in women over 38 years of age and in those with elevated basal FSH levels [37]. However, the benefit of AH in the older age group remains unclear [38]. An unselected group of ET patients showed similarity between the outcomes of AH performed using

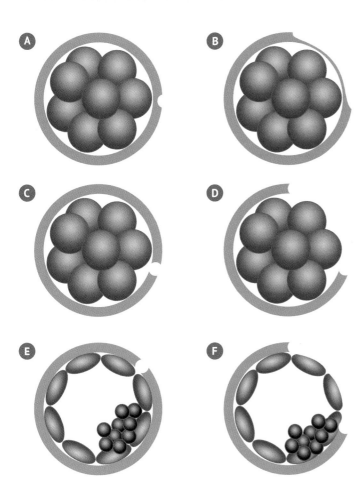

Figure 11.3 Assisted hatching of cleavage embryo and blastocyst. (A–B) Partial dissection of ZP in cleavage-stage embryo; (C–D) ZP-drilled embryos; (E–F) ZP-drilled blastocysts.

partial ZP dissection [39] or acidic Tyrode ZP drilling [40] versus non-treated. However, it has to be noted that AH might effectively increase embryo implantation rates in humans, but only in selected cases. Recommendation of the European Society for Human Reproduction and Embryology (ESHRE) and the American Society for Reproductive Medicine (ASRM) for this procedure remains unclear and has become even fainter over the years.

Embryo Transfer Procedure

The ET procedure is one of the most critical steps in the process of IVF (Figure 11.4). The success rate of ART directly depends on embryo quality and uterine receptivity.

The first step in ET is the "time-out" process, during which identification and matching of patients and embryos are performed. A double identity check of the patient, the patient's file, and the culture dish(es) is mandatory immediately before the transfer. To perform ET the preparation of patient is required that includes positioning the patient, introducing the speculum, cleaning the cervix, and manipulating the uterus. There is no compelling evidence that patient position affects the outcome of ET [41], and it is recommended to choose a position most comfortable for both patient and therapist. A bivalve speculum is then gently introduced into the vagina to expose the cervix. Maneuvering the speculum can improve cervical–uterine alignment to allow easier access by the catheter. Removing mucus from the endocervical canal using sterile cotton swabs, or aspiration with a catheter improves clinical outcomes [42]. Also, it has been reported that passive bladder distension results in significantly higher pregnancy rates in contrast to patients with an empty bladder

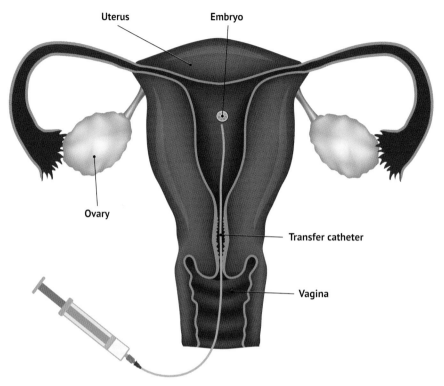

Figure 11.4 Embryo transfer procedure.

[43]. The ET procedure requires abdominal ultrasound for monitoring of catheter placement. Limited centers have utilized transvaginal ultrasound for ET, which has been associated with improved patient comfort relative to transabdominal ultrasound due to the lack of bladder filling [44]. Cervical dilatation can be performed in patients with cervical stenosis, where the passage of the catheter is challenging. The cervix can be cleaned by swabbing, vigorous rinsing, or aspiration to remove excess mucus; there is no clear agreement on the best method. To gain a better understanding of the patient's anatomy, a "mock" ET (trial run that allows determining the best route and the ideal location to place the embryo in the uterus) can be performed [45]. Mock ET has been shown to minimize the problems associated with the actual ET procedure and to improve pregnancy and implantation rates. Usually, the ET procedure is performed without any anesthesia. Local or general anesthesia is sometimes required if the ET procedure is complicated.

ET pregnancy rates depend on the physician performing the procedure [46–47]. Examples of difficult transfers, retained embryos, or other mishaps can be recounted, many with happy endings [46].

Microbial contamination of the ET catheter tip is correlated with a significant reduction in pregnancy rate [48]. Prophylactic antibiotics administered during oocyte retrieval and on the day of ET significantly reduce the incidence of positive microbial cultures from ET catheter tips 48 hours after antibiotic administration [49], but have not been shown to improve clinical pregnancy rates.

There is insufficient evidence regarding the effect of acupuncture, analgesics, traditional Chinese medicine, or massage therapy on ET pregnancy rates.

Catheters

Many different catheters are commercially available for ET. Catheters are classified according to their tip structure, flexibility, and presence of a separate outer sheath, location of the distal port (end- or side-loading), degree of stiffness, thickness, length, diameter, and echogenic visibility. However, they are generally grossly classified as soft or stiff (or firm). There is little difference in concept and technology between ET catheters and so there is no distinctly superior catheter. The main characteristic required of a transfer catheter is the ability to maneuver it into the uterine cavity without causing trauma to the embryos and endometrium. Some advantage was shown with an increased chance of clinical pregnancy when soft ET catheters are used [50]. Soft catheters can more easily follow the contour of the endometrial cavity, reducing the risk of endometrial trauma or of plugging the catheter tip. However, at the same time, soft catheters are more difficult to insert and pass. In some cases, the insertion of the catheter is difficult due to cervical stenosis. An operable stylet device can be used with some soft catheters to negotiate a difficult internal os. In technically difficult ETs, mainly where difficulties are encountered in negotiating the internal cervical os, there is often a need for the stiffer firm catheters. The switch from soft to firm catheters for these transfers may account for help in ET and pregnancy rate. There is sufficient evidence demonstrating that soft ET catheters improve IVF-ET pregnancy rates.

Catheter Loading

The critical part of the ET process is embryo loading into the transfer catheter. The type of syringes and catheters selected for ET and how they are handled are very important. Three main options exist for transfer syringes: 1 ml glass Hamilton syringes, 1 ml rubber-free syringes, and 1 ml syringes with rubber stoppers. No clear advantage of one syringe type over another has been shown. Critical factors considered for selection of a particular device include the preferred amount of resistance when depressing the plunger and the type of plunger with regard to chemical toxicity concerns. Glass Hamilton syringes require sterilization between cases and can wear out over time.

Rinsing of the catheter, to remove any substances or debris that may be present inside the catheter before loading embryos for transfer, is recommended by some specialists. However, such rinsing can form air bubbles inside the catheter wall and may affect the smoothing of the medium flow during aspiration and embryo loading.

Once the catheter and syringe are selected, and catheters are prepped, various embryo loading methods can be used (Figure 11.5). Wide debate exists over the impact of air loading in the ET catheter. Alternation of medium–air loading can help with ultrasound visualization during the transfer. Various studies failed to show a clear advantage of the medium–air catheter loading method compared with medium only, in terms of pregnancy, implantation, miscarriage, or live birth rates [51]. Furthermore, the embryo can be stuck to an air

bubble in the uterine cavity after ET and degenerate. An additional disadvantage of air in the catheter/uterus is the possible pH change of the expelled medium. Moreover, air is not generally found in the uterus and should not be present in the uterine cavity.

The volume of media in the catheter may be an important factor impacting pregnancy and implantation rates. More fluid (50 µl) yielded superior pregnancy and implantation rates than smaller fluid volumes (20 µl) [52].

Time Frame of an Embryo in the Catheter

The timing of each ET step may also be involved in success rates. The interval between catheter loading and embryo discharge into the uterine cavity may affect IVF outcomes. At intervals of more than 120 seconds, both implantation and pregnancy rates were lower [53]. This phenomenon may be related to environmental stress caused by exposure of the embryo outside the incubator. Thus, minimizing the time between loading and transfer of embryos is highly recommended.

Depth of Catheter Placement in the Uterus

There is no consensus to the depth of placement of the ET catheter within the uterus. It is widely accepted that contact with the uterine fundus can stimulate contractions that may be responsible for ET failure or ectopic gestation [54–55]. High-frequency uterine contractions on the day of ET have been found to decrease implantation and clinical pregnancy rates, possibly by expelling embryos from the uterine cavity [56].

Embryos placed too high in the uterine space may increase the probability of endometrial trauma and may induce uterine contractions with potentially adverse effects. Significantly higher pregnancy rates were obtained when the selected location was approximately 2 cm from the uterine fundus compared with 1 cm from the fundus [57]. Results of others show no difference in implantation and pregnancy rates when embryos were placed in the upper versus lower half of the endometrial cavity [58–59].

Uterine movements must be distinguished from uterine contractions. Ultrasound assessments have shown that endometrial wave movements flowing from the cervix to fundus and from fundus to cervix

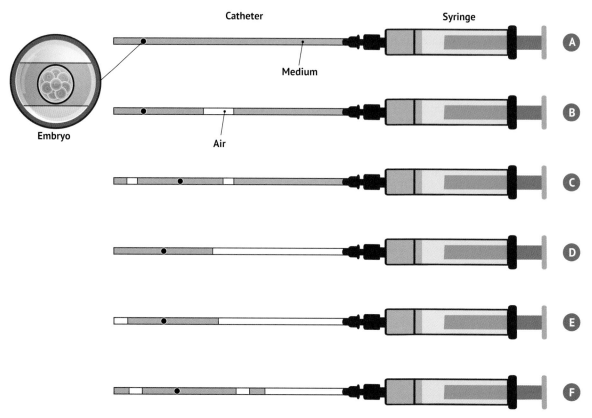

Figure 11.5 Embryo loading options. (A) medium loading; (B–F) variants in medium/air proportion.

begin at both ends simultaneously. The intensity of the endometrial movements differs in every patient at different times. The uterine wave movements help the embryo implant into the "right place." We can conclude that expulsion of the embryo during ET to the exact point is not really necessary.

Complications during ET may be related to inability or difficult ability to insert the catheter into the uterine cavity leading to trauma of the embryo and/or endometrium. That is one of the critical determinants of success. Easy or intermediate transfers resulted in approximately two-fold higher pregnancy rate than complicated transfers. In order to assist more accurate catheter placement within the uterus, ultrasound-guided ET is highly recommended instead of relying on clinician "feel" [60]. Improvements in both implantation and clinical pregnancy rates can be achieved by using ultrasound-guided ET [61]. Transabdominal and transvaginal ultrasound appear to be similarly effective in terms of pregnancy outcomes [62].

Embryo Expulsion Speed

The exact speed of embryo–fluid expulsion into the uterus is unknown and may also impact ET outcome. Rapid expulsion increases the rates of shrunken and/or collapsed embryos and the apoptotic index of rapidly injected embryos is higher than those injected slower [63]. A pump-regulated ET device provided reliable and reproducible injection speeds, whereas manual injection showed considerable variation in speed even with a standardized protocol [64]. Great caution is required with expulsion speed to avoid embryo trauma. To prevent embryonic damage inject the fluid as slow as possible. During the ET procedure, the syringe plunger should be gently pushed to the end of a syringe without depression; negative pressure built up by depression may suck the embryo back.

To minimize potential embryo expulsion from the uterus following ET, biological glue (hyaluronic acid [HA]- or hyaluronan-enriched medium) has been used to attach the embryo to the endometrium at the site of embryo deposition. However, the hatched blastocyst continues to move within the uterine cavity and routine use of embryo glue, as ET medium, does not improve the ART outcomes [65]. From another side, HA improves clinical pregnancy rates in patients with previous IVF failures [66], and the use of HA-enriched ET medium is beneficial [67], increasing the live birth rate by 8% [68]. The potential positive complimentary effect of HA on IVF outcome cannot be denied. HA is a member of the glycosaminoglycan family, secreted into the extracellular matrix from the cell surface. HA has a wide variety of physiological functions in the body, including maintenance of a viscoelastic cushion to protect tissues, control of tissue hydration and water transport, lubrication of bio-interfaces, the formation of large protein and proteoglycan assemblies, and receptor-mediated signaling roles in cell detachment, mitosis, migration, and inflammation. HA secretion is regulated by interleukins and gonadal steroids [69]. HA presents in follicular, oviductal, and uterine fluids. Human embryos at all stages of development possess HA receptors [70], and HA and its receptor are present in the uterine endometrium with the most abundant expression at the time of implantation. HA may directly stimulate the embryo growth or provides the nourishing environment. Cell–cell adhesion and cell–matrix adhesion have been shown to be increased by HA, which may facilitate the apposition and attachment of the embryo. HA and its receptor CD44 have both been implicated in the angiogenesis of endometrium. HA can promote angiogenesis by both degradation products and interaction with epidermal growth factor. On the day of implantation, uterine HA levels increase significantly and appear to be associated with regions that contain stromal cells that are proliferating in preparation for embryo implantation.

Once the embryo is discharged from the embryo catheter, the physician can immediately withdraw the transfer catheter or pause before doing so. Immediate withdrawal and a 30-second delay were found to have no difference in pregnancy rates [71].

It was noted that the presence of mucus on the ET catheter, once it is withdrawn, is not associated with a lower clinical pregnancy rate or live birth rate [72]. The presence of blood on the catheter following ET was also not adversely associated with pregnancy rates [73]. However, others have reported that the presence of blood on the catheter has been related to poorer results [74–75]. Intrauterine blood coagulating with

the embryo inside the uterus may lead to the adverse effects. To summarize, the success rate of IVF depends on factors such as patient preparation, medication, mock ET, type of catheter, and optimal transfer technique.

After ET, the catheter should be carefully examined to rule out embryo retention; this should be done by gently rinsing the catheter, avoiding bubbles.

Bed Rest

Historically, in the past, bed rest following ET has been advised. During the early years of IVF, there were significant variations in the time recommended to remain in a supine position, practiced in hope of avoiding uterine contractions and "premature expulsion" of embryos from the uterus. Anecdotal reports have included durations of bed rest for 24 hours to as long as 2 weeks. To date, there is no significant evidence that bed rest improves the implantation rates [76–77]. Moreover, some works have even indicated a possible detrimental effect of bed rest [78]. Thus, although recommendations should be individualized to patient preference and anxiety levels, bed rest after ET has no proven benefit.

When Should the Embryo Be Transferred?

Embryos can be transferred on day 2, day 3, day 4, or day 5 postfertilization. The highest pregnancy and implantation rates were reported when embryos were transferred on day 3 rather than on day 2 [79]. Another report showed no changes in implantation or live birth rates when delaying transfer from day 2 to day 3 [80]. Delaying ET until day 4 resulted in similar implantation and pregnancy rates to those achieved following ET on day 2 or day 3 [81]. No significant difference in pregnancy and implantation rates was determined when ET was performed on either day 3 or day 5 [82]. However, delay of ET to day 5 enabled the identification of embryos with very high implantation potential. Clinical pregnancy rates were almost double those recorded for day 3 transfers when exclusively cavitating embryos were transferred on day 5 [25; 83–84]. The number of ET cycles necessary until achieving the first live birth was significantly lower for embryos transferred on day 5 compared with day 3. However, the cumulative live birth rates were the same for cleavage-stage and blastocyst-stage transfers.

One of the disadvantages of delaying ET to day 5 is that ET may be canceled if the cleavage-stage embryo will not develop to blastocyst in culture. It should be noted that in patients with a high number of embryos, blastocyst transfer is desirable. Overall, blastocyst transfer has advantages over cleavage ET, in both higher implantation rates and lower miscarriage rates, but with an increased risk of monozygotic and monochorionic twins.

Transfer of the Frozen-Thawed Embryo

Frozen–thawed ET (FET) is a procedure used for the transfer of cryopreserved embryos. FET prevents embryo waste and increases the chance of pregnancy in a single stimulated cycle. FET in a "more physiologic," non-stimulated endometrium may not only result in higher pregnancy rates [85–86], but may also decrease maternal and neonatal morbidity [87–88]. It is suggested that the natural cycle (NC) is superior to hormonal replacement treatment because the NC is close to the physiology of a natural process. In terms of ET timing, initiation of P_4 intake (luteal support) should preferably be on the theoretical day of oocyte retrieval, and blastocyst transfer should be at human chorionic gonadotropin (trigger) + 7 days or luteinizing hormone (surge) + 6 days in modified or true NC, respectively.

Hence, FET should be performed at optimal window time when the embryo seeking implantation matches to the receptive/selective endometrial stage. Although FET is increasingly used for multiple indications, the optimal protocol has not yet been determined.

FET and fresh ET appear to result in similar pregnancy outcomes [89]. Singletons born after cryopreservation of embryos had a significantly higher birth weight (macrosomia) than those conceived after fresh ET [90]. This increased risk of higher than gestational age weight cannot be explained by intrinsic maternal factors or birth order [91]. The increase in birth weight ranged from 50 g to 250 g [92]. This phenomenon may also be the result of the epigenetic effect of freezing–thawing procedures, manifested by abnormal methylation of the *H19* gene in both maternal and paternal alleles.

Whether fresh or frozen ETs yield the best clinical outcomes is still under discussion. Elective freeze-all embryo cycles are growing in popularity due to increasing evidence of success rates of FET [93]. However, FETs have added benefits only for patients who produced large numbers of oocytes (15 or more at collection). Such patients had slightly higher birth rates for frozen compared with fresh embryos. Patients who produced low (1 to 5) or intermediate (6 to 14) numbers of oocytes had higher birth rates with fresh compared with frozen embryos [94]. In addition, freezing can also lead to another 1 or 2 months of waiting without knowing if the procedure will work, which can be emotionally draining for patients.

How Many Embryos Should Be Transferred?

When considering how many embryos to transfer, several variables must be taken into account, i.e., prognosis for live birth, the health risks for the children, the costs to the couples and society. A few decades ago, the implantation rate was low, but was considered acceptable for an IVF clinic. Taking into account the low implantation rate, transferring two or more embryos was considered necessary to achieve an acceptable implantation rate or pregnancy rate. Although high success with multiple blastocyst transfer leads to a high multiple pregnancy rate (MPR), the high MPR has been a problem for ART (pregnancy complications, premature delivery, and health of newborns) over the past two decades. Multiple pregnancy is associated with well-documented increases in maternal morbidity and mortality as a result of gestational diabetes, hypertension, cesarean delivery, pulmonary emboli, and postpartum bleeding. It also increases the risk of premature birth, resulting in fetal, neonatal, and childhood complications as a result of neurological insults, ocular and pulmonary damage, learning disabilities, retardation, and congenital malformations [95–96]. Reducing the MPR has become a crucial public health requirement in IVF practices. The most effective method to avoid multiple pregnancies (aside from monozygotic twinning [MZT]) is the transfer of a single embryo [84].

MZT is a rare phenomenon in humans, occurring in 0.42% of spontaneous pregnancies. MZT occurs more frequently after single blastocyst transfer compared with cleavage-stage ET [97]. Several studies also reported monozygotic twins and triplets following single blastocyst transfer [98–99].

A cumulative live birth rate following single ET (SET) is not substantially lower than that of double ET

(DET) [100], but the multiple birth rate is markedly reduced. If no live birth occurs in the fresh SET cycle, a SET of a cryopreserved–thawed embryo is performed. The SET strategy is better than the DET strategy when considering a number of deliveries with at least one live-born child, the incremental cost-effectiveness ratio, and maternal and pediatric complications [101].

After SET, the prevalence of multiple pregnancies with splitting is 1.36% [102]. Splitting pregnancies are associated with frozen–warmed ET cycles, blastocyst culture, or AH. In fresh SET cycles, the prevalence of splitting pregnancy after single blastocyst transfer is significantly higher than after SET cycles with cleavage embryos [102]. However, there is no evidence that splitting is a result of ovarian stimulation and fertilization methods.

In summary, the single embryo transfer is more beneficial than multiple embryo transfer.

Endometrial Suitability for Embryo

Embryo implantation is the result of successful interaction between the embryo and the endometrium. Successful implantation is determined both by the quality of the embryo and by the receptiveness of the endometrium. The interaction between a competent embryo and a receptive endometrium involves complex molecular activities indispensable for successful implantation [103]. Decidualization, the secretory transformation that the endometrial stromal compartment undergoes to accommodate pregnancy, plays a vital role in endometrium receptivity as it is thought to contribute to the active selection of embryos attempting implantation [104]. In IVF it is a trick to determine the exact time of the "implantation window." This window occurs between days 20 and 24 of a normal menstrual cycle [105–106]. However, this window may not be absolute and considerable individual variability may exist. Hence, confirmation that the endometrium is adequately prepared at the time of ET must be performed for each patient individually.

It is generally accepted that the endometrium has to be at least 7 mm thick on the day of ovulation trigger in fresh IVF cycles and before the start of P_4 in frozen–thaw ET cycles [107–108]. Some differences in endometrial thickness are natural and some are subjective; the fluctuations of thickness depend on variations in measurement techniques, ultrasound equipment, ART protocols, and patient age. The accepted optimal endometrial thickness threshold of more than 10 mm has been correlated with maximized live birth and minimized pregnancy loss rates [109]. Although clinical pregnancy and live birth rates are lower when the endometrial thickness is below 8 mm at the time of ET, they are still within a reasonably acceptable range [110].

The human microbiota, i.e., the community of microorganisms that populate human tissue, may contribute to endometrial receptivity for embryo implantation. Most bacterial communities coexist in relationships with the human host, and it is known that the microbiota evolved together with our genome [111]. Successful ET depends upon many factors, including the presence of microbial colonization of the upper genital tract [112].

Transcervical procedures, such as hysterosalpingography and hysteroscopy, and transvaginal procedures, such as oocyte retrieval, may potentially contaminate the endometrium, Fallopian tubes, or peritoneal cavity with microorganisms from the endocervix or upper vagina. Intrauterine infection has been observed in many cases of premature birth. Correlations between bacterial infiltration via an ET catheter tip and pregnancy outcomes have been reported [113]. Moreover, microbial contamination at ET may influence implantation rates [114]. To date, the use of antibiotics during and after IVF treatments has been associated with reduced risk of infection in these procedures.

Intercourse during a Peri-transfer Period

Hypothetically, intercourse may impair implantation by introducing infection or initiating uterine contractions. During an IVF cycle, the uterine cavity is vulnerable to intercourse-related infection since the passage of the ET catheter disrupts the cervical mucus barrier. Furthermore, uterine myometrial activity is increased during intercourse, especially in the event of female orgasm [115]. These contractions may interfere with the implantation of the early embryo since high levels of spontaneous uterine activity are associated with poor IVF-ET outcomes [116]. On the other hand, intercourse during the peri-transfer period of an IVF cycle is not detrimental to early pregnancy and women exposed to semen via sexual intercourse during this period showed a significant improvement in early embryo implantation and development [117].

Endometrial Injury (Pipelle)

Over the last two decades, endometrial injury has been studied to improve implantation rates and decrease the incidence of implantation failure in IVF cycles. Endometrial injury is an intentional infliction of damage to the endometrium, usually produced by a Pipelle catheter. The capacity of the female reproductive tract to remodel after an injury is similar to that which occurs during every menstrual cycle, involving the balanced activity of inflammation, associated with vascular, connective tissue, and epithelial cell remodeling. Morphological studies demonstrated similarities between endometrial regeneration after normal menses and the recovery from endometrial injury [118]. Endometrial injury, resulting in inflammation [119–120], is characterized by the upregulation of cytokines and chemokines, followed by the recruitment of immune cells to the injured tissue. These cells, in turn, secrete a range of cytokines that induce tissue remodeling by stimulating cell proliferation and differentiation. The specific cellular differentiation occurring during the window of implantation includes the transformation of the fibroblast-like endometrial stromal cells into larger and rounded decidual cells [121] and the emergence of large apical protrusions (pinopodes) and microvilli on the luminal epithelium [122].

Endometrial injury performed between day 7 of the previous cycle and day 7 of the ET cycle is associated with improved clinical pregnancy rates in women with repeated implantation failures (more than two prior failed ETs) [123]. However, there is still insufficient evidence to support the use of endometrial injury in women with implantation failure [124].

References

1. Barnes FL. The effects of the early uterine environment on the subsequent development of embryo and fetus. *Theriogenology* 2000; **53**:649–658.

2. Gardner DK, Lane M, Calderon I, Leeton J. Environment of the preimplantation human embryo in vivo: metabolite analysis of oviduct and uterine fluids and metabolism of cumulus cells. *Fertil. Steril.* 1996; **65**:349–353.

3. Tay JI, Rutherford AJ, Killick SR, et al. Human tubal fluid: production, nutrient composition and response to adrenergic agents. *Hum. Reprod.* 1997; **12**:2451–2456.

4. Fischer B, Bavister BD. Oxygen tension in the oviduct and uterus of rhesus monkeys, hamsters and rabbits. *J. Reprod. Fertil.* 1993; **99**:673–679.

5. Kaufman DL, Mitchell JA. Intrauterine oxygen tension during the oestrous cycle in the hamster: patterns of change. *Comp. Biochem. Physiol. Comp. Physiol.* 1994; **107**:673–678.

6. Ottosen LD, Hindkaer J, Husth M, et al. Observations on intrauterine oxygen tension measured by fibre-optic microsensors. *RBM Online* 2006; **13**:380–385.

7. Macdonald RR, Lumley IB. Endocervical pH measured in vivo through the normal menstrual cycle. *Obstet. Gynecol.* 1970; **35**:202–206.

8. Will MA, Clark NA, Swain JE. Biological pH buffers in IVF: help or hindrance to success. *J. Assist. Reprod. Genet.* 2011; **28**:711–724.

9. Simic N, Ravlic A. Changes in basal body temperature and simple reaction times during the menstrual cycle. *Arh. Hig. Rada Toksikol.* 2013; **64**:99–106.

10. Zuspan FP, Rao P. Thermogenic alterations in the woman. I. Interaction of amines, ovulation, and basal body temperature. *Am. J. Obstet. Gynecol.* 1974; **118**:671–678.

11. Hunter RH. Temperature gradients in female reproductive tissues. *RBM Online* 2012; **24**:377–380.

12. Wong JJ, Au AY, Gao D, et al. RBM3 regulates temperature sensitive miR-142-5p and miR-143 (thermomiRs), which target immune genes and control fever. *Nucleic Acids Res.* 2016; **44**:2888–2897.

13. Parsons JH, Bolton VN, Wilson L, Campbell S. Pregnancies following in vitro fertilization and ultrasound-directed surgical embryo transfer by perurethral and transvaginal techniques. *Fertil. Steril.* 1987; **48**:691–693.

14. Kato O, Takatsuka R, Asch RH. Transvaginal-transmyometrial embryo transfer: the Towako method; experiences of 104 cases. *Fertil. Steril.* 1993; **59**:51–53.

15. Desai NN, Goldstein J, Rowland DY, Goldfarb JM. Morphological evaluation of human embryos and derivation of an embryo quality scoring system specific for day 3 embryos: a preliminary study. *Hum. Reprod.* 2000; **15**:2190–2196.

16. Ziebe S, Petersen K, Lindenberg S, et al. Embryo morphology or cleavage stage: how to select the best embryos for transfer after in-vitro fertilization. *Hum. Reprod.* 1997; **12**:1545–1549.

17. Kahraman S, Yakin K, Dönmez E, et al. Relationship between granular cytoplasm of oocytes and pregnancy outcome following intracytoplasmic sperm injection. *Hum. Reprod.* 2000; **15**:2390–2393.

18. Von Royen E, Mangelschots K, De Neubourg D, et al. Characterization of a top quality embryo, a step towards single-embryo transfer. *Hum. Reprod.* 1999; **14**:2345–2349.

19. Giorgetti C, Terriou P, Auquier P, et al. Embryo score to predict implantation after in-vitro fertilization: based on 957 single embryo transfers. *Hum. Reprod.* 1995; **10**:2427–2431.

20. Antczak M, Van Blerkom J. Temporal and spatial aspects of fragmentation in early human embryos: possible effects on developmental competence and association with the differential elimination of regulatory proteins from polarized domains. *Hum. Reprod.* 1999; **14**:429–447.

21. Shoukir Y, Campana A, Farley T, Sakkas D. Early cleavage of in-vitro fertilized human embryos to the 2-cell stage: a novel indicator of embryo quality and viability. *Hum. Reprod.* 1997; **12**:1531–1536.

22. Magli MC, Gianaroli L, Ferraretti AP, et al. Embryo morphology and development are dependent on the chromosomal complement. *Fertil. Steril.* 2007; **87**:534–541.

23. Murakoshi Y, Sueoka K, Takahashi K, et al. Embryo developmental capability and pregnancy outcome are related to the mitochondrial DNA copy number and ooplasmic volume. *J. Assist. Reprod. Genet.* 2013; **30**:1367–1375.

24. Braude P, Bolton V, Moore S. Human gene expression first occurs between the four- and eight-cell stages of preimplantation development. *Nature* 1988; **332**:459–461.

25. Gardner DK, Vella P, Lane M, et al. Culture and transfer of human blastocysts to increase implantation rate and eliminate high order multiple gestations: a prospective randomised trial. *Fertil. Steril.* 1998; **69**:84–88.

26. Dokras A, Sargent IL, Barlow DH. Human blastocyst grading: an indicator of developmental potential? *Hum. Reprod.* 1993; **8**:2119–2127.

27. Gardner DK, Lane M, Stevens J, Schlenker T, Schoolcraft WB. Blastocyst score affects implantation and pregnancy outcome: towards a single blastocyst transfer. *Fertil. Steril.* 2000; **73**:1155–1158.

28. Shapiro BS, Daneshmand ST, Desai J, et al. The risk of embryo-endometrium asynchrony increases with maternal age after ovarian stimulation and IVF. *RBM Online* 2016; **33**:50–55.

29. Cohen J, Malter H, Fehilly C, et al. Implantation of embryos after partial opening of oocyte zona pellucida to facilitate sperm penetration. *Lancet* 1988; **2**:162.

30. De Vos A, Van Steirteghem A. Zona hardening, zona drilling and assisted hatching: new achievements in assisted reproduction. *Cell Tissues Organs* 2000; **166**:220–227.

31. Kim HJ, Kim CH, Lee SM, et al. Outcomes of preimplantation genetic diagnosis using either zona drilling with acidified Tyrode's solution or partial zona dissection. *Clin. Exp. Reprod. Med.* 2012; **39**:118–124.

32. Obruca A, Strohmer H, Blaschitz A, et al. Ultrastructural observations in human oocytes and preimplantation embryos after zona opening using an erbium–yttrium–aluminium–garnet (Er: YAG) laser. *Hum Reprod.* 1997; **12**:2242–2245.

33. Mahadevan MM, Miller MM, Maris MO, Moutos D. Assisted hatching of embryos by micromanipulation for human in vitro fertilization, UAMS experience. *J. Ark. Med. Soc.* 1998; **94**:529–531.

34. Feng HL, Hershlag A, Scholl GM, Cohen MA. A retroprospective study comparing three different assisted hatching techniques. *Fertil. Steril.* 2009; **91**:1323–1325.

35. Grace J, Bolton V, Braude P, Khalaf Y. Assisted hatching is more effective when embryo quality was optimal in previous failed IVF/ICSI cycles. *J. Obstet. Gynaecol.* 2007; **27**:56–60.

36. Meldrum DR, Wisot A, Yee B, et al. Assisted hatching reduces the age-related decline in IVF outcome in women younger than age 43 without increasing miscarriage or monozygotic twinning. *J. Assist. Reprod. Genet.* 1998; **15**:418–421.

37. Cohen J, Alikani M, Trowbridge J, Rosenwaks Z. Implantation enhancement by selective assisted hatching using zona drilling of human embryos with poor prognosis. *Hum. Reprod.* 1992; **7**:685–691.

38. Lanzendorf SE, Nehchiri F, Mayer JF, Oehninger S, Muasher SJ. A prospective, randomized, double-blind study for the evaluation of assisted hatching in patients with advanced maternal age. *Hum. Reprod.* 1998; **13**:409–413.

39. Hellebaut S, De Sutter P, Dozortsev D, et al. Does assisted hatching improve implantation rates after in vitro fertilization or intracytoplasmic sperm injection in all patients? A prospective randomized study. *J. Assist. Reprod. Genet.* 1996; **13**:19–22.

40. Tucker MJ, Morton PC, Wright G, et al. Enhancement of outcome from intracytoplasmic sperm injection: does co-culture or assisted hatching improve implantation rates? *Hum. Reprod.* 1996; **11**:2434–2437.

41. Agarwal SK, Coe S, Buyalos RP. The influence of uterine position on pregnancy rates with in vitro fertilization-embryo transfer. *J. Assist. Reprod. Genet.* 1994; **11**:323–324.

42. Moini A, Kiani K, Bahmanabadi A, Akhoond M, Akhlaghi A. Improvement in pregnancy rate by removal of cervical discharge prior to embryo transfer in ICSI cycles: a randomised clinical trial. *Aust. N. Z. J. Obstet. Gynaecol.* 2011; **51**:315–320.

43. Lewin A, Schenker JG, Avrech O, et al. The role of uterine straightening by passive bladder distension

before embryo transfer in IVF cycles. *J. Assist. Reprod. Genet.* 1997; **14**:32–34.

44. Bodri D, Colodron M, Garcia D, et al. Transvaginal versus transabdominal ultrasound guidance for embryo transfer in donor oocyte recipients: a randomized clinical trial. *Fertil. Steril.* 2011; **95**:2263–2268.

45. Mansour R, Aboulghar M, Serour G. Dummy embryo transfer: a technique that minimizes the problems of embryo transfer and improves the pregnancy rate in human in vitro fertilization. *Fertil. Steril.* 1990; **54**:678–681.

46. Hearns-Stokes RM, Miller BT, Scott L, et al. Pregnancy rates after embryo transfer depend on the provider at embryo transfer. *Fertil. Steril.* 2000; **74**:80–86.

47. Angelini A, Brusco GF, Barnocchi N, et al. Impact of physician performing embryo transfer on pregnancy rates in an assisted reproductive program. *J. Assist. Reprod. Genet.* 2006; **23**:329–332.

48. Fanchin R, Harmas A, Benaoudia F, et al. Microbial flora of the cervix assessed at the time of embryo transfer adversely affects in vitro fertilization outcome. *Fertil. Steril.* 1998; **70**:866–870.

49. Egbase PE, Udo EE. Al Sharhan M, Grudzinskas JG. Prophylactic antibiotics and endocervical microbial inoculation of the endometrium at embryo transfer. *Lancet* 1999; **354**:651–652.

50. Buckett W. A review and meta-analysis of prospective trials comparing different catheters used for embryo transfer. *Fertil. Steril.* 2006; **85**:728–734.

51. Abou-Setta AM. Air fluid versus fluid-only models of embryo catheter loading: a systematic review and meta-analysis. *RBM Online* 2007; **14**:80–84.

52. Montag M, Kupka M, van der Ven K, van der Ven H. ET on day 3 using low versus high fluid volume. *Eur. J. Obstet. Gynecol. Reprod. Biol.* 2002; **102**:57–60.

53. Matorras R, Mendoza R, Exposito A, Rodriguez-Escudero FJ. Influence of the time interval between embryo catheter loading and discharging on the success of IVF. *Hum. Reprod.* 2004; **19**:2027–2030.

54. Lesny P, Killick SR, Tetlow RL, Robinson J, Maguiness SD. Uterine junctional zone contractions during assisted reproduction cycles. *Hum. Reprod. Update* 1998; **4**:440–445.

55. Waterstone J, Curson R, Parsons J. Embryo transfer to low uterine cavity. *Lancet* 1991; **337**:1413.

56. Fanchin R, Righini C, Olivennes F, et al. Uterine contractions at the time of embryo transfer alter pregnancy rates after in-vitro fertilization. *Hum. Reprod.* 1998; **13**:1968–1974.

57. Coroleu B, Barri PN, Carreras O, et al. The influence of the depth of embryo replacement into the uterine cavity on implantation rates after IVF: a controlled, ultrasound-guided study. *Hum. Reprod.* 2002; **17**:341–346.

58. Franco JG Jr, Martins AM, Baruffi RL, et al. Best site for embryo transfer: the upper or lower half of endometrial cavity? *Hum. Reprod.* 2004; **19**:1785–1790.

59. Kwon H, Choi DH, Kim EK. Absolute position versus relative position in embryo transfer: a randomized controlled trial. *Reprod. Biol. Endocrinol.* 2015; **13**:78.

60. Sallam HN, Sadek SS. Ultrasound-guided embryo transfer: a meta-analysis of randomized controlled trials. *Fertil. Steril.* 2003; **80**:1042–1046.

61. Wood EG, Batzer FR, Go KJ, Gutmann JN, Corson SL. Ultrasound-guided soft catheter embryo transfers will improve pregnancy rates in in-vitro fertilization. *Hum. Reprod.* 2000; **15**:107–112.

62. Porat N, Boehnlein LM, Schouweiler CM, Kang J, Lindheim SR. Interim analysis of a randomized clinical trial comparing abdominal versus transvaginal ultrasound-guided embryo transfer. *J. Obstet. Gynaecol. Res.* 2010; **36**:384–392.

63. Grygoruk C, Pietrewicz P, Modlinski JA, et al. Influence of embryo transfer on embryo preimplantation development. *Fertil. Steril.* 2012; **97**:1417–1421.

64. Groeneveld E, de Leeuw B, Vergouw CG, et al. Standardization of catheter load speed during embryo transfer: comparison of manual and pump-regulated embryo transfer. *RBM Online* 2012; **24**:163–169.

65. Safari S, Razi MH, Razi Y. Routine use of EmbryoGlue (®) as embryo transfer medium does not improve the ART outcomes. *Arch. Gynecol. Obstet.* 2015; **291**:433–437.

66. Singh N, Gupta M, Kriplani A, Vanamail P. Role of Embryo Glue as a transfer medium in the outcome of fresh non-donor *in-vitro* fertilization cycles. *J. Hum. Reprod. Sci.* 2015; **8**:214–217.

67. Friedler S, Schachter M, Strassburger D, et al. A randomized clinical trial comparing recombinant hyaluronan/recombinant albumin versus human tubal fluid for cleavage stage embryo transfer in patients with multiple IVF-embryo transfer failure. *Hum. Reprod.* 2007; **22**:2444–2448.

68. Bontekoe S, Heineman MJ, Johnson N, Blake D. Adherence compounds in embryo transfer media for assisted reproductive technologies. *Cochrane Database Syst. Rev.* 2014; **25**:CD007421.

69. Uchiyama T, Sakuta T, Kanayama T. Regulation of hyaluronan synthases in mouse uterine cervix. *Biochem. Biophys. Res. Commun.* 2005; **327**:927–932.

70. Furnus CC, Valcarcel A, Dulout FN, Errecalde AL. The hyaluronic acid receptor (CD44) is expressed in bovine

oocytes and early stage embryos. *Theriogenology* 2003; **60**:1633–1644.

71. Sroga JM, Montville CP, Aubuchon M, Williams DB, Thomas MA. Effect of delayed versus immediate embryo transfer catheter removal on pregnancy outcomes during fresh cycles. *Fertil. Steril.* 2010; **93**:2088–2090.

72. Tiras B, Korucuoglu U, Polat M, et al. Effect of blood and mucus on the success rates of embryo transfers. *Eur. J. Obstet. Gynecol. Reprod. Biol.* 2012; **165**:239–242.

73. Plowden TC, Hill MJ, Miles SM, et al. Does the presence of blood in the catheter or the degree of difficulty of embryo transfer affect live birth? *Reprod. Sci.* 2017; **24**:726–730.

74. Alvero R, Hearns-Stokes RM, Catherino WH, Leondires MP, Segars JH. The presence of blood in the transfer catheter negatively influences outcome at embryo transfer. *Hum. Reprod.* 2003; **18**:1848–1852.

75. Goudas VT, Hammitt DG, Damario MA, et al. Blood on the embryo transfer catheter is associated with decreased rates of embryo implantation and clinical pregnancy with the use of in vitro fertilization-embryo transfer. *Fertil. Steril.* 1998; **70**:878–882.

76. Sharif K, Afnan M, Lashen H, et al. Is bed rest following embryo transfer necessary? *Fertil. Steril.* 1998; **69**:478–481.

77. Bar-Hava I, Kerner R, Yoeli R, et al. Immediate ambulation after embryo transfer: a prospective study. *Fertil. Steril.* 2005; **83**:594–597.

78. Gaikwad S, Garrido N, Cobo A, Pellicer A, Remohi J. Bed rest after embryo transfer negatively affects in vitro fertilization: a randomized controlled clinical trial. *Fertil. Steril.* 2013; **100**:729–735.

79. Carrillo AJ, Lane B, Pridman DD, et al. Improved clinical outcomes for in vitro fertilization with delay of embryo transfer from 48 to 72 hours after oocyte retrieval: use of glucose- and phosphate-free media. *Fertil. Steril.* 1998; **69**:329–334.

80. Ertzeid G, Dale PO, Tanbo T, et al. Clinical outcome of day 2 versus day 3 embryo transfer using serum-free culture media: a prospective randomized study. *J. Assist. Reprod. Genet.* 1999; **16**:529–534.

81. Huisman GJ, Alberda AT, Leerentveld RA, Verhoeff A, Zeilmaker GH. A comparison of in vitro fertilization results after embryo transfer after 2, 3, and 4 days of embryo culture. *Fertil. Steril.* 1994; **61**:970–971.

82. Scholtes MC, Zeilmaker GH. A prospective, randomized study of embryo transfer results after 3 or 5 days of embryo culture in in vitro fertilization. *Fertil. Steril.* 1996; **65**:1245–1248.

83. Milki AA, Hinckley MD, Fisch JD, Dasig D, Behr B. Comparison of blastocyst transfer with day 3 embryo transfer in similar patient populations. *Fertil. Steril.* 2000; **73**:126–129.

84. Stillman RJ, Richter KS, Banks NK, Graham JR. Elective single embryo transfer: a 6-year progressive implementation of 784 single blastocyst transfers and the influence of payment method on patient choice. *Fertil. Steril.* 2009; **92**:1895–1906.

85. Shapiro BS, Daneshmand ST, Garner FC, et al. Evidence of impaired endometrial receptivity after ovarian stimulation for in vitro fertilization: a prospective randomized trial comparing fresh and frozen-thawed embryo transfer in normal responders. *Fertil. Steril.* 2011; **96**:344–348.

86. Roque M, Lattes K, Serra S, et al. Fresh embryo transfer versus frozen embryo transfer in in vitro fertilization cycles: a systematic review and meta-analysis. *Fertil. Steril.* 2013; **99**:156–162.

87. Evans J, Hannan NJ, Edgell TA, et al. Fresh versus frozen embryo transfer: backing clinical decisions with scientific and clinical evidence. *Hum. Reprod. Update* 2014; **20**:808–821.

88. Ishihara O, Araki R, Kuwahara A, et al. Impact of frozen-thawed single-blastocyst transfer on maternal and neonatal outcome: an analysis of 277,042 single-embryo transfer cycles from 2008 to 2010 in Japan. *Fertil. Steril.* 2014; **101**:128–133.

89. Maheshwari A, Raja EA, Bhattacharya S. Obstetric and perinatal outcomes after either fresh or thawed frozen embryo transfer: an analysis of 112,432 singleton pregnancies recorded in the Human Fertilisation and Embryology Authority anonymized dataset. *Fertil. Steril.* 2016; **106**:1703–1708.

90. Shih W, Rushford DD, Bourne H, et al. Factors affecting low birth weight after assisted reproduction technology: difference between transfer of fresh and cryopreserved embryos suggests an adverse effect of oocyte collection. *Hum. Reprod.* 2008; **23**:1644–1653.

91. Pinborg A, Henningsen AA, Loft A, et al. Large baby syndrome in singletons born after frozen embryo transfer (FET): is it due to maternal factors or the cryotechnique? *Hum. Reprod.* 2014; **29**:618–627.

92. Shapiro BS, Daneshmand ST, Bedient CE, Garner FC. Comparison of birth weights in patients randomly assigned to fresh or frozen-thawed embryo transfer. *Fertil. Steril.* 2016; **106**:317–321.

93. Roque M, Valle M, Kostolias A, Sampaio M, Geber S. Freeze-all cycle in reproductive medicine: current perspectives. *JBRA Assist. Reprod.* 2017; **21**:49–53.

94. Acharya KS, Acharya CR, Bishop K, et al. Freezing of all embryos in in vitro fertilization is beneficial in high responders, but not intermediate and low responders: an analysis of 82,935 cycles from the Society for

Assisted Reproductive Technology registry. *Fertil. Steril.* 2018; **110**:880–887.

95. Kogan MD, Alexander GR, Kotelchuck M, et al. Trends in twin birth outcomes and prenatal care utilization in the United States, 1981–1997. *JAMA* 2000; **284**:335–341.

96. Scher AI, Petterson B, Blair E, et al. The risk of mortality or cerebral palsy in twins: a collaborative population-based study. *Pediatr. Res.* 2002; **52**:671–681.

97. Guerif F, Lemseffer M, Bidault R, et al. Single day 2 embryo versus blastocyst-stage transfer: a prospective study integrating fresh and frozen embryo transfers. *Hum. Reprod.* 2009; **24**:1051–1058.

98. Yanaihara A, Yorimitsu T, Motoyama H, Watanabe H, Kawamura T. Monozygotic multiple gestation following *in vitro* fertilization: analysis of seven cases from Japan. *J. Exp. Clin. Assist. Reprod.* 2007; **4**:4.

99. Lee SF, Chapman M, Bowyer L. Monozygotic triplets after single blastocyst transfer: case report and literature review. *Aust. N. Z. J. Obstet. Gynaecol.* 2008; **48**:583–586.

100. Thurin A, Hausken J, Hillensjö T, et al. Elective single-embryo transfer versus double-embryo transfer in in-vitro fertilization. *N. Engl. J. Med.* 2004; **351**:2392–2402.

101. Kjellberg AT, Carlsson P, Bergh C. Randomized single versus double embryo transfer: obstetric and paediatric outcome and a cost-effectiveness analysis. *Hum. Reprod.* 2006; **21**:210–216.

102. Ikemoto Y, Kuroda K, Ochiai A, et al. Prevalence and risk factors of zygotic splitting after 937 848 single embryo transfer cycles. *Hum. Reprod.* 2018; **33**:1984–1991.

103. Tabibzadeh S. Molecular control of the implantation window. *Hum. Reprod. Update* 1998; **4**:465–471.

104. Brosens JJ, Salker MS, Teklenburg G, et al. Uterine selection of human embryos at implantation. *Sci. Rep.* 2014; **4**:3894.

105. Achache H, Revel A. Endometrial receptivity markers, the journey to successful embryo implantation. *Hum. Reprod. Update* 2006; **12**:731–746.

106. Karizbodagh MP, Rashidi B, Sahebkar A, Masoudifar A, Mirzaei H. Implantation window and angiogenesis. *J. Cell Biochem.* 2017; **118**:4141–4151.

107. Shufaro Y, Simon A, Laufer N, Fatum M. Thin unresponsive endometrium – a possible complication of surgical curettage compromising ART outcome. *J. Assist. Reprod. Genet.* 2008; **25**:421–425.

108. El-Toukhy T, Coomarasamy A, Khairy M, et al. The relationship between endometrial thickness and outcome of medicated frozen embryo replacement cycles. *Fertil. Steril.* 2008; **89**:832–839.

109. Gallos ID, Khairy M, Chu J, et al. Optimal endometrial thickness to maximize live births and minimize pregnancy losses: analysis of 25,767 fresh embryo transfers. *RBM Online* 2018; **37**:542–548.

110. Liu KE, Hartman M, Hartman A, Luo ZC, Mahutte N. The impact of a thin endometrial lining on fresh and frozen–thaw IVF outcomes: an analysis of over 40 000 embryo transfers. *Hum. Reprod.* 2018; **33**:1883–1888.

111. Moran NA, Sloan DB. The hologenome concept: helpful or hollow? *PLoS Biol.* 2015; **13**: e1002311.

112. Kroon B, Hart RJ, Wong BM, Ford E, Yazdani A. Antibiotics prior to embryo transfer in ART. *Cochrane Database Syst. Rev.* 2012; **3**:CD008995.

113. Moore DE, Soules MR, Klein NA, Fujimoto VY, Agnew KJ, Eschenbach DA. Bacteria in the transfer catheter tip influence the live-birth rate after in vitro fertilization. *Fertil. Steril.* 2000; **74**:1118–1124.

114. Garsia-Velasco JA, Menabrito M, Catalan IB. What fertility specialists should know about the vaginal microbiome: a review. *RBM Online* 2017; **35**:103–112.

115. Fox CA, Wolff HS, Baker JA. Measurement of intra-vaginal and intra-uterine pressures during human coitus by radio-telemetry. *J. Reprod. Fertil.* 1970; **22**:243–251.

116. Franchin R, Righini C, Olivennes F, et al. Uterine contractions at the time of embryo transfer alter pregnancy rates after in-vitro fertilization. *Hum. Reprod.* 1998; **13**:1968–1974.

117. Tremellen KP, Valbuena D, Landeras J, et al. The effect of intercourse on pregnancy rates during assisted human reproduction. *Hum. Reprod.* 2000; **15**:2653–2658.

118. Salamonsen LA. Tissue injury and repair in the female human reproductive tract. *Reproduction* 2003; **125**:301–311.

119. Gnainsky Y, Aldo PB, Barash A, et al. Local injury of the endometrium induces an inflammatory response that promotes successful implantation. *Fertil. Steril.* 2010; **94**:2030–2036.

120. Granot I, Gnainsky Y, Dekel N. Endometrial inflammation and effect on implantation improvement and pregnancy outcome. *Reproduction* 2012; **144**:661–668.

121. Dunn CL, Kelly RW, Critchley HO. Decidualization of the human endometrial

stromal cell: an enigmatic transformation. *RBM Online* 2003; **7**:151–161.

122. Paria BC, Reese J, Das SK, Dey SK. Deciphering the cross-talk of implantation: advances and challenges. *Science* 2002; **296**:2185–2188.

123. Siristatidis C, Kreatsa M, Koutlaki N, et al. Endometrial injury for RIF patients undergoing IVF/ICSI: a prospective nonrandomized

controlled trial. *Gynecol. Endocrinol.* 2017; **33**:297–300.

124. Gui J, Xu W, Yang J, Feng L, Jia J. Impact of local endometrial injury on in vitro fertilization/ intracytoplasmic sperm injection outcomes: a systematic review and meta-analysis. *J. Obstet. Gynaecol. Res.* 2018; **45**:57–68. doi:10.1111/ jog.13854.

Chapter 12

Cryopreservation

Cryopreservation involves the cooling of cells and tissues to subzero temperatures to stop all biological activity and preserve them for future use. Initial cryopreservation methods were ineffective as simple cooling techniques led to cellular damage due to the altered concentration of solutes within the cells, ice formation, and excessive dehydration.

Cryopreservation is an adjacent and useful procedure of assisted reproductive technology (ART). In 1948, Dr. Chris Polge serendipitously discovered that glycerol, in a mislabeled bottle of sugar solutions, is an effective cryoprotective agent for sperm. The first human delivery from frozen sperm was reported in 1953. In the 1970s, additional cryoprotectants such as propanediol (propylene glycerol [PrOH]), dimethyl sulfoxide (DMSO) and ethylene glycol (EG) were identified and established to minimize cellular damage (Figure 12.1). Since the 1970s, oocytes and embryos of more than 30 mammalian species have been successfully cryopreserved, bringing about the birth of millions of normal offspring. The first human birth from a cryopreserved embryo was in 1984 [1]. Oocytes and embryos have been cryopreserved by slow freezing or vitrification methods. The slow-freezing method uses relatively low concentrations of 10% cryoprotective additives (CPAs), cooling rates higher than 1°C/min, and warming rates higher than 250°C/min. In contrast, vitrification, or the reversible transition of a liquid into an amorphous noncrystalline glass [2], uses high CPA concentrations (30–40%), saccharides as supplements, cooling rates much higher than 2000°C/min, and very speedy warming rates. Often, extremely high cooling rates more than 10 000°C/min are used.

Mechanism of Cryopreservation

One of the major causes of cell destruction during freezing and thawing is the formation of intracellular ice crystals. Treatment of the cells with cryoprotectants forces osmotic water movement and leads to dehydration of the cell. While shifting water out of a cell may help reduce the amount of intracellular ice crystal formation, it may result in osmotic shock and a detrimental change in volume. The basic concepts of slow cryopreservation are to protect the cells from the effect of intracellular ice crystal formation, drastic changes in solute concentrations, and cellular dehydration at both high and low temperatures. Cryoprotectant is thought to protect cells by reducing or eliminating lethal intracellular ice formation, by stabilizing intracellular proteins, and by moderating the impact of concentrated intracellular and extracellular electrolytes [3]. One major factor affecting the response of a cell to freezing is the ratio of its surface area to volume. In general, the larger the cell, the slower the cooling process must be to ensure survival. Additionally, at temperature around 0°C, special care must be taken to avoid extreme fluctuations in cell volume during CPA equilibration, as rapid volume change can immediately damage cells and make them more sensitive to stress during subsequent cooling or thawing procedures [4]. At the same time, exposure to CPAs should be minimized due

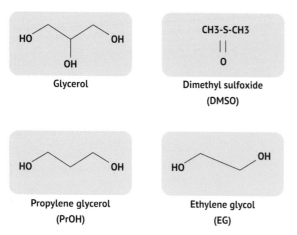

Figure 12.1 Types of regular cryoprotective additives.

to their potentially toxic effect. For example, DMSO induces plasma membrane pore formation and initiates caspase-3-independent apoptotic processes upon translocation of apoptosis-inducing factor from the mitochondria to the nucleus [5]. Cryoprotectant toxicity can be lowered by reducing the temperature of exposure, but this may require a longer exposure time. Although many investigators attribute cellular damage during freezing solely to the toxicity of the CPAs, others argue that cellular damage is due entirely to osmotic shock.

When aqueous solutions are frozen, water is removed, causing the components within the cell to become increasingly concentrated as the temperature falls; the reverse occurs during thawing. As the cells are frozen, they respond osmotically to massive changes in extracellular fluid concentrations. It has also been claimed that cells can be damaged upon extended exposure to high electrolyte concentrations, excessive cell dehydration, and the mechanical effects of external ice.

Vitrification is a cryopreservation method in which the biological material and the surrounding liquid solution become an amorphous glass-like solid, free of all crystalline structures when plunged in liquid nitrogen (LN_2) [2]. Vitrification requires much higher concentrations of cryoprotectants, which may elicit toxic and osmotic effects. Since the development of the first vitrification solution in the 1970s, which contained DMSO, PrOH and acetamide [2], various CPAs have been found to be effective. The most extensively used CPAs are composed of permeable agents that penetrate the cell (such as EG, DMSO, PrOH or glycerol) as well as non-permeable, low-molecular-weight, non-penetrating CPAs (such as raffinose, sucrose, trehalose, egg yolk citrate, albumin). Also, CPA solutions contain high-molecular-weight polymers such as Ficoll (PM 70 or 400).

Many "open" and "closed" carrier devices are currently utilized to load the biological material before storage in LN_2, and their design can indirectly impact outcomes by causing alterations in the cooling and warming rates. However, the variety of vitrification methods, carrier devices, and hypertonic CPAs may introduce complexities when oocytes or embryos at different stages of development are transferred to other in vitro fertilization (IVF) centers that routinely use different techniques to perform vitrification.

The success of a vitrification protocol is based on effective dehydration upon cell exposure to hypertonic conditions, as well as on the penetration rate of a CPA, which should be sufficient to generate an intracellular environment that will vitrify and remain vitrified for a defined cooling–warming rate. Also, CPA removal causes successive phases of shrinkage and re-expansion, due to movement of water and CPA across the cell membranes.

In the vitrification process, oocytes or embryos are exposed to a non-vitrifying CPA solution, containing only permeable CPAs, and then to a vitrifying CPA solution, containing both permeable and non-permeable CPAs. The CPA concentration and composition vary between commercial kits. During exposure to the non-vitrifying CPAs, the cell immediately adjusts its osmolarity by losing water and shrinking. The CPAs then enter the cell slowly due to their low membrane permeability [6]. The duration of exposure to the non-vitrifying solutions at a defined temperature is of critical importance, as it determines the intracellular CPA concentration. Depending on the CPA used and the type and developmental stage of the biological material, exposure time may range between 3 and 15 minutes. The biological material is then exposed to vitrifying CPAs for 30–90 seconds. This solution causes further cellular dehydration, which concentrates the intracellular CPA. The overall goal of this procedure is to create an intracellular environment that will remain vitrified for a defined cooling–warming rate.

The transition of water and CPAs across cell membranes is crucial for cell survival during cryopreservation, and the degree of membrane permeability depends upon the stage of embryo development (Figure 12.2). While it is possible visually to detect the shrinkage and swelling of cells under a stereomicroscope, it is not possible to estimate the proportion of CPA that enters the cells. Only full expansion of oocytes or embryos, representing full equilibration with CPA, may be assessed. Water and CPAs can move across the plasma membrane of oocytes and embryos by simple, slow diffusion through the lipid bilayer membrane, in which case, permeability is low and temperature-dependent energy activation is high. In parallel, aquaporins, a variety of water channels expressed by mammalian oocytes and embryos, play a role in CPA transport [7]. Permeability via the channels is high and temperature-dependent energy activation is low [8]. The movement of water across each unit of the cell surface as a function of time is a function of the cell volume.

Oocytes and zygotes have the lowest surface/volume ratio compared with an embryo, so they are less effective than cleavage-stage embryos at losing water and taking up CPAs, and thus are more susceptible to intracellular ice formation if the exposure time to CPAs is not well adapted [9]. The ideal duration of exposure to CPA solutions may differ between stages of development. For example, in ultra-rapid vitrification, an average time of 5–15 minutes is necessary to protect oocytes from cryoinjury, while a maximum 5-minute exposure is required for collapsed blastocysts. Also, each CPA has its own cell penetration characteristics. During slow freezing, each CPA is intended to be adapted to different stages of embryonic development: PrOH for zygote and cleavage-stage embryos, DMSO for cleavage-stage embryos, and glycerol for day 5 embryos. Similarly, during vitrification, mixtures of DMSO/EG or PrOH/EG are used for oocytes as well as for the early stages of cleavage embryo development and blastocysts. In morulae and blastocysts, glycerol, EG, and DMSO move rapidly through the cell membrane by facilitated diffusion through channels, whereas PrOH enters only slowly by simple diffusion [8].

The transformation of a solution into a glassy state occures when the temperature is very rapidly lowered to below the glass transition temperature. To reach ultra-rapid cooling rates of more than 20 000°C/min, open embryo carriers (e.g., Cryoloop, Cryoleaf, Cryotop, Cryolock) were designed to allow direct contact of the biological material with LN_2 (Figure 12.3). The advantage of ultra-rapid cooling is that although the cells are exposed to increasing CPA concentrations for a short time, enabling the extraction of the intracellular water, only a limited amount of CPA permeates the cells. Another alternative is hermetically closed carrier devices, allowing full isolation and protection of the sample from direct contact with LN_2 during the cooling procedure and subsequent long-term storage. In a closed system, the specimen is not allowed to come in contact with the LN_2. Therefore, a carrier is obligatory to deliver the maximum heat transfer rate to the contained specimen.

Cryopreservation of Embryos (Zygote/Cleavage-Stage/Blastocyst)

Since the first birth from a cryopreserved embryo, cryopreservation has been considered a routine and important component of IVF treatment.

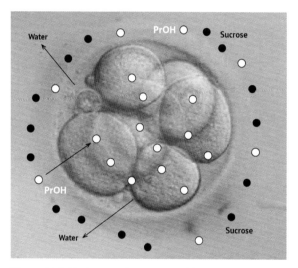

Figure 12.2 Mechanism of preparation (dehydration) of embryo for cryopreservation.

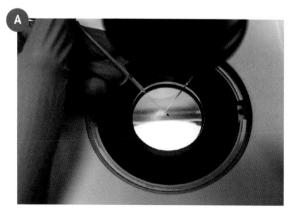

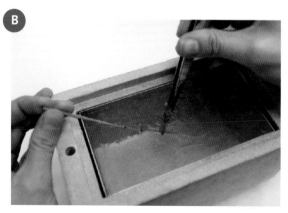

Figure 12.3 Process of vitrification (A) Transfer of embryo on the tip of carrier device. (B) Plunging of carrier device into LN2 followed by closing with device cover.

Zygote cryopreservation. It has been suggested that freezing at the zygote stage provides for improved results compared with freezing at the cleavage stage [10]. This is probably due to the reason that a zygote is a single cell, like the oocyte, but without the complexities arising from the sensitive meiotic spindle. Zygote vitrification is a routine method in ART [11], with survival rates at least as high as with slow freezing. However, vitrification and warming can have a significant impact on zygote morphology; about 15% of zygotes do not show pronuclear appearance after warming, which has been associated with poorer outcomes [12]. This type of morphological change is uncommon after a slow freezing.

Cleavage embryo cryopreservation. Cryopreservation of embryos optimizes the IVF cycle by enabling the storage of all excess embryos, and reducing the risk of multiple pregnancies. Frozen embryos also allow the patient to achieve pregnancies without requiring subsequent stimulation of a new IVF cycle. In cycles with hyperstimulated ovaries, cryopreservation can reduce the risk of ovarian hyperstimulation syndrome [13]. Cryopreservation of the embryo has been successfully achieved at the cleavage (day 2 or day 3) and blastocyst (day 5) stages. Embryos are initially maintained in an equilibration solution comprising Ham's F-10 medium, supplemented with 7.5% EG, 7.5% DMSO, and 20% patient serum, for 5–15 minutes, at room temperature (~20–25°C) [14]. After the initial shrinkage and recovery, the embryos are aspirated and placed in the vitrification solution (15% EG, 15% DMSO, and 0.5 M sucrose) at room temperature (~20–25°C), for at least 50 seconds but no longer than 60 seconds. After visually confirming that cellular shrinkage has occurred, the embryos are aspirated and placed on the tip of the loading device (carrier) and directly in contact with the LN_2.

Embryo survival rates are the primary parameter used to assess the efficiency of a freezing program. The survival rate is accepted as a function of the number of vital embryos thawed, as assessed by morphological evaluation immediately after thawing. The final selection of thawed embryo for transfer can be based on a range of factors, including the number of intact blastomeres and resumption of mitosis. Pregnancies from damaged embryos have been achieved and required a threshold of 50% blastomere survival [15]. Later reports demonstrated the importance of obtaining fully intact embryos, which were associated with significantly higher implantation rates than embryos with cell loss [16].

Blastocyst cryopreservation. Blastocyst vitrification is conventionally performed on collapsed or non-collapsed blastocysts. Applying assisted hatching before blastocyst vitrification allows better permeation of the cryoprotectants and better blastocoele dehydration [17]. No statistical differences in survival, implantation, or clinical pregnancy rates were noted between blastocysts that had undergone laser pulse opening or micro-needle puncture [18]. Collapsed blastocysts have to be exposed to equilibration solution, which generally contains 7.5% DMSO/EG, for 2–5 minutes, while non-collapsed blastocysts require a ~10-minute incubation in DMSO-free glycerol solution. After that, samples are incubated in vitrification solution (15% DMSO/EG and 0.5 M sucrose) for 1 minute. At the time of vitrification, the blastocyst is placed in a loading device surrounded by vitrification media. The device is then plunged into and stored in LN_2. Embryos frozen at the expanded blastocyst stage exhibited equal viability, implantation potential, and pregnancy outcome [19].

During the thaw, the embryo is subjected to a three-step warming procedure. First, it is immediately immersed in 1 M sucrose for 1–1.5 minutes, then transferred to 0.5 M sucrose two times for 2 minutes each, and then washed three times in buffer MOPS or HTF (human tubal fluid) for 3 minutes each and then cultured in medium.

Frozen–thawed blastocysts undergo multiple morphological changes that include the collapse of the blastocoele cavity along with cellular lysis and degeneration. Morphological assessments of thawed blastocysts are necessary to estimate the survival of individual cells and the whole embryo. By visual examination of the extent and locale of cellular degeneration, a skilled embryologist can estimate the proportion of viable cells. Blastocysts that develop to at least grade 2 in expansion, with at least grade B inner cell mass (ICM) and TE, and with no signs of degeneration, according to Gardner's grading system [20], are vitrified on day 5. All remaining embryos are assessed on day 6 and vitrified if they reach at least grade 4 in expansion, at least grade B ICM and TE both, and show no signs of degeneration. These assessment criteria are associated with successful cryopreservation of at least one blastocyst in 36% of cycles. The pregnancy and implantation rates using vitrified blastocysts are comparable to those associated with the use of fresh blastocysts [21]. Biopsied embryos cryopreserved at the blastocyst stage have demonstrated better survival following vitrification than following slow freezing.

The vitrification outcome (embryo survival) is highly operator dependent and requires entirely different skills than those needed for slow freezing. For example, the embryologist must rapidly handle the embryos in micro-volumes of extremely viscous media. Also, because there are a variety of loading devices available, specific training on the use and storage of each device and standardization of quality control procedures is mandatory.

Singletons born after cryopreservation of embryos (cleavage-stage or blastocyst) had a significantly higher birth weight than both those conceived by fresh embryo transfer and naturally conceived singletons [22]. The reason for this occurrence could be explained by the epigenetic effect of increased methylation at the imprinting control region of the *H19* gene in embryos during cryopreservation.

Cryopreservation of Oocytes

Oocyte cryostorage is indicated in various situations, for both subfertile and fertile patients. For example, it is recommended for women at risk of losing their reproductive function due to oncological treatment or premature ovarian failure. Women, who wish to delay motherhood for "social reasons," including career, absence of a partner, or adverse social and economic conditions, could also benefit from oocyte vitrification. Christopher Chen reported the first successful attempt at freezing and thawing a human oocyte in 1983, and the first human birth from standard inseminated frozen oocyte was reported in 1986 [23].

Oocytes are extremely sensitive to cryoinjury, and the meiotic spindle, cytoskeleton, cortical granules, and zona pellucida (ZP) are at particular risk. The initial success of oocyte cryopreservation was limited by the fragility of the metaphase II (MII) oocyte, rooted in its size, water content, and chromosomal arrangement. Oocyte cryopreservation requires that cells tolerate three nonphysiological conditions: exposure to molar concentrations of CPAs, cooling to subzero temperature, and removal of almost all liquid cell water or its conversion to a solid state. Vitrification of human oocytes has proven effective, and usually superior compared with standard slow freezing, with functional survival of cryopreserved oocytes, i.e., the ability to go through fertilization and embryo development,

approaching 100%. The ability of the extracellular solution to form glass when cooled at high rates is considered essential to successful oocyte cryopreservation. The key to survival is the vitrification capacity of the oocyte contents.

The first step is to equilibrate the cells with a CPA. One of the keys to the success of oocyte cryopreservation appears to be reaching adequate permeation of CPAs across the oocyte membrane. Because EG readily permeates oocytes, its use lessens the likelihood of osmotic shock when oocytes are diluted out of even very concentrated solutions.

High-quality MII oocytes suitable for cryopreservation are colorless and of regular shape, with regular ZP and a small perivitelline space without debris, homogeneous cytoplasm, and no vacuoles or granulations [24–25]. Also, the presence of an intact, round or ovoid polar body (PB) with a smooth surface should be considered a selection criterion [26]. Furthermore, an excessive extension of the culture period before freezing could affect oocyte competence after cryopreservation, since oolema permeability changes over time [27]; therefore, oocyte cryopreservation should be carried out as soon as possible after retrieval (~3–4 hours). Current best practice denudes oocytes immediately before cryopreservation. For slow freezing, this should be completed within 38 hours after human chorionic gonadotropin (hCG), with intracytoplasmic sperm injection (ICSI) performed 2–3 hours post-thaw to allow the spindle reorganization. For vitrification, oocytes should be vitrified 38–40 hours post-hCG, with ICSI performed at the equivalent of 40–41 hours post-hCG (i.e., between 1 and 3 hours post-warming).

MII oocytes are sensitive to cryoinjury because the meiotic spindle is acutely temperature sensitive. Transient cooling of oocytes to 20°C can irreversibly disrupt the spindle apparatus, whereas rapid depolarization occurs when the temperature is lowered to 0°C [28–29]. The appropriate organization of spindle microtubules is crucial for the correct alignment and segregation of chromosomes. Oocyte freezing can, therefore, increase the rate of aneuploidy during extrusion of the second PB, through nondisjunction of sister chromatids. In addition to the cytogenetic effect of cryopreservation, there is an increased risk of parthenogenetic activation of the oocytes after thermal shock and exposure to CPAs.

There are some oocyte behaviors during vitrification that may predict the outcome of a later warming procedure [14]. For example, during exposure to the equilibration solution, the oocytes should be completely shrunken within 3–6 minutes, depending on the dilution of the equilibration solution. From this time, oocyte shape starts to recover, with full recovery expected within 9–15 minutes. For human oocytes, full-size recovery seems to be highly important for the success of the warming procedure: if they are still smaller than before the process, an additional equilibration time is strongly recommended. During exposure to the vitrification solution, the oocytes initially shrink very quickly and float on the surface. They then partially recover but are not able to completely reshape before being loaded onto the carrier and vitrified.

Cryopreserved specimens should be transported between clinics/laboratories at a temperature below -132°C (ideally below -150°C), which should be verified by a temperature logging device.

Social oocyte preservation. Delayed marriage and late childbearing have led to a dramatic decline in birth rate and population. Nothing has changed in women's physiology that can support the deliberate delay of childbearing. Pregnancies and deliveries should ideally be completed before a woman reaches the age of 35, at which point, fertility tends to drop at a faster rate. Women who freeze their eggs before the age of 35 preserve the fertility at the age of freezing. Social oocyte freezing is a procedure lacking indication. The target population is all single women of almost all age groups. The intense debate about the role of "social" egg freezing repeats many of the assertions made initially about IVF itself. Women who wish to freeze their eggs for their future use face many hurdles. Vitrification of oocytes and the accumulated experience with frozen donor egg banks have shown that "young" frozen eggs thawed, fertilized, and transferred as blastocysts have the same reproductive potential as "fresh" eggs [30]. The recommended number of eggs to be frozen to give a fair chance of success differs with age. Statistics show that, in general, only 1 out of 20–25 eggs collected (4–5%) will result in the delivery of a baby [31]. The regular number of eggs collected in a single cycle is 8–12, requiring two to four cycles at the cost of 6–15 000 US$ per cycle, plus variable annual storage cost, to freeze 20–25 mature eggs [32]. To suggest that women who freeze their eggs are likely to be too "choosy" when seeking a suitable partner is demeaning of women who decide to avail themselves of this technology. Those who do choose to freeze at an ideal time, i.e., under the age of 35 (or even earlier), may be faced with the intolerable dilemma of allowing their eggs to stay frozen or creating embryos with donor sperm, which may then be stored for additional years.

Thawing Oocytes/Zygotes/Embryos

Warming is a "reversal" of the cooling process and aims to rehydrate the cell and to remove the cryoprotectant that has permeated the cell. In order to avoid osmotic shock, gradual, stepwise removal of cryoprotectant is essential [33]. When frozen cells are warmed rapidly, melting of the cell suspension is equivalent to a rapid dilution of the CPA that turns out to be concentrated during the freezing process. The rapid influx of water into cells as the extracellular milieu begins to melt can cause an osmotic shock at subzero temperature. Sensitivity to osmotic shock is, therefore, a function of the cell's permeability to water and solutes. This shock can be decreased by the use of a nontoxic, impermeable substance as an osmotic buffer, such as sucrose [34]. Warming is usually initiated by the immediate transfer of the device with a sample to a prewarmed environment.

The first warming step for oocytes is generally performed at 37°C, in a 1 M sucrose solution for 1 minute (Figure 12.4); as soon as the oocytes are released from the carrier, they tend to float and appear "vitreous." In the next warming solution, generally 0.5 M sucrose for 2 minutes, the oocytes shrink and look as if clear and very bright. During the following warming steps, 0.25 M sucrose and/or subsequent three sets of washing for 3 minutes each, the oocytes slowly recover their original shape. If the oocytes appear dark or flat or quickly recover their shape at the first stages of warming, they are possibly damaged and will degenerate.

When thawing cleavage-stage embryos, some remain intact, while others are fully degenerated or partially survive, with a mix of necrotic and normal blastomeres within the same embryo. The embryo transfer of partially damaged cleaving embryos is associated with decreased implantation rates as well as lowered pregnancy rates when compared with the transfer of fully intact embryos [35]. Integration of assisted hatching with lysed cell removal has been proposed to improve the implantation potential of such embryos [36]. If fragments can be reabsorbed by embryonic cells of fresh embryos, the same thing or

149

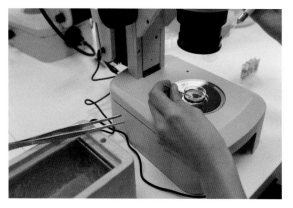
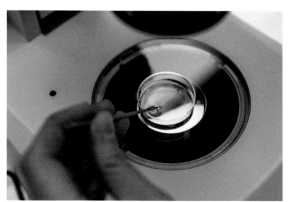

Figure 12.4 Process of thawing after cryopreservation.

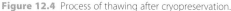

the same mechanism can be observed in thawed intact embryos [37]. In contrast, degenerated cells in frozen–thawed embryos will not or cannot be reabsorbed by the remaining living cells of the embryo; therefore, the removal of necrotic cells could be recommended [38]. Poor-quality thawed embryos (<50% intact blastomeres after thawing) resulted in a zero implantation rate [39].

Survival of human oocytes/zygotes/embryos after cryopreservation can be affected by their stage of development, their quality, or biophysical factors resulting from the cryopreservation procedure used. The combined elements of freezing and thawing represent a dynamic process during which many physical and chemical factors, such as osmotic and hydrostatic pressure, intracellular ionic content, pH, and temperature, fluctuate over a wide nonphysiological range and may impact genomic integrity.

After warming, viable blastocysts re-expand and are usually incubated for 4–6 hours to regain their vitality before being transferred. Re-expansion is the sign of viability. The timing of blastocyst re-expansion is an important predictor of vitrified–warmed blastocyst transfer outcomes; the earlier the blastocyst expands, the better it is expected to perform transfer [40].

Cryopreservation of Ovarian Tissue

In prepubertal girls, adolescents, and women who cannot delay the start of chemotherapy or radiotherapy, cryopreservation of ovarian tissue is the only available fertility preservation option. The ovarian tissue is obtained before the onset of the gonadotoxic anticancer therapy and can be autotransplanted to the patient after she has been cured of her disease. This technology may also be used to preserve fertility in girls with mosaic Turner syndrome, who experience premature menopause, and subsequently lose their ability to conceive during the regular fertile years [41]. This procedure could be useful for female-to-male transgender [42].

Different types of cells exhibit different optimum warming rates. This phenomenon is especially relevant to the cryopreservation of ovarian cortex, a tissue composed of diverse types of cells, each with its characteristic shape, size, and permeability properties. Therefore, cooling and warming conditions that are optimum for one cell type within the ovarian cortex may be harmful to others. More importantly, the survival of frozen tissues is dependent on the rate and method by which CPAs are removed from cryopreserved tissues. The recently reported successful cryopreservation of whole human ovaries represents a new method in considering whole ovary autotransplantation for the clinical way of cryopreservation [43].

Ovarian tissue can be picked up at any time during the menstrual cycle. Cryopreservation of ovarian tissue means cryopreservation of ovarian cortex due to the follicle localization in the cortex of the ovary. The primordial and primary follicles are located at a mean depth of 271 μm in infants and 460–500 μm in women. The majority of secondary follicles are located less than 1000 μm from the ovarian surface (mean depth: 639 μm). In women with premature ovarian insufficiency (POI), the mean depth of primordial and primary follicles is 566 μm, whereas 70% of secondary follicles are located at depths of more than 1000 μm [44]. These measures suggest that an optimum ovarian tissue thickness of less than 1 mm should be chosen

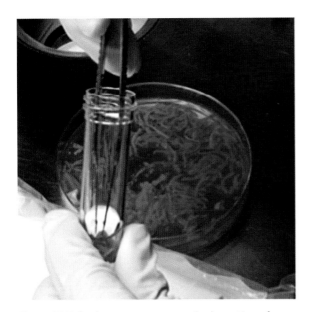

Figure 12.5 Ovarian cortex cryopreservation by portions of fragments.

for cryopreservation in regular patients and thicker ovarian cortices, which include secondary follicles, should be subjected for cryopreservation in POI patients (Figure 12.5). Primordial follicles, which comprise about 90% of the follicular population of each ovary, are less cryosensitive than maturing follicles, mature oocytes, and embryos, primarily due to their structureless cytoplasm and cryosensitive cytoplasmic components, lack of ZP, fewer granulosa cells, as well as the low metabolic rate associated with their dormancy. Primordial oocytes appear to be less sensitive to cryoinjury than mature oocytes as they are smaller, lack a ZP and cortical granules, and are relatively metabolically quiescent and undifferentiated.

Various protocols are used worldwide for the cryopreservation of ovarian tissue for fertility preservation purposes. The efficiency and efficacy of the majority of these protocols have not been extensively evaluated. A practical method for the preservation of the human ovarian cortex is based on Gosden's slow-freezing protocol and involves equilibration of thin slices (~1.5 mm thick) for 1 hour at 4°C, in a freezing solution containing cryoprotectant plus sucrose [45]. This protocol ensures a maximal surface area for rapid CPA (EG or DMSO) penetration. Ovarian specimens are cooled at 0.5°C/min to approximately -55°C and then at 2°C/min to approximately -140°C, and plunged into LN_2. Then, ovarian tissue is stored in LN_2 at -196°C.

Vitrification of ovarian tissue fragments can be completed using a two-step vitrification procedure, with equilibration first in 7.5% DMSO, 7.5% EG, and 20% synthetic serum substitute (SSS), followed by incubation in a final vitrification medium containing 15% DMSO, 15% EG, and 20% SSS [46]. Another successful vitrification protocol involves equilibration of slices in a solution of 7.5% DMSO and 20% SSS followed by a vitrification solution containing 15% DMSO, 15% EG, 20% SSS, and 0.5 M sucrose [47].

Ovarian cortex specimens are thawed rapidly by being swirled in a water bath at ~25–37°C, and the CPA is diluted out of the tissue by repeated rinses with fresh medium, under continuous agitation. DMSO is a known epimutagen and EG has been reported to be toxic at high concentrations, therefore, it has to be removed in a short time. DMSO requires a more prolonged and more elaborate thawing procedure than EG, as well as continuous dilution. CPA traces can remain in the warmed/thawed ovarian tissue before transplantation [48] and their impact on the mother and the baby must be considered.

After cryopreservation/thawing, the majority of ovarian follicles are in the primordial or primary stages [49]. Most of the follicles (more than 90%) in the antral stage show some signs of degeneration after freezing and thawing [49]. Stromal cells, which are essential for the neovascularization of an ovarian graft after autotransplantation [50], are more vulnerable to the damaging effects of the freeze–thaw procedure than follicles.

A comparison of slow-freezing and vitrification of ovarian tissue showed that the number of secondary follicles was lower in the vitrified group. At the same time, *AXIN1* (a gene encoding a cytoplasmic protein which contains a regulation of G protein signaling domain and an axin domain) expression was significantly lower in slow-frozen samples compared with vitrified samples [51]. The expression of apoptotic genes, excluding *CASP3*, was significantly reduced in slow-frozen samples. Conversely, *BAX/BCL2* expression was significantly higher in vitrification versus slow freezing. Follicles in slow-frozen samples displayed nuclear and cytoplasmic β-catenin staining, while control and vitrification groups only showed β-catenin protein in the cytoplasm. Slow freezing results in superior preservation, regardless of the type of follicle. Although slow freezing of ovarian cortical fragments is currently used in clinical settings, vitrification offers a more cost-effective and

151

ice-free alternative for preserving ovarian tissue. Improvements in the outcome of transplantation of ovarian tissue are further anticipated, particularly concerning revascularization.

Transplantation of ovarian tissue restores both fertility and endocrine function. Transplantation of ovarian tissue resulted in a remarkably consistent return of menstrual cycling and normal follicle-stimulating hormone (FSH) levels within 4–5 months [52]. The finding that as FSH decreased, ovulation resumed, with anti-Müllerian hormone (AMH) initially rising to high levels followed by a return to very low levels, indicated that a massive over-recruitment of primordial follicles led to subsequent depletion in the ovarian reserve [52]. Despite low AMH levels, the grafts sustained ovarian function for long periods of time. Transplanted slices of ovarian cortex continued to function normally for several years, likely due to the smaller ovarian reserve and the decreased rate of primordial follicle recruitment. However, cryopreserved stock of ovarian cortex slices may play an important role as a reservoir for fertility preservation for a long time. The first human live birth from orthotopic transplantation of frozen ovarian tissue was reported in 2004, with another successful live birth achieved in 2005 [52–53].

The disadvantage of the ovarian cryopreservation method includes the risk of malignant cell contamination. The solid fibrous tissue of the ovarian cortex controls follicle development and represents a relatively inhospitable location for cancer cells. Storage of ovarian tissue for cancer patients has a risk of reintroducing malignant cells in the tissue graft [54]. Most cancer diseases do not display specific cancer markers. Therefore, in most cases, it is not possible to test for potential malignant cell contamination in the ovarian tissue. Furthermore, even if markers were available, testing of one or two ovarian pieces for cell contamination does not necessarily represent the real status of cancer cells in the remaining ovarian pieces due to be transplanted.

Cryopreservation of Sperm

Sperm cryopreservation is the most operative way to preserve male fertility and has become one of the essential elements of ART. Sometimes, the male partner of a couple undergoing IVF is unable to collect semen for oocyte fertilization on the day of the oocyte retrieval. Backup of his frozen sperm resolves this problem. Cryopreservation is also widely used to

preserve spermatozoa obtained from azoospermic patients who have undergone testicular sperm extraction. Cytotoxic treatments, such as radiotherapy and chemotherapy, as well as surgical treatments may lead to testicular failure or ejaculatory dysfunction. In such situations, freezing of spermatozoa can be a suitable solution to preserve fertility. Banking of frozen donor sperm provides solutions for men with nonobstructive azoospermia and women with no partner.

The pioneer in cryopreservation of sperm was the Italian priest and scientist Lazzaro Spallanzani (1776), who attempted to preserve spermatozoa by chilling them in snow, followed by their successful rewarming. Survival of human spermatozoa was already observed in 1866 by Italian physician Paolo Mantegazza, who cooled them to -15°C and proposed the concept of a human sperm bank to store semen specimens. Further scientific progress led to the discovery of glycerol's cryoprotectant properties [55]. The first human pregnancies and births resulting from artificial insemination with semen samples that had been frozen and stored in dry ice, at -70°C, for up to 6 weeks, were reported in 1953. Several years later, births resulting from artificial insemination with human spermatozoa, frozen and stored for 5 months in nitrogen vapor, were reported [56].

The lipid configuration of the sperm plasma membrane is a significant factor influencing the cryotolerance and cold sensitivity of spermatozoa. CPAs for sperm cryopreservation include glycerol, DMSO, EG, in some cases supplemented with sucrose, raffinose, and glycine. Glycerol is preferred over DMSO, as it protects sperm structures [57]. Extenders contain glycerol and egg yolk, and protect the apical segment of the acrosome and circular mitochondria as could be found after thawing [58]. Glycerol supplemented with citrate or egg yolk acts as a cryobuffer because this composition contains macromolecules that do not infiltrate the cell membranes of the sperm. Glycerol serves as an energy source for the sperm cell and also maintains osmotic pressure by forming hydrogen bonds with membrane phospholipids and sugars. This action increases membrane stability and reduces the overall damage to the membrane. Innovative cryoprotective supplements, such as soybean lecithin and low-density lipoprotein, have been evaluated in human and animal sperm freezing [59]. These new CPAs have lipid properties that can directly combat reactive oxygen species (ROS). Antifreeze proteins and antifreeze glycoproteins are agents found in various species that have adapted to extreme temperature conditions, such as polar fish, as well as some insects and plants [60–61]. These components act at a low freezing point and inhibit ice crystal formation, and stabilize phospholipids and unsaturated fatty acids in plasma membranes.

Cryopreservation of spermatozoa usually involves the following steps: cells are rinsed in a suspension and then placed in a solution, into which the CPA is slowly added to minimize osmotic shock to the sperm membranes. The sperm cells are then gradually cooled to 4°C and then to subzero temperature at a moderately low rate of ~5–10°C/min, after that to an intermediate subzero temperature of ~-75°C, and then plunged into LN_2 at -196°C, for storage. A gradual drop of temperature decreases the rate at which cells can lose water. Spermatozoa are particularly sensitive to fluctuations of temperature and in osmolalities of solutions because of the delicate nature of the acrosome. Vitrification without the use of a permeable cryoprotectant is an alternative method used for the storage of human spermatozoa [62].

On average, 50% of sperm cells are damaged or destroyed by freezing and thawing, limiting the overall efficiency and efficacy of semen preservation. What makes sperm freezing even less efficient is the fact that spermatozoa from different males exhibit widely variable responses to the same freezing conditions [63]. Such differences may be rooted in the variations in saturated and unsaturated fatty acid composition in the sperm membrane. Sperm membrane composition may also be influenced by lifestyle, hormonal status, and the season of the year. These variations likely impact permeability characteristics, as has been suggested by fluorescence anisotropy of spermatozoa before and after cryopreservation, performed to determine the fluidity of sperm membranes [64]. Anisotropy, which refers to the rotational motion of a membrane probe distributed throughout the hydrophobic core of the lipid bilayer of the cell membrane, varied among different men, and sperm membranes of all individuals were rendered less fluid following cryopreservation. Measurements of lipid dynamics in the plasma membrane of human spermatozoa showed that lipid diffusion in the acrosome and midpiece of spermatozoa was reduced after cryopreservation, compared with that of fresh sperm cells [65]. A characteristic feature of sperm membranes is the extremely high proportion of ether-linked fatty acids, instead of the more typical ester links seen in

membranes of other cells. Many of the phospholipids contain a docosahexaenoic acid side chain, which may result in increased membrane fluidity. Sperm plasma membrane lipids exist in two phases, fluid and gel. At physiological temperature, the two forms coexist, but as the temperature is lowered, a phase transition occurs in turn of the gel form [66].

Acrosome disintegration and partial elimination of the outer acrosomal membrane with depletion of acrosomal content are common alterations attributed to freezing events [67]. These defects are likely the result of ice crystal formation during the freezing of extracellular fluids, which leads to the expansion of the subacrosomal region. Alternatively, osmotic changes may cause injury to the lipid membrane structure, leading to tension changes in water canal proteins and ionic leakage across plasma membranes. Sperm cells are less likely to decondense after cryopreservation, indicating that freezing and thawing of sperm induces changes in disulfide bonds and/or causes denaturation. Destabilizing effects of cryopreservation on the nucleo-protein union, i.e., disruption of disulfide bonds might result in a subsequent increase in DNA fragmentation.

A spermatozoon delivers paternal mRNA to the oocyte during fertilization [68] and thus plays a vital role in early embryo development [69]. During the freezing process, transcripts and mRNA–protein interactions in spermatozoa can be lost, which may directly influence embryo development [70]. DNA integrity is a concern during cell freezing since cryopreservation quickly changes mitochondrial membrane properties and increases the production of ROS, which may subsequently have a consequence in the oxidation of DNA, producing high frequencies of single- and double-strand DNA breaks [71]. For this reason of additional sperm DNA damage, repeated freezing and thawing should be avoided [72].

Many studies have shown that similar clinical outcomes were achieved after ICSI using frozen–thawed motile sperm from an ejaculate, percutaneous epididymal sperm aspiration (PESA) [73], or testicular aspiration (TESA) [74] compared to fresh motile sperm. Full-term human pregnancies have been achieved by ICSI with frozen–thawed epididymal spermatozoa [75]. In clinical practice, only motile spermatozoa, including those from ejaculate, PESA, and TESA, are used for cryopreservation in most centers worldwide [76].

It has been suggested that a minimum of 40 million motile spermatozoa are needed for cryopreservation for intrauterine insemination purposes [77]. However, it could be less. In the past a single (or small numbers of) human spermatozoon was injected into an empty ZP prior to cryopreservation [78] and was subsequently used for fertilization by ICSI [79]. A novel sperm vitrification device provides an efficient means of freezing a small number of human spermatozoa from men suffering from nonobstructive azoospermia [80].

Frozen human semen is reportedly stable for 3 years only [81]. However, the birth of two healthy baby girls from the use of semen stored for 40 years was described [82]. It is a known fact that only 5–10% of patients that bank their semen before treatment come back for IVF treatment using their cryopreserved specimens. Possible reasons for this situation include the recovery of spermatogenesis after cessation of chemotherapy, frustration in IVF treatment, financial constraints, no plans for more children, death of the patient, and patient uncertainty regarding long-term prognosis. However, even though relatively few patients may return for treatment, cryopreservation should continue to be offered by healthcare professionals as standard care to all patients at risk for iatrogenic infertility.

Gender identity disorder (GID) is a condition in which a person experiences a discrepancy between the sex assigned at birth and the gender they identify with. Transsexualism is considered the most extreme form of GID and characterized by the desire to live and be treated as a member of the opposite gender. In the majority of cases, hormone therapy is administered. After at least 1 year of hormonal therapy, sex reassignment surgery can be offered, which includes orchidectomy and penectomy in combination with vaginoplasty [83]. Both hormonal and surgical interventions negatively affect the male reproductive system. Hormone therapy itself leads to decreased spermatogenesis and eventually to azoospermia. Current reproductive techniques can offer adult transsexual women the possibility of having genetically related children [84]. They can store their sperm for long-term cryopreservation before undergoing hormonal therapy, for future use in ART.

Testicular Tissue Banking

Semen cryopreservation is the first option for preserving male fertility; this cannot help out prepubertal boys. Nevertheless, these boys do have spermatogonial stem cells (SSCs) that are able to produce sperm at the start of puberty, which allows them to safeguard their fertility through testicular tissue cryopreservation. In vitro spermatogenesis has opened new possibilities to restore fertility in humans. However, these techniques are still at a research stage and banking of testicular tissue in prepubertal boys is still in experimental phases [85]. However, with the promising results accepted in animal models, the preservation of SSCs is now being introduced in more and more centers worldwide. Vitrification seems to be a convenient method for cryopreservation of immature human testicular tissue [86–87]. During the past few decades, several groups showed the feasibility of cryopreservation of human testicular tissue from both adult and immature individuals. Cryopreservation of testicular biopsied tissue provides several options after thawing: (a) autologous SSCs transplantation; (b) grafting of testicular tissue to the testis or a heterotopic area; (c) in vitro spermatogenesis.

References

1. Zeilmaker GH, Alberda AT, van Gent I, Rijkmans CM, Drogendijk AC. Two pregnancies following transfer of intact frozen-thawed embryos. *Fertil. Steril.* 1984; **42**:293–296.

2. Rall WF, Fahy GM. Ice-free cryopreservation of mouse embryos at -196°C by vitrification. *Nature* 1985; **313**:573–575.

3. Mazur P. Kinetics of water loss from cells at subzero temperatures and the likelihood of intracellular freezing. *J. Gen. Physiol.* 1963; **47**:347–369.

4. Newton HJ, Pegg DE, Barrass R, Gosden RG. Osmotically inactive volume, hydraulic conductivity, and permeability to dimethyl sulphoxide of human mature oocytes. *Reprod. Fertil.* 1999; **117**:27–33.

5. Galvao J, Davis B, Tilley M, et al. Unexpected low-dose toxicity of the universal solvent DMSO. *FASEB J.* 2014; **28**:1317–1330.

6. Schneider U, Mazur P. Osmotic consequences of cryoprotectant permeability and its relation to the survival of frozen-thawed embryos. *Theriogenology* 1984; **21**:68–79.

7. Edashige K, Tanaka M, Ichimaru N, et al. Channel dependent permeation of water and glycerol in mouse morulae. *Biol. Reprod.* 2006; **74**:625–632.

8. Kasai M, Edashige K. Movement of water and cryoprotectants in mouse oocytes and embryos at different stages: relevance to cryopreservation. In: Chian RC, Quinn P, eds., *Fertility Cryopreservation*. Cambridge: Cambridge University Press. 2010; 16–23.

9. Maneiro E, Ron-Corzo A, Julve J, Goyanes VJ. Surface area/volume ratio and growth equation of the human early embryo. *Int. J. Dev. Biol.* 1991; **35**:139–143.

10. Senn A, Vozzi C, Chanson A, De Grandi P, Germond M. Prospective randomized study of two cryopreservation policies avoiding embryo selection: the pronucleate stage leads to a higher cumulative delivery rate than the early cleavage stage. *Fertil. Steril.* 2000; **74**:946–952.

11. Al-Hasani S, Ozmen B, Koutlaki N, et al. Three years of routine vitrification of human zygotes: is it still fair to advocate slow-rate freezing? *RBM Online* 2007; **14**:288–293.

12. Isachenko V, Todorov P, Dimitrov Y, Isachenko E. Integrity rate of pronuclei after cryopreservation of pronuclear-zygotes as a criteria for subsequent embryo development and pregnancy. *Hum. Reprod.* 2008; **23**:819–826.

13. Oehninger S, Mayer J, Muasher S. Impact of different clinical variables on pregnancy outcome following embryo cryopreservation. *Mol. Cell. Endocrinol.* 2000; **169**:73–77.

14. Kuwayama M, Vajta G, Kato O, Leibo SP. Highly efficient vitrification method for cryopreservation of human oocytes. *RBM Online* 2005; **11**:300–308.

15. Hartshorne GM, Wick K, Elder K, Dyson H. Effect of cell number at freezing upon survival and viability of cleaving embryos generated from stimulated IVF cycles. *Hum. Reprod.* 1990; **5**:857–861.

16. Edgar DH, Bourne H, Spiers AL, McBain JC. A quantitative analysis of the impact of cryopreservation on the implantation potential of human early cleavage stage embryos. *Hum. Reprod.* 2000; **15**:175–179.

17. Zech NH, Lejeune B, Zech H, Vanderzwalmen P. Vitrification of hatching and hatched human blastocysts: effect of an opening in the zona pellucida before vitrification. *RBM Online* 2005; **11**:355–361.

18. Mukaida T, Oka C, Goto T, Takahashi K. Artificial shrinkage of blastocoeles using either a micro-needle or a laser pulse prior to the cooling steps of vitrification improves survival rate and pregnancy outcome of vitrified human blastocysts. *Hum. Reprod.* 2006; **21**:3246–3252.

19. Richter KS, Shipley SK, McVearry I, Tucker MJ, Widra EA. Cryopreserved embryo transfers suggest that endometrial receptivity may contribute to reduced success rates of later developing embryos. *Fertil. Steril.* 2006; **86**:862–866.

20. Gardner DK, Schoolcraft WB. In vitro culture of human blastocysts. In: Jansen R, Mortimer D, eds.,

Toward Reproductive Certainty: Fertility and Genetics Beyond. London: Parthenon Publishing. 1999; 378–388.

21. Takahashi K, Mukaida T, Goto T, Oka C. Perinatal outcome of blastocyst transfer with vitrification using cryoloop: a 4-year follow-up study. *Fertil. Steril.* 2005; **84**:88–92.

22. Pinborg A, Henningsen AA, Loft A, et al. Large baby syndrome in singletons born after frozen embryo transfer (FET): is it due to maternal factors or the cryotechnique? *Hum. Reprod.* 2014; **29**:618–627.

23. Chen C. Pregnancy after human oocyte cryopreservation. *Lancet* 1986; **1**:884–886.

24. Alpha Scientists in Reproductive Medicine; ESHRE Special Interest Group Embryology. Istanbul consensus workshop on embryo assessment: proceedings of an expert meeting. *RBM Online* 2011; **22**:632–646.

25. Alpha Scientists in Reproductive Medicine and ESHRE Special Interest Group Embryology. Istanbul consensus workshop on embryo assessment: proceedings of an expert meeting. *Hum. Reprod.* 2011; **26**:1270–1283.

26. Ebner T, Yaman C, Moser M, et al. Prognostic value of first polar body morphology on fertilization rate and embryo quality in intracytoplasmic sperm injection. *Hum. Reprod.* 2000; **15**:427–430.

27. Hunter JE, Bernard A, Fuller BJ, McGrath JJ, Shaw RW. Measurements of the membrane water permeability (Lp) and its temperature dependence (activation energy) in human fresh and failed-to-fertilize oocytes and mouse oocyte. *Cryobiology* 1992; **29**:240–249.

28. Pickering SJ, Braude PR, Johnson MH, Cant A, Currie J. Transient cooling to room temperature can cause irreversible disruption of the meiotic spindle in the human oocyte. *Fertil. Steril.* 1990; **54**:102–108.

29. Zenzes MT, Bielecki R, Casper RF, Leibo SP. Effects of chilling to 0 degrees C on the morphology of meiotic spindles in human metaphase II oocytes. *Fertil. Steril.* 2001; **75**:769–777.

30. Cobo A, Kuwayama M, Pérez S, et al. Comparison of concomitant outcome achieved with fresh and cryopreserved donor oocytes vitrified by the Cryotop method. *Fertil. Steril.* 2007; **89**:1657–1664.

31. Doyle JO, Richter KS, Lim J, et al. Successful elective and medically indicated oocyte vitrification and warming for autologous in vitro fertilization, with predicted birth probabilities for fertility preservation according to number of cryopreserved oocytes and age at retrieval. *Fertil. Steril.* 2016; **105**:459–466.

155

32. Ben Rafael Z. The dilemma of social oocyte freezing: usage rate is too low to make it cost-effective. *RBM Online* 2018; **37**:443–448.

33. Leibo SP, Mazur P, Jackowski SC. Factors affecting survival of mouse embryos during freezing and thawing. *Exp. Cell Res.* 1974; **89**:79–88.

34. Leibo SP, Oda K. High survival of mouse zygotes and embryos cooled rapidly or slowly in ethylene glycol plus polyvinylpyrrolidone. *Cryo Letters* 1993; **14**:133–134.

35. Van den Abbeel E, Camus M, Van Waesberghe L, Devroey P, Van Steirteghem A. Viability of partially damaged human embryos after cryopreservation. *Hum. Reprod.* 1997; **12**:2006–2010.

36. Rienzi L, Nagy ZP, Ubaldi F, et al. Laser-assisted removal of necrotic blastomeres from cryopreserved embryos that were partially damaged. *Fertil. Steril.* 2002; **77**:1196–1201.

37. Hardarson T, Lofman C, Coull G, et al. Internalization of cellular fragments in a human embryo: time-lapse recordings. *RBM Online* 2002; **5**:36–38.

38. Rienzi L, Ubaldi F, Iacobelli M, et al. Developmental potential of fully intact and partially damaged cryopreserved embryos after laser-assisted removal of necrotic blastomeres and post-thaw culture selection. *Fertil. Steril.* 2005; **84**:888–894.

39. Nagy ZP, Taylor T, Elliott T, et al. Removal of lysed blastomeres from frozen-thawed embryos improves implantation and pregnancy rates in frozen embryo transfer cycles. *Fertil. Steril.* 2005; **84**:1606–1612.

40. Leoni GG, Berlinguer F, Succu S, et al. A new selection criterion to assess good quality ovine blastocysts after vitrification and to predict their transfer into recipients. *Mol. Reprod. Dev.* 2008; **75**:373–382.

41. Huang JY, Tulandi T, Holzer H, et al. Cryopreservation of ovarian tissue and in vitro matured oocytes in a female with mosaic Turner syndrome: case report. *Hum. Reprod.* 2008; **23**:336–339.

42. De Roo P, Lierman S, Tilleman K, et al. Ovarian tissue cryopreservation in female-to-male transgender people: insights into ovarian histology and physiology after prolonged androgen treatment. *RBM Online* 2017; **34**:557–566.

43. Westphal JR, Gerritse R, Braat DDM, Beerendonk CCM, Peek RJ. Complete protection against cryodamage of cryopreserved whole bovine and human ovaries using DMSO as a cryoprotectant. *Assist. Reprod. Genet.* 2017; **34**:1217–1229.

44. Haino T, Tarumi W, Kawamura K, et al. Determination of follicular localization in human ovarian cortex for vitrification. *J. Adolesc. Young Adult Oncol.* 2018; **7**:46–53.

45. Newton H, Fisher J, Arnold JR, et al. Permeation of human ovarian tissue with cryoprotective agents in preparation for cryopreservation. *Hum. Reprod.* 1998; **13**:376–380.

46. Kagawa N, Kuwayama M, Nakata K, et al. Production of the first offspring from oocytes derived from fresh and cryopreserved preantral follicles of adult mice. *RBM Online* 2007; **14**:693–699.

47. Hasegawa A, Mochida N, Ogasawara T, Koyama K. Pup birth from mouse oocytes in preantral follicles derived from vitrified and warmed ovaries followed by in vitro growth, in vitro maturation, and in vitro fertilization. *Fertil. Steril.* 2006; **86**:1182–1192.

48. Nakamura Y, Obata R, Okuyama N, et al. Residual ethylene glycol and dimethyl sulphoxide concentration in human ovarian tissue during warming/thawing steps following cryopreservation. *RBM Online* 2017; **35**:311–313.

49. Bastings L, Westphal JR, Beerendonk CCM, et al. Clinically applied procedures for human ovarian tissue cryopreservation result in different levels of efficacy and efficiency. *J. Assist. Reprod. Genet.* 2016; **33**:1605–1614.

50. Demeestere I, Simon P, Emiliani S, Delbaere A, Englert Y. Orthotopic and heterotopic ovarian tissue transplantation. *Hum. Reprod. Update* 2009; **15**:649–665.

51. Dalman A, Deheshkar Gooneh Farahani NS, Totonchi M, et al. Slow freezing versus vitrification technique for human ovarian tissue cryopreservation: an evaluation of histological changes, WNT signaling pathway and apoptotic genes expression. *Cryobiology* 2017; **79**:29–36.

52. Meirow D, Levron J, Eldar-Geva T, et al. Pregnancy after transplantation of cryopreserved ovarian tissue in a patient with ovarian failure after chemotherapy. *N. Engl. J. Med.* 2005; **353**:318–321.

53. Donnez J, Dolmans MM, Demylle D, et al. Live birth after orthotopic transplantation of cryopreserved ovarian tissue. *Lancet* 2004; **364**:1405–1410.

54. Shaw J, Trounson AO. Ovarian banking for cancer patients – oncological implications in the replacement of ovarian tissue. *Hum. Reprod.* 1997; **12**:403–405.

55. Polge C, Smith AU, Parkes AS. Revival of spermatozoa after vitrification and dehydration at low temperatures. *Nature* 1949; **164**:666.

56. Perloff WH, Steinberger E, Sherman JK. Conception with human spermatozoa frozen by nitrogen vapor technic. *Fertil. Steril.* 1964; **15**:501.

57. Serafini P, Hauser D, Moyer D, Marrs R. Cryopreservation of human spermatozoa: correlations of ultrastructural sperm head configuration with

sperm motility and ability to penetrate zona-free hamster ova. *Fertil. Steril.* 1986; **46**:691–695.

58. Woolley D, Richardson D. Ultrastructural injury to human spermatozoa after freezing and thawing. *J. Reprod. Fertil.* 1978; **53**:389–394.

59. Emamverdi M, Zhandi M, Shahneh AZ, et al. Flow cytometric and microscopic evaluation of post-thawed ram semen cryopreserved in chemically defined home-made or commercial extenders. *Anim. Prod. Sci.* 2015; **55**:551–558.

60. Cheung RCF, Ng TB, Wong JH. Antifreeze proteins from diverse organisms and their applications: an overview. *Curr. Protein Pept. Sci.* 2017; **18**:262–283.

61. Kim HJ, Lee JH, Hur YB, et al. Marine antifreeze proteins: structure, function, and application to cryopreservation as a potential cryoprotectant. *Mar. Drugs* 2017; **15**:27.

62. Isachenko E, Isachenko V, Katkov II, Dessole S, Nawroth F. Vitrification of mammalian spermatozoa in the absence of cryoprotectants: From past practical difficulties to present success. *RBM Online* 2003; **6**:191–200.

63. Centola GM, Raubertas RF, Mattox JH. Cryopreservation of human semen. Comparision of cryopreservatives, sources of variability, and prediction of post-thaw survival. *J. Andrology* 1992; **13**:283–288.

64. Giraud MN, Motta C, Boucher D, Grizard G. Membrane fluidity predicts the outcome of cryopreservation of human spermatozoa. *Hum. Reprod.* 2000; **15**:2160–2164.

65. James PS, Wolfe CA, Mackie A, et al. Lipid dynamics in the plasma membrane of fresh and cryopreserved human spermatozoa. *Hum. Reprod.* 1999; **14**:1827–1832.

66. Holt WV. Basic aspects of frozen storage of semen. *Anim. Reprod. Sci.* 2000; **62**:3–22.

67. Barthelemy C, Royere D, Hammahah S, et al. Ultrastructural changes in membranes and acrosome of human sperm during cryopreservation. *Syst. Biol. Reprod. Med.* 1990; **25**:29–40.

68. Lalancette C, Miller D, Li Y, Krawetz SA. Paternal contributions: new functional insights for spermatozoal RNA. *J. Cell. Biochem.* 2008; **104**:1570–1579.

69. Jodar M, Selvaraju S, Sendler E, Diamond MP, Krawetz SA. The presence, role and clinical use of spermatozoal RNAs. *Hum. Reprod.* 2013; **19**:604–624.

70. Valcarce DG, Carton-Garcia F, Herraez MP, Robles V. Effect of cryopreservation on human sperm messenger RNAs crucial for fertilization and early embryo development. *Cryobiology* 2013; **67**:84–90.

71. Said TM, Gaglani A, Agarwal A. Implication of apoptosis in sperm cryoinjury. *RBM Online* 2010; **21**:456–462.

72. Liu T, Gao J, Zhou N, et al. The effect of two cryopreservation methods on human sperm DNA damage. *Cryobiology* 2016; **72**:210–215.

73. Sukcharoen N, Sithipravej T, Promviengchai S, Chinpilas V, Boonkasemsanti W. Comparison of the outcome of intracytoplasmic sperm injection using fresh and frozen-thawed epididymal spermatozoa obtained by percutaneous epididymal sperm aspiration. *J. Med. Assoc. Thai.* 2001; **84**(Suppl. 1): S331–S337.

74. Hessel M, Robben JC, D'Hauwers KW, Braat DD, Ramos L. The influence of sperm motility and cryopreservation on the treatment outcome after intracytoplasmic sperm injection following testicular sperm extraction. *Acta Obstet. Gynecol. Scand.* 2015; **94**:1313–1321.

75. Devroey P, Silber S, Nagy Z, et al. Ongoing pregnancies and birth after intracytoplasmic sperm injection with frozen-thawed epididymal spermatozoa. *Hum. Reprod.* 1995; **10**:903–906.

76. Tongdee P, Sukprasert M, Satirapod C, Wongkularb A, Choktanasiri W. Comparison of cryopreserved human sperm between ultra rapid freezing and slow programmable freezing: effect on motility, morphology and DNA integrity. *J. Med. Assoc. Thai.* 2015; **98**:S33–S42.

77. Bordson BL, Ricci E, Dickey RP, et al. Comparison of fecundability with fresh and frozen semen in therapeutic donor insemination. *Fertil. Steril.* 1986; **46**:466–469.

78. Cohen J, Garrisi GJ, Congedo-Ferrara TA, et al. Cryopreservation of single human spermatozoa. *Hum. Reprod.* 1997; **12**:994–1001.

79. Liu J, Zheng XZ, Baramki TA, et al. Cryopreservation of a small number of fresh human testicular spermatozoa and testicular spermatozoa cultured in vitro for 3 days in an empty zona pellucida. *J. Androl.* 2000; **21**:409–413.

80. Berkovitz A, Miller N, Silberman M, Belenky M, Itsykson P. A novel solution for freezing small numbers of spermatozoa using a sperm vitrification device. *Hum. Reprod.* 2018; **33**:1975–1983.

81. Smith KD, Steinberger E. Survival of spermatozoa in a human sperm bank. Effects of long-term storage in liquid nitrogen. *J. Am. Med. Assoc.* 1973; **223**:774–777.

82. Szell AZ, Bierbaum RC, Hazelrigg WB, Chetkowski RJ. Live births from frozen human semen stored for 40 years. *J. Assist. Reprod. Genet.* 2013; **36**:743–744.

83. Selvaggi G, Ceulemans P, De Cuypere G, et al. Gender identity disorder: general overview and surgical

157

treatment for vaginoplasty in male-to-female transsexuals. *Plast. Reconstr. Surg.* 2005; **116**:135–145.

84. De Sutter P. Gender reassignment and assisted reproduction: present and future options for transsexual people. *Hum. Reprod.* 2001; **16**:612–614.

85. Onofre J, Baert Y, Faes K, Goossens E. Cryopreservation of testicular tissue or testicular cell suspensions: a pivotal step in fertility preservation. *Hum. Reprod. Update* 2016; **22**:744–761.

86. Curaba M, Poels J, van Langendonckt A, Donnez J, Wyns C. Can prepubertal human testicular tissue be cryopreserved by vitrification? *Fertil. Steril.* 2011; **95**:2123.e9–2123.e12.

87. Zarandi NP, Galdon G, Kogan S, Atala A, Sadri-Ardekani H. Cryostorage of immature and mature human testis tissue to preserve spermatogonial stem cells (SSCs): a systematic review of current experiences toward clinical applications. *Stem Cells Cloning* 2018; **11**:23–38.

Chapter 13

In Vitro Maturation (IVM)

In vitro maturation (IVM) systems have been developed to support the growth and development of oocytes, from their most immature stages to developmentally competent oocytes [1–2]. The IVM technique has been in veterinary practice for a long time. The first reported study of IVM in humans dates back to 1965 [3]; however, the first pregnancy resulting from IVM in humans was only reported in 1991 and involved the use of donated oocytes from unstimulated ovaries from women undergoing gynecological surgery [4]. A 1994 report described a pregnancy in an anovulatory woman with polycystic ovary syndrome (PCOS) after IVM of her oocytes [5]. Initial reports concentrated on the development of specific culture conditions [6], variations in stimulation and priming protocols [7], and patient selection [8], as well as fertilization techniques [9]. Traditionally, cycles of IVM are followed by intracytoplasmic sperm injection (ICSI) for fertilization, although similar fertilization rates have been reported for IVM-in vitro fertilization (IVF), rendering IVM-IVF an optional method, due to its cost-effectiveness and lower invasiveness [10]. Earlier studies that compared the results after IVM with those after conventional IVF (in vivo-matured oocytes) reported significantly lower pregnancy rates with IVM. The majority of the treatment protocols involved human chorionic gonadotropin (hCG) priming, which led to the early resumption of meiosis. The adoption of a "freeze-all" IVF protocol, with the transfer of a single blastocyst in a subsequent frozen embryo transfer cycle, has led to live birth rates that approximate those of traditional IVF cycles, with the avoidance of ovarian hyperstimulation syndrome (OHSS) [11]. These improvements have generated a renewed interest in IVM research, particularly for PCOS patients.

To develop IVM methodologies, we must fully understand the physiological processes that occur in vivo.

Oocyte Maturation In Vivo

The prolonged arrest in meiosis occurs in the primary oocyte (germinal vesicle [GV]-arrested oocyte at prophase I) before birth. Years later, meiosis is reinitiated just before ovulation and is again halted at metaphase II (MII) until fertilization. Fertilization activates the completion of meiosis and is followed by successive mitotic divisions of the newly formed embryo.

Before resumption of meiosis, the oocyte undergoes a growth phase, during which it accumulates both mRNA and regulatory proteins required for the completion of meiosis. Meiotic progression depends upon the precise control of these essential regulatory proteins and any alteration in this control could result in maturation failure. These proteins are controlled via regulation of their production, phosphorylation, localization, and degradation.

The extended meiotic arrest of the oocyte at the GV stage is maintained by several external factors, including cAMP, most of which are transferred to the oocyte from the cumulus cells (CCs) via gap junctions. Elevated cAMP levels downregulate meiosis promoting factor (MPF), which is a heterodimer, composed of p34cdc2 kinase (known also as CDK1) and cyclin B. Granulosa cells (GCs) produce natriuretic peptide precursor type C (NPPC) that binds the NPPC receptor (NPR2) on CCs, resulting in the production of cGMP, which is then transferred to the oocyte via gap junctions [12] to inhibit phosphodiesterase 3A (PDE3A), thereby preventing hydrolysis of cAMP [13–14]. cGMP is also nitric oxide (NO) dependent, and supplementation of NO inhibits meiotic resumption [15].

The oocyte meiotic resumption is an incredibly complex chain of reactions (Figure 13.1). There are many molecular cascades maintaining meiotic resumption in the oocyte, all of which are orchestrated by multiple molecules produced by the pituitary gland and follicular cells. Meiosis reinitiation is stimulated by gonadotropins, luteinizing hormone

(LH) and follicle-stimulating hormone (FSH), preovulatory peaks. While LH receptors are located on GCs and CCs [16], CCs have been shown to be insensitive to direct LH stimulation [17]. A surge in LH induces reprogramming of the mural GCs in the follicle and the expression of epidermal growth factor-like peptides, including amphiregulin and epiregulin, that are needed to propagate the LH stimulus from the mural GC to the CC [17]. FSH binds to its receptors on both GCs and CCs. The transition from GV to GV breakdown (also known as the metaphase I [MI] stage) is the first morphological marker of meiotic resumption in the oocyte. The breakdown of the nuclear envelope occurs about 2 hours after LH exposure [18]. LH interrupts cell-to-cell interactions in the ovarian follicle (expansion and disconnection of the cells). Connexin 43, the ovarian gap junction protein, is dramatically phosphorylated during the LH and FSH surges, leading to gap junction closure between CCs, thereby reducing the supply of cGMP to the oocyte within 2 hours. This event, in turn, leads to the activation of intra-oocyte PDE3A that reduces intra-oocyte cAMP. Disconnection of the gap junctions between cells also reduces the cAMP supply to the oocyte. A low level of cAMP reinitiates meiosis and oocyte maturation. LH also inhibits adenylate cyclase, leading to a drop in the production of cAMP, which has an added effect on oocyte maturation. cAMP acts as a primary negative regulator of meiosis by inhibiting p34cdc2 kinase dephosphorylation. Dephosphorylation of p34cdc2 kinase on Thr-14 and Tyr-15 by cdc25 results in MPF activation, which drives meiosis resumption via an increase in the activity of mitogen-activated protein (MAP) kinase (MAPK; MAPK1/2 known also as MEK1/2 and MAPK3 known as ERK) that remains elevated until the completion of the second meiotic division. Active MAPK is required to maintain the oocyte in the second metaphase arrest. The upstream regulator of MAPK in the oocyte is Moloney sarcoma (MOS) kinase, the product of the c-mos protooncogene (Figure 13.2). In most cases, the subsequent inactivation of MPF is brought about by the ubiquitin–proteasome pathway activated by anaphase-promoting complex/cyclosome (APC/C directs the destruction of cell cycle regulatory proteins at the metaphase–anaphase transition of first and second meiosis). APC/C activation results in a release of separase (also known as separin), which is necessary for chromatid separation (Figure 13.3). At the transition from stage MI to stage MII, actin-related protein 2/3 regulates migration of the MI spindle to the oocyte membrane, which is necessary for extrusion of the first polar body (PB).

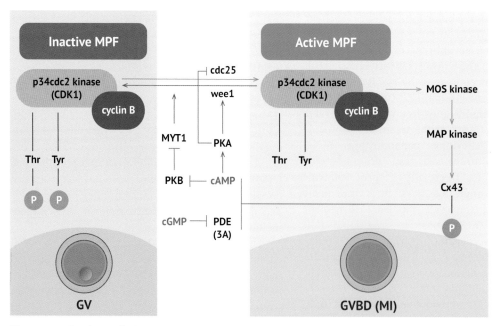

Figure 13.1 Regulation of MPF inactivation and activation. Cx43; connexin 43; GVBD, germinal vesicle breakdown; MAP kinase, mitogen activated protein kinase; MOS kinase, Moloney sarcoma kinase; MYT1, myelin transcription factor 1; PKA, protein kinase A; PKB, protein kinase B.

A global analysis of the number of active genes detected in oocytes showed a progressive decrease in the number of genes expressed during oocyte nuclear maturation, with the lowest number of genes expressed in MII oocytes compared with GV or MI oocytes [16]. The translation of all three zona pellucida glycoproteins decreases dramatically during oocyte maturation, while genes involved in meiosis, such as MPF, APC/C, and spindle checkpoint complexes, are markedly overexpressed.

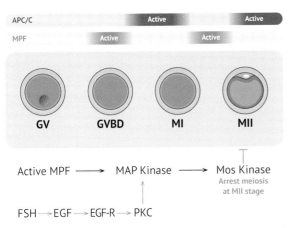

Figure 13.2 Oocyte maturation and the arrest of meiosis at second metaphase.

Full achievement of meiosis is only accomplished after fecundation because metaphase exit is prevented by the activity of cytostatic factor (CSF), which is only relieved by gamete fusion [16]. The endpoint of activation with any activating agent (i.e., penetration of the sperm cell into the oocyte) eliciting Ca^{2+} release is the physical destruction of cyclin B1, which leads to inactivation of p34cdc2 kinase and to a drop in MPF and CSF activity (CSF reduces cyclin B1 degradation) [19].

Approximately 8.6–15.2% of all infertility patients produce at least one meiotically incompetent oocyte. Women who are showing more than 25% immature oocytes suffer from significantly lower fertilization with lower clinical pregnancy rates [20]. Oocyte maturation failure is occasionally absolute, i.e., no mature oocytes are produced. Oocyte maturation arrest can occur at any of its development stages: GV arrest, MI arrest, or MII arrest.

Type I (GV arrest). The activation of MPF controls the resumption of meiosis from the diplotene arrest. Morphologically, reinitiation of meiosis I and entry into the M phase is marked by the breakdown of the GV. Disruption of the key signaling events leading up to MPF activation results in the arrest of the oocyte before MI. In an animal model, cdc25b (-/-) female mice (cdc25 dephosphorylates and activates MPF)

Figure 13.3 Active APC/C inactivates MPF and induces chromatid separation. EGF, epidermal growth factor; PKC, protein kinase C.

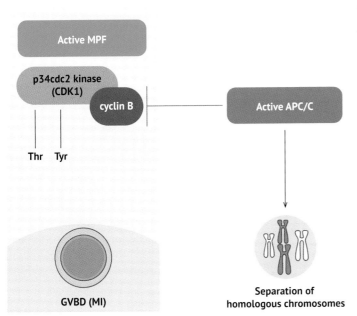

GVBD (MI)

Separation of homologous chromosomes

bear oocytes arrested in the GV stage [21]. Women who produce oocytes arrested at GV possess a defect in the signaling cascade responsible for the activation of MPF. Regulation of oocyte cAMP expression has also been found to be essential for oocyte maturation. PDE3A is primarily responsible for oocyte cAMP hydrolysis. PDE3A-deficient female mice are entirely infertile because ovulated oocytes contain increased cAMP levels and are arrested at the GV stage [22].

Type II (MI arrest). Progression through meiosis MI to MII arrest requires chromosome condensation, the formation of the metaphase spindle, and chromosome alignment along with the first metaphase plate, followed by the separation and segregation of the homologous chromosomes. The completion of the first meiotic division is marked by the formation of the first PB. Oocyte arrest before the formation of the first PB is morphologically classified as MI arrest. MI arrest could occur because of either a defect in the signal transduction pathway mediating meiotic progression or any abnormality in the meiotic spindle, which results in activation of the spindle assembly checkpoint. APC/C mediates the metaphase-to-anaphase transition. Disruption of the critical signaling events leading up to APC/C activation results in the arrest of the oocyte at the MI stage. Targeted degradation of securin by APC/C releases separase, which cleaves cohesin and results in chromosome segregation [23]. APC/C also triggers the destruction of cyclin B, leading to the inactivation of MPF and exit from meiosis I [24]. Additional oocyte factors can be involved in MI arrest. The knockdown of H1foo (an oocyte-specific subtype of the linker histone H1) resulted in oocyte arrest at MI [25]. In vivo, H1foo function is mediated through methylation; therefore, it is possible that epigenetic modification of H1foo may result in altered gene expression and oocyte maturation competence. Mei1 and Mlh1 mediate recombination during meiosis [26] and Mei1-deficient oocytes demonstrate severe synapsis defects and unpaired and disorganized chromosomes and undergo MI arrest [27].

Type III (MII arrest). MII oocytes are generally described as "mature" and arrested in MII; they are presumed to be capable of fertilization. However, there are subsets of women who produce oocytes with MII morphology that are not capable of embryo formation after fertilization. Some of these women may be carrying oocytes arrested at MII due to their

inability to complete meiosis. They may be carrying immature oocytes arrested at any stage between first PB formation and MII, which match the MII morphological classification but are still unable to be fertilized. Arrest at MII has initiated inhibition of APC/C by Emi2 and maintained inhibition of the MOS/MAPK pathway and spindle assembly checkpoint by Emi2 [28]. Oocytes deficient in Emi2 protein are not able to form a spindle complex during the second meiosis and are arrested at MII [29]. Similarly, MOS-null mutant oocytes that progressed to MII could not complete second meiosis after fertilization [30]. Release from MII arrest is dependent upon sperm-specific phospholipase C zeta and downstream activation of APC/C [31]. APC/C activation results in the inactivation of MPF and the release of separase, which is necessary for sister chromatid separation [32]. Proteins involved in this pathway include calmodulin-dependent protein kinase II (CamKII) and protein kinase C (PKC). CamKII and PKC inhibitors block exit from meiosis, resulting in MII arrest [33]. Maturation arrest is characterized by incapacity of the oocyte to progress through meiosis due to either signaling errors or aberrations in chromosomal/spindle formation. These aberrations can be a reason for aneuploidy. Aneuploidy was found in 41.9% of oocytes after first meiosis (homologous chromosomes) and 37.3% of oocytes after second meiosis (sister chromosomes), with 29.1% of these oocytes having both first meiosis and second meiosis errors [34].

Although nuclear maturation and cytoplasmic maturation are linked, cytoplasmic maturation can occur independently of full nuclear maturation. During the initial growth phase of the oocyte, nuclear chromatin is decondensed and is transcriptionally active. As folliculogenesis progresses, the oocyte acquires meiotic competence, as identified by the condensing and nuclear association of chromatin, and the formation of microtubule organizing centers, necessary for spindle formation. Developmental competence requires a series of nuclear and cytoplasmic cellular events that take place alongside meiotic stages, to enable fertilization, DNA replication, and zygote ploidy.

At present, the use of donor oocytes is the only option available for women with oocyte maturation failure after several unsuccessful stimulation cycles.

Oocyte Metabolism during Maturation

Anaerobic glycolysis is a major pathway for glucose metabolism in the mammalian follicle, consuming glucose and producing lactate as the growing follicle undergoes luteinization [35–36]. The oocyte, however, has a low glucose metabolism capacity due, in part, to low phosphofructokinase activity [37]. Instead, CCs with high glycolytic activity metabolize glucose into pyruvate, which is transferred to the oocyte as an energy source. In the oocyte, pyruvate is converted, in the mitochondria, to acetyl CoA, which enters the tricarboxylic acid cycle and electron transport system to produce ATP [36]. The oocyte, in turn, ensures receipt of pyruvate by upregulating glycolytic genes in CCs [38].

During ovulation, the maturing oocyte supports the increased energy expenditure through mitochondrial oxidation of free fatty acids, a more efficient source of ATP than glycolysis [39]. Fatty acids within the cumulus–oocyte complex enter the mitochondria, where they are converted to acetyl CoA and continue to produce ATP through beta-oxidation [40]. With increased oxygen and pyruvate consumption during oocyte maturation, the oocyte also regulates the delivery of amino acids and cholesterol from CCs for other cellular processes.

Free radicals that can damage cellular macromolecules during follicle growth and oocyte maturation include reactive oxygen species (ROS) and reactive nitrogen species. High ROS levels and low antioxidant capacity in follicular fluid predict lower pregnancy outcomes following IVF [41–42].

Oocyte Maturation In Vitro

IVM offers a number of potential benefits when compared with standard IVF, principally related to the avoidance of high doses of hormonal stimulation with gonadotropins and gonadotropin-releasing hormone (GnRH) analogs. In patients with PCOS, this avoids the risk of OHSS [43]. Moreover, IVM can also be offered in other cases, such as gonadotropin-resistant ovary to stimulation by FSH [44].

For the follicle aspiration technique employed in an IVM cycle, most centers use a small-gauge size (16 or 17 gauge) with either a single- or double-lumen needle, with suction pressures in the range of 52–200 mm Hg [45–46]. The aspiration of oocytes, when the leading follicle is 10–12 mm in diameter, and the transfer of a single blastocyst-stage embryo performed under hormone therapy to assist endometrial development demonstrated excellent implantation and pregnancy rates [47]. To synchronize the development of the fertilized oocyte and endometrium, estradiol (E_2) is

first administered at a dose of 2 mg, three times a day, from the day of oocyte collection, followed by progesterone (P_4) administration from the next day after oocyte collection. The dosage of P_4 depends on the formulations, which include oral, vaginal, rectal, subcutaneous, and intramuscular preparations. The dosage of E_2 depends on the endometrial thickness. If the endometrial thickness is less than 6 mm, 10–12 mg of E_2 are given; if the endometrial thickness is between 6 and 8 mm, 8–10 mg of E_2 are administered in divided doses.

The effectiveness of IVM relies on the successful synchronization of the meiotic and cytoplasmic maturation of oocytes [48]. There are several types of IVM: classic IVM (maturation of COC in vitro with gonadotropins from GV stage), hCG-primed IVM (truncated IVF, followed by IVM), and rescue IVM (maturation of denuded immature oocytes after regular IVF).

Sample of classic protocol for IVM: in vivo FSH priming (150 IU daily for 3 days) from day 3 of the cycle, then coasting for 2–5 days, followed by hCG priming. Since smaller follicles do not express LH receptors, they are insensitive to hCG. GCs respond to LH once follicles reached 9–10 mm, therefore CC-oocyte complexes retrieved from 10 mm follicles (dominance is not established at this stage) resulted in recovery with most oocytes at the GV stage. Recovered CC-oocyte complexes are cultured in medium with gonadotropins for 30–48 hours. IVM culture media are based on culture media, hormonal additives, and a source of protein. For successful resumption of meiosis, the combination of FSH with either hCG or LH in the culture media is necessary to promote the proliferation and expansion of the coronal cells and aid in the final stages of oocyte maturation. The combination of FSH with hCG improved clinical pregnancy rates and implantation rates in a randomized trial [49].

The timing of oocyte aspiration is not so critical when hCG priming is used; however, it is critical when no trigger is used. Improved clinical outcomes were obtained upon transfer of single vitrified warmed embryos in a non-hCG-primed IVM cycle to PCOS patients, compared with fresh embryo transfer [50]. These effects are mainly attributed to low endometrial receptivity in fresh embryo transfer cycles. Embryos transferred in a vitrified–warmed cycle are associated with clinical pregnancy rates identical to those after IVF cycles in women with PCOS

[51]. The first IVM baby was born in October 2003. A 33-year-old woman became pregnant from an oocyte that had been matured in vitro, fertilized, frozen as a blastocyst, and then thawed [52].

Immature human oocytes are able to mature in vitro, particularly those from gonadotropin-stimulated ovaries; however, they are developmentally incompetent when compared with oocytes matured in vivo. Oocyte size is associated with maturation in most species examined, which may indicate that a specific size is necessary to initiate the molecular cascade of normal nuclear and cytoplasmic maturation. The loss of developmental competence in oocytes cultured to MII in vitro is associated with the absence of specific proteins. The presence of follicle support cells in culture is necessary for the gonadotropin-mediated response required to mature oocytes in vitro. Gonadotropin concentration and the sequence of FSH and FSH–LH exposure may be significant for human oocytes, particularly those not exposed to the gonadotropin surge in vivo. Exposure of immature oocytes to high FSH levels during IVM accelerates nuclear maturation and disrupts chromosomal alignment on the spindle during first meiosis, causing an increase in aneuploid MII oocytes [53]. The co-culture of CCs with non-mature oocytes improves the maturation of the oocytes, possibly due to the accumulation of a protein critical for spindle assembly [54]. Complete maturation of oocytes is essential for the developmental competence of embryos.

IVM is certainly no panacea for poor-prognosis patients with low levels of anti-Müllerian hormone (AMH) and antral follicle count (AFC). On the contrary, IVM success rates are highly correlated with AMH and AFC levels. IVM oocytes differ from in vivo-matured oocytes, including reduced protein content in the former compared with the latter oocytes [55]. In addition, differential gene expression was found between in vivo maturation and IVM [56]. Over 2000 genes are expressed at more than two-fold higher levels in IVM oocytes compared with in vivo-matured oocytes [57]. Transmission electron microscopy showed that IVM oocytes have normal ooplasm, with uniform distribution of organelles. However, large mitochondria–vesicle complexes partially replaced mitochondria–smooth endoplasmic reticulum aggregates in IVM oocytes. Vacuoles were found in all oocytes and were frequently associated with lysosomes. [58]. Multinucleation rates following

ICSI also are higher in IVM than in in vivo-matured MII oocytes [59]. The IVM oocytes also had lower normal fertilization rates than the MII-aspirated oocytes [60]. In addition, embryos derived from oocytes that failed to mature in vivo under standard treatment of ovarian stimulation may show a different morphokinetic profile than their sibling oocytes aspirated at the MII stage after completing maturation in vivo [60]. Rescue IVM produced ~1.5 more additional embryos for transfer [61] compared with embryos from in vivo-matured oocytes. However, pregnancy rates with IVM remain lower than with conventional IVF, and higher miscarriage rates have been reported with IVM. As research of IVM expands, success rates are slowly improving, but still remain lower than regular IVF.

High rates of chromosomal aberrations have been reported in rescue IVM embryos [62]. A comparison of IVM with classic IVF and/or ICSI has found no differences in the incidence of congenital anomalies [63]. Although there is currently limited evidence of the long-term outcomes of children born following IVM, studies have demonstrated that the outcomes are similar to conventional IVF controls [64].

IVM suggests a valuable alternative for assisted reproductive technology in select patient populations, such as those at high risk of OHSS, delivering improved pregnancy outcomes and more efficient bench-time management compared with traditional IVM laboratory techniques. IVM is also significantly cheaper than conventional hormonal alternatives [43].

Follicle Maturation In Vitro

Primordial follicles can be grown to produce oocytes that can be fertilized. In a mouse model live offspring have been produced from such in vitro-grown oocytes [65]. A two-step culture system has been developed for human primordial follicle activation and growth to the second stage within cortical pieces [66]. Other groups have demonstrated the developmental potential of growing isolated human multilaminar follicles in vitro [67] and have confirmed that they can develop from the preantral to the antral stage in a two-step culture system, where they resume meiosis and reach MII [68]. An in vitro model of ovarian follicle development is characterized by accelerated follicular maturation, which is associated with improved developmental competence of the oocyte, compared with follicles recovered in vivo [69]. A four-step combined (in vitro follicle growth and oocyte IVM) culture system was developed. The system requires the removal of growing follicles, which are then cultured in a serum-free medium for 8 days (Step 1). At the end of this period, the secondary/multilaminar follicles are dissected from the strips, and intact 100–150 μm in diameter follicles are selected for further culture. Isolated follicles are cultured individually in serum-free medium in the presence of 100 ng/ml human recombinant activin A (Step 2). Individual follicles are monitored and after 8 days, and cumulus–oocyte complexes are retrieved by application of gentle pressure on the cultured follicles. Complexes with complete CCs and adherent mural GCs are selected and cultured in the presence of FSH and activin A for an additional 4 days (Step 3). At the end of Step 3, complexes containing oocytes more than 100 μm in diameter are selected for IVM in medium (Step 4). In vitro-grown human oocytes progress to MII after a total of 20 days in culture, starting from primordial/unilaminar follicles [70].

Significantly more genes involved in "response to stimulus," "secretion," and "extracellular matrix" are identified in CCs, suggesting that CCs are more active in cell-to-cell communication processes than the oocyte. Conversely, genes annotated "reproduction," "ubiquitin ligase complex," "microtubule-associated complex," "microtubule motor activity," "nucleic acid binding," and "ligase activity" are significantly more frequently associated with genes overexpressed in oocytes, in agreement with the major processes involved in meiosis and implying attachment of microtubules to chromosomes and APC/C regulation [14].

APC/C regulates the migration of the MI spindle to the oocyte membrane, which is necessary for the extrusion of the first PB, which expresses the maturity status of the oocyte. An oocyte displaying a first PB is not necessarily expressed at the MII stage, because still immature telophase I oocytes may show a first PB as well. Both the proximity of the spindle to the oocyte cortex and the interchromosomal spacing within MII spindles influence PB size [71]. Wider spacing of chromosomes and loss of spindle contact with the oocyte cortex leads to extrusion of PBs of unusually large sizes compared with controls [72].

In Vitro Activation (IVA) of Ovary

A recently developed technology of IVA can be implemented in women with primary ovarian insufficiency (POI), diminishing ovarian reserve (DOR), and in low responders with healthy dormant follicles.

Suggested IVA procedure: resected ovarian tissue is dissected to remove residual medulla from the cortex. The cortical layer is cut into strips (10×10 mm, 1–2 mm thick) and fragmented into 1–2 mm^3 cubes. Ovarian splitting could disrupt the ovarian Hippo signaling pathway (the major suppressor of tissue overgrowth), and also lead to ovarian follicle growth [73]. The cortical tissue cubes are then treated with a phosphatase and tensin (PTEN) homolog inhibitor (PTEN inhibition results in activation of primordial follicles) and activators of phosphatidylinositol-3-kinase (PI3K) and serine/threonine-specific protein kinase (AKT) for 2 days to generate massive dormant follicles growth [74]. Both PI3K and AKT interact with intracellular signaling pathways involved in cellular growth, proliferation, and differentiation. Activated ovarian cubes are then transplanted into tubal serosa or an intact ovary [75]. After IVA, the first sign of follicle growth is an elevation of E_2 levels. When growing follicles reach 14–18 mm in diameter, patients are injected with 10 000–20 000 IU hCG to induce oocyte maturation before oocyte retrieval. Doses of hCG used are higher than in regular IVF stimulation protocols due to poor vasculature of grafts.

Early stages of POI and DOR patients show spontaneous activation of dormant primordial follicles reaching the secondary stage, secondary follicle growth, and could be promoted to patients using drug-free IVA without tissue culture [76]. For patients with ovaries containing residual secondary follicles, it is likely that the fragmentation step (Hippo signaling disruption) alone is enough to promote follicle growth [77]. Pregnancy was achieved in a patient with POI, following drug-free IVA without tissue culture. After the ovarian tissue transplantation, treatment with a GnRH agonist and human menopausal gonadotropin led to the growth of preovulatory follicles, followed by retrieval of oocytes [78].

References

1. Eppig JJ, Telfer EE. Isolation and culture of oocytes. *Methods Enzymol.* 1993; **225**:77–84.

2. Eppig JJ, O'Brien MJ. Development in vitro of mouse oocytes from primordial follicles. *Biol. Reprod.* 1996; **54**:197–207.

3. Edwards RG. Maturation in vitro of human ovarian oocytes. *Lancet.* 1965; **2**:926–929.

4. Cha KY, Koo JJ, Ko JJ, et al. Pregnancy after in vitro fertilization of human follicular oocytes collected from nonstimulated cycles, their culture in vitro and their transfer in a donor oocyte program. *Fertil. Steril.* 1991; **55**:109–113.

5. Trounson A, Wood C, Kausche A. In vitro maturation and the fertilization and developmental competence of oocytes recovered from untreated polycystic ovarian patients. *Fertil. Steril.* 1994; **62**:353–362.

6. Benkhalifa M, Demirol A, Ménézo Y, et al. Natural cycle IVF and oocyte in-vitro maturation in polycystic ovary syndrome: a collaborative prospective study. *RBM Online* 2009; **18**:29–36.

7. Son WY, Tan SL. Laboratory and embryological aspects of hCG-primed in vitro maturation cycles for patients with polycystic ovaries. *Hum. Reprod. Update* 2010; **16**:675–689.

8. Hreinsson J, Rosenlund B, Fridén B, et al. Recombinant LH is equally effective as recombinant hCG in promoting oocyte maturation in a clinical in-vitro maturation programme: a randomized study. *Hum. Reprod.* 2003; **18**:2131–2136.

9. Söderström-Anttila V, Mäkinen S, Tuuri T, Suikkari AM. Favourable pregnancy results with insemination of in vitro matured oocytes from unstimulated patients. *Hum. Reprod.* 2005; **20**:1534–1540.

10. Walls ML, Junk S, Ryan JP, Hart R. IVF versus ICSI for the fertilization of in-vitro matured human oocytes. *RBM Online* 2012; **25**:603–607.

11. Walls ML, Douglas K, Ryan JP, Tan J, Hart R. In-vitro maturation and cryopreservation of oocytes at the time of oophorectomy. *Gynecol. Oncol. Rep.* 2015; **13**:79–81.

12. Sela-Abramovich S, Edry I, Galiani D, Nevo N, Dekel N. Disruption of gap junctional communication within the ovarian follicle induces oocyte maturation. *Endocrinology* 2006;**147**:2280–2286.

13. Mehlmann L. Signaling for meiotic resumption in granulosa cells, cumulus cells, and oocyte. In: Coticchio G, Albertini DF, De Santis L, eds., *Oogenesis*. London: Springer. 2013; 171–182.

14. Matzuk M, Li Q. How the oocyte influences follicular cell function and why. In: Coticchio G, Albertini DF, De Santis L, eds., *Oogenesis*. London: Springer. 2013; 75–92.

15. Wang S, Ning G, Chen X, et al. PDE5 modulates oocyte spontaneous maturation via cGMP-cAMP but not cGMP-PKG signaling. *Front. Biosci.* 2008;**13**:7087–7095.

16. Assou S, Anahory T, Pantesco V, et al. The human cumulus-oocyte complex gene-expression profile. *Hum. Reprod.* 2006; **21**:1705–1719.

17. Conti M, Hsieh M, Zamah AM, Oh JS. Novel signaling mechanisms in the ovary during oocyte maturation and ovulation. *Mol. Cell. Endocrinol.* 2012; **356**:65–73.

18. Robinson JW, Zhang M, Shuhaibar LC, et al. Luteinizing hormone reduces the activity of the NPR2 guanylyl cyclase in mouse ovarian follicles, contributing to the cyclic GMP decrease that promotes resumption of meiosis in oocytes. *Dev. Biol.* 2012; **366**:308–316.

19. Hyslop LA, Nixon VL, Levasseur M, et al. Ca(2+)-promoted cyclin B1 degradation in mouse oocytes requires the establishment of a metaphase arrest. *Dev. Biol.* 2004; **269**:206–219.

20. Bar-Ami S, Zlotkin E, Brandes JM, Itskovitz-Eldor J. Failure of meiotic competence in human oocytes. *Biol. Reprod.* 1994; **50**:1100–1107.

21. Lincoln AJ, Wickramasinghe D, Stein P, et al. Cdc25b phosphatase is required for resumption of meiosis during oocyte maturation. *Nat. Genet.* 2002; **30**:446–449.

22. Masciarelli S, Horner K, Liu C, et al. Cyclic nucleotide phosphodiesterase 3A-deficient mice as a model of female infertility. *J. Clin. Invest.* 2004; **114**:196–205.

23. Fan HY, Sun QY, Zou H. Regulation of separase in meiosis: separase is activated at the metaphase I-II transition in *Xenopus* oocytes during meiosis. *Cell Cycle* 2006; **5**:198–204.

24. Winston NJ. Stability of cyclin B protein during meiotic maturation and the first mitotic cell division in mouse oocytes. *Biol. Cell* 1997; **89**:211–219.

25. Furuya M, Tanaka M, Teranishi T, et al. H1foo is indispensable for meiotic maturation of the mouse oocyte. *J. Reprod. Dev.* 2007; **53**:895–902.

26. Nasmyth K. How do so few control so many? *Cell* 2005; **120**:739–746.

27. Libby BJ, De La Fuente R, O'Brien MJ, et al. The mouse meiotic mutation mei1 disrupts chromosome synapsis with sexually dimorphic consequences for meiotic progression. *Dev. Biol.* 2002; **242**:174–187.

28. Madgwick S, Jones K. How eggs arrest at metaphase II: MPF stabilisation plus APC/C inhibition equals cytostatic factor. *Cell Div.* 2007; **2**:4.

29. Shoji S, Yoshida N, Amanai M, et al. Mammalian Emi2 mediates cytostatic arrest and transduces the signal for meiotic exit via Cdc20. *EMBO J.* 2006; **25**:834–845.

30. Araki K, Naito K, Haraguchi S, et al. Meiotic abnormalities of c-mos knockout mouse oocytes: activation after first meiosis or entrance into third meiotic metaphase. *Biol. Reprod.* 1996; **55**:1315–1324.

31. Saunders CM, Larman MG, Parrington J, et al. PLC zeta: a sperm-specific trigger of Ca(2+) oscillations in

eggs and embryo development. *Development* 2002; **129**:3533–3544.

32. Madgwick S, Nixon VL, Chang HY, et al. Maintenance of sister chromatid attachment in mouse eggs through maturation-promoting factor activity. *Dev. Biol.* 2004; **275**:68–81.

33. Madgwick S, Levasseur M, Jones KT. Calmodulin-dependent protein kinase II, and not protein kinase C, is sufficient for triggering cell-cycle resumption in mammalian eggs. *J. Cell Sci.* 2005; **118**:3849–3859.

34. Kuliev A, Verlinsky Y. Meiotic and mitotic nondisjunction: lessons from preimplantation genetic diagnosis. *Hum. Reprod. Update* 2004; **10**:401–407.

35. Gull I, Geva E, Lerner-Geva L, et al. Anaerobic glycolysis. The metabolism of the preovulatory human oocyte. *Eur. J. Obstet. Gynecol. Reprod. Biol.* 1999; **85**:225–228.

36. Sutton-McDowall ML, Gilchrist RB, Thompson JG. The pivotal role of glucose metabolism in determining oocyte developmental competence. *Reproduction* 2010; **139**:685–695.

37. Cetica P, Pintos L, Dalvit G, Beconi M. Activity of key enzymes involved in glucose and triglyceride catabolism during bovine oocyte maturation in vitro. *Reproduction* 2002; **124**:675–681.

38. Sugiura K, Su YQ, Diaz FJ, et al. Oocyte-derived BMP15 and FGFs cooperate to promote glycolysis in cumulus cells. *Development* 2007; **134**:2593–2603.

39. Paczkowski M, Silva E, Schoolcraft W, Krisher R. Comparative importance of fatty acid beta-oxidation to nuclear maturation, gene expression, and glucose metabolism in mouse, bovine, and porcine cumulus oocyte complexes. *Biol. Reprod.* 2013; **88**:111.

40. Dunning KR, Anastasi MR, Zhang VJ, Russell DL, Robker RL. Regulation of fatty acid oxidation in mouse cumulus-oocyte complexes during maturation and modulation by PPAR agonists. *PLoS One* 2014; **9**: e87327.

41. Bedaiwy MA, Elnashar SA, Goldberg JM, et al. Effect of follicular fluid oxidative stress parameters on intracytoplasmic sperm injection outcome. *Gynecol. Endocrinol.* 2012; **28**:51–55.

42. Palini S, Benedetti S, Tagliamonte MC, et al. Influence of ovarian stimulation for IVF/ICSI on the antioxidant defence system and relationship to outcome. *RBM Online* 2014; **29**:65–71.

43. Ellenbogen A, Shavit T, Shalom-Paz E. IVM results are comparable and may have advantages over standard IVF. *Facts Views Vis. Obgyn.* 2014; **6**:77–80.

44. Flageole C, Toufaily C, Bernard DJ, et al. Successful in vitro maturation of oocytes in a woman with gonadotropin-resistant ovary syndrome associated with a novel combination of FSH receptor gene

variants: a case report. *J. Assist. Reprod. Genet.* 2019; **36**:425–432. doi:10.1007/s10815-018-1394-z.

45. Gremeau AS, Andreadis N, Fatum M, et al. In vitro maturation or in vitro fertilization for women with polycystic ovaries? A case-control study of 194 treatment cycles. *Fertil. Steril.* 2012; **98**:355–360.

46. Guzmán L, Adriaenssens T, Ortega-Hrepich C, et al. Human antral follicles <6 mm: a comparison between in vivo maturation and in vitro maturation in non-hCG primed cycles using cumulus cell gene expression. *Mol. Hum. Reprod.* 2013; **19**:7–16.

47. Junk SM, Yeap D. Improved implantation and ongoing pregnancy rates after single-embryo transfer with an optimized protocol for in vitro oocyte maturation in women with polycystic ovaries and polycystic ovary syndrome. *Fertil. Steril.* 2012; **98**:888–892.

48. Sánchez F, Lolicato F, Romero S, et al. An improved IVM method for cumulus-oocyte complexes from small follicles in polycystic ovary syndrome patients enhances oocyte competence and embryo yield. *Hum. Reprod.* 2017; **32**:2056–2068.

49. Fadini R, Dal Canto MB, Renzini MM, et al. Effect of different gonadotrophin priming on IVM of oocytes from women with normal ovaries: a prospective randomized study. *RBM Online* 2009; **19**:343–351.

50. Ortega-Hrepich C, Stoop D, Guzmán L, et al. A "freeze-all" embryo strategy after in vitro maturation: a novel approach in women with polycystic ovary syndrome? *Fertil. Steril.* 2013; **100**:1002–1007.

51. Walls ML, Hunter T, Ryan JP, et al. In vitro maturation as an alternative to standard in vitro fertilization for patients diagnosed with polycystic ovaries: a comparative analysis of fresh, frozen and cumulative cycle outcomes. *Hum. Reprod.* 2015; **30**:88–96.

52. Menezo Y, Nicollet B, Rollet J, Hazout A. Pregnancy and delivery after in vitro maturation of naked ICSI-GV oocytes with GH and transfer of a frozen thawed blastocyst: case report. *J. Assist. Reprod. Genet.* 2006; **23**:47–49.

53. Roberts R, Iatropoulou A, Ciantar D, et al. Follicle-stimulating hormone affects metaphase I chromosome alignment and increases aneuploidy in mouse oocytes matured in vitro. *Biol. Reprod.* 2005; **72**:107–118.

54. Chen J, Torcia S, Xie F, et al. Somatic cells regulate maternal mRNA translation and developmental competence of mouse oocytes. *Nat. Cell Biol.* 2013; **15**:1415–1423.

55. Trounson A, Anderiesz C, Jones G. Maturation of human oocytes in vitro and their developmental competence. *Reproduction* 2001; **121**:51–75.

56. Camargo LSA, Munk M, Sales JN, et al. Differential gene expression between in vivo and in vitro

maturation: a comparative study with bovine oocytes derived from the same donor pool. *JBRA Assist. Reprod.* 2019; **23**:7–14. doi:10.5935/1518-0557.20180084.

57. Jones GM, Cram DS, Song B, et al. Gene expression profiling of human oocytes following in vivo or in vitro maturation. *Hum. Reprod.* 2008; **23**:1138–1144.

58. Coticchio G, Dal Canto M, Fadini R, et al. Ultrastructure of human oocytes after in vitro maturation. *Mol. Hum. Reprod.* 2016; **22**:110–118.

59. De Vincentiis S, De Martino E, Buffone MG, Brugo-Olmedo S. Use of metaphase I oocytes matured in vitro is associated with embryo multinucleation. *Fertil. Steril.* 2013; **99**:414–421.

60. Margalit T, Ben-Haroush A, Garor R, et al. Morphokinetic characteristics of embryos derived from in-vitro-matured oocytes and their in-vivo-matured siblings after ovarian stimulation. *RBM Online* 2019; **38**:7–11.

61. Lee HJ, Barad DH, Kushnir VA, et al. Rescue in vitro maturation (IVM) of immature oocytes in stimulated cycles in women with low functional ovarian reserve (LFOR). *Endocrine* 2016; **52**:165–171.

62. Zhang XY, Ata B, Son WY, et al. Chromosome abnormality rates in human embryos obtained from in-vitro maturation and IVF treatment cycles. *RBM Online* 2010; **21**:552–559.

63. Chian RC, Xu CL, Huang JY, Ata B. Obstetric outcomes and congenital abnormalities in infants conceived with oocytes matured in vitro. *Facts Views Vis. Obgyn.* 2014; **6**:15–18.

64. Roesner S, von Wolff M, Elsaesser M, et al. Two-year development of children conceived by IVM: a prospective controlled single-blinded study. *Hum. Reprod.* 2017; **32**:1341–1350.

65. O'Brien MJ, Pendola JK, Eppig JJ. A revised protocol for in vitro development of mouse oocytes from primordial follicles dramatically improves their developmental competence. *Biol. Reprod.* 2003; **68**:1682–1686.

66. Telfer EE, McLaughlin M, Ding C, Thong KJ. A two-step serum-free culture system supports development of human oocytes from primordial follicles in the presence of activin. *Hum. Reprod.* 2008; **23**:1151–1158.

67. Xu M, Barrett SL, West-Farrell E, et al. In vitro grown human ovarian follicles from cancer patients support oocyte growth. *Hum. Reprod.* 2009; **24**:2531–2540.

68. Xiao S, Zhang J, Romero MM, et al. In vitro follicle growth supports human oocyte meiotic maturation. *Sci. Rep.* 2015; **5**:17323.

69. Cadoret V, Frapsauce C, Jarrier P, et al. Molecular evidence that follicle development is accelerated *in vitro* compared to *in vivo*. *Reproduction* 2017; **153**:493–508.

70. McLaughlin M, Albertini DF, Wallace WHB, Anderson RA, Telfer EE. Metaphase II oocytes from human unilaminar follicles grown in a multi-step culture system. *Mol. Hum. Reprod.* 2018; **24**:135–142.

71. Barrett SB, Albertini DF. Cumulus cell contact during oocyte maturation in mice regulates meiotic spindle positioning and enhances developmental potential. *J. Assist. Reprod. Genet.* 2010; **27**:29–39.

72. Coticchio G, Guglielmo MC, Dal Canto M, et al. Mechanistic foundations of the metaphase II spindle of human oocytes matured in vivo and in vitro. *Hum. Reprod.* 2013; **28**:3271–3282.

73. Li J, Kawamura K, Cheng Y, et al. Activation of dormant ovarian follicles to generate mature eggs. *Proc. Natl.Acad. Sci. U. S. A.* 2010, **107**:10280–10284.

74. Reddy P, Liu L, Adhikari D, et al. Oocyte-specific deletion of *Pten* causes premature activation of the primordial follicle pool. *Science* 2008; **319**:611–613.

75. Kawamura K, Kawamura N, Hsueh A. Activation of dormant follicles: a new treatment for premature ovarian failure? *Curr. Opin. Obstet. Gynecol.* 2016; **28**:217–222.

76. Kawamura K, Ishizuka B, Hsueh A. Drug-free in-vitro activation of follicles for infertility treatment in poor ovarian response patients with decreased ovarian reserve. *RBM Online* 2020; **40**:245–253.

77. Kawashima I, Kawamura K. Regulation of follicle growth through hormonal factors and mechanical cues mediated by Hippo signaling pathway. *Syst. Biol. Reprod. Med.* 2018; **64**:3–11.

78. Fabregues F, Ferreri J, Calafell JM, et al. Pregnancy after drug-free in vitro activation of follicles and fresh tissue autotransplantation in primary ovarian insufficiency patient: a case report and literature review. *J. Ovarian Res.* 2018; **11**:76.

Chapter 14

Biopsy of Testicles

Testicular Spermatozoa

Historically, the absence or a small number of sperm cells in the ejaculate often precluded men from fathering their genetic progeny and relegated couples to the use of donor spermatozoa insemination or adoption or childlessness. With the development of intracytoplasmic sperm injection (ICSI), men with azoospermia (absence of sperm cells in the ejaculate) or severe oligozoospermia (less than 5×10^6 spermatozoa in the ejaculate) are able to father a child following single sperm cell injection into the cytoplasm of a single oocyte. In the years after the development of ICSI, it was discovered that sperm cells retrieved directly from testicular tissue can also be used for oocyte fertilization and enable healthy embryo development.

Azoospermia is defined by a lack of spermatozoa in ejaculate identified in two separate semen specimens directly examined following centrifugation and volume condensation. While azoospermia is rare, affecting approximately 1% of the male population [1], approximately 10–15% of all infertile men are diagnosed as azoospermic [2]. Azoospermia can result due to a blockage anywhere along the sperm transit path, i.e., the efferent ducts, epididymis, vas deferens, ejaculatory duct, and urethra. When these problems in sperm cells delivery occur, azoospermia is classified as obstructive azoospermia (OA). The majority of OA cases can be determined by the patient's medical history and physical examination alone. Other conditions that can be determined based on a review of readily available clinical evidence include vasal obstruction from prior hernia repair, congenital vassal agenesis, prior extirpative pelvic surgery, and ejaculatory duct obstruction.

Azoospermia can be classified into three categories: pre-testicular, testicular, and post-testicular. Pre-testicular causes of azoospermia include endocrine abnormalities with adverse effects on spermatogenesis (secondary testicular failure). Testicular causes of azoospermia (primary testicular failure) include disorders of spermatogenesis intrinsic to the testes. Post-testicular reasons of azoospermia relate to ejaculatory dysfunction or ductal obstruction that impairs sperm cell transit (Figure 14.1).

Cases in which the testicles do not produce spermatozoa at all or produce too few sperm cells are classified as nonobstructive azoospermia (NOA). NOA is due to defective spermatogenesis and can be classified as hypospermatogenesis, maturation arrest, or Sertoli cell-only syndrome. Defective spermatogenesis may be due to genetic abnormalities such as Y chromosome microdeletions or karyotype abnormalities but is largely idiopathic (Figure 14.2) [3]. Thus, men with NOA have fewer therapeutic options and reproduction relies on surgical spermatozoa retrieval. Common conditions that cause NOA include current or prior usage of exogenous testosterone, history of undescended testes, history of malignancy and chemotherapy, current malignancy, genetic anomalies, environmental exposures, and pituitary dysfunction.

The ability to use limited numbers of testicular or epididymal sperm cells for ICSI brought a dramatic revolution in the management of couples with azoospermia. However, low embryo quality and incidence of direct uneven cleavage of embryos have been observed to be higher after ICSI with sperm cell biopsy retrieved from azoospermic males [4], compared with normozoospermic males.

The important difference of OA from NOA is that sperm cell retrieval techniques are always successful in locating sperm cells from OA patients, while locating sperm cells from NOA patients is challenging, in the best circumstances, and can be impossible in some.

Examination of several preoperative variables, including follicle-stimulating hormone (FSH) and luteinizing hormone (LH) levels, and testicular size and volume, was initially employed to diagnose the category of azoospermia and predict the outcome of sperm cell retrieval. However, later, these factors were demonstrated to have low sensitivity and specificity in

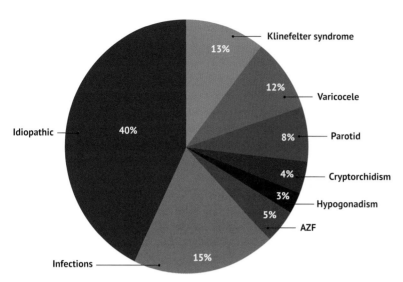

Figure 14.1 Etiology of azoospermia. AZF, azoospermia factor.

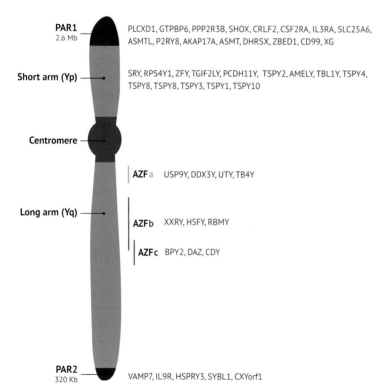

Figure 14.2 Genetic composition of chromosome Y.

predicting the success of sperm cell retrieval [5]. Testosterone, while not very useful as an isolated test, is helpful in relation to FSH, LH, prolactin, and estradiol levels in determining the overall function of the male reproductive gonadal–pituitary system. Analyses of FSH (most experts consider FSH >7.6 mIU/ml as abnormal for spermatogenesis) and LH levels have been shown to differentiate OA from NOA with some degree of accuracy. While a semen analysis is, in most cases, a crude indicator of a man's fertility potential, the consistent finding of a total absence of sperm cells on multiple analyses indicates that the man is infertile. Semen parameters such as pH, semen volume, and the presence/absence of fructose are additional and useful clinical data [6].

Men with low ejaculate volume should repeat the semen analysis, paying close attention to complete and proper collection after a 2–3-day abstinence [7]. In men with low ejaculate volume (less than 1.5 ml) and normal FSH and testis volume, evaluation of the collection process, and post-ejaculate urine analysis to evaluate possible retrograde ejaculation are essential first steps. Usually, millions of sperm cells found in the post-ejaculate urine manifest retrograde ejaculation. When men with low ejaculate volume, oligozoospermia or azoospermia, and palpable vasa do not suffer from retrograde ejaculation and semen pH is <7.2, a transrectal ultrasound (TRUS) to evaluate dilation of seminal vesicles or ejaculatory ducts is a useful diagnostic test to identify ejaculatory duct obstruction [8]. TRUS is a vital tool in the evaluation of men with azoospermia. Ejaculatory duct obstruction is an unusual and difficult-to-diagnose disorder. On transrectal ultrasonography, one can often, but by no means always, see dilated seminal vesicles and a dilated ejaculatory duct. While there are no absolute diagnostic features for this condition, when a patient has sufficient findings (e.g., midline prostatic cyst, dilation of the seminal vesicle, and seminal vesicle agenesis), obstruction is likely to have occurred. Additional seminal indicators of ejaculatory duct obstruction are seminal acidic pH (<7.2) and fructose absence, whereas at normal status seminal vesicle secretions are alkaline and contain fructose.

Because normal vas (ductus) can be easily palpated within the scrotum, the diagnosis of unilateral or bilateral vasal agenesis is made by physical examination. Approximately 25% of men with unilateral vasal agenesis and about 10–15% with congenital bilateral absence of the vas deferens (CBAVD) usually have unilateral renal agenesis, which can be identified by ultrasonography [9]. In azoospermic men with unilateral vasal agenesis, TRUS may assist in demonstrating a related contralateral segmental atresia of the seminal vesicle or vas deferens [10]. There is a robust association between CBAVD and mutations of the cystic fibrosis transmembrane conductance regulator (CFTR) gene [11]; almost all men with clinical cystic fibrosis have CBAVD. Conversely, at least three-quarters of men with CBAVD have mutations of the CFTR gene [12]. However, failure to detect a CFTR abnormality in a man with CBAVD does not completely rule out a mutation entirely, because 10–40% are undetectable using conventional clinically available methods. Rates of CFTR mutations are not higher in patients with renal anomalies and unilateral or bilateral vassal agenesis compared with the overall population [13–14]; these patients likely have a non-CFTR etiology for these anomalies. Most men with CBAVD have regular spermatogenesis, but other potential coexisting causes of impaired spermatogenesis must be investigated before collecting sperm cells for assisted reproduction [15].

In azoospermic men with average semen volume, serum FSH and testicular volume are the most important determinants of whether a diagnostic testicular biopsy may help assess spermatogenesis. A marked increase in serum FSH and low testicular volume strongly suggest NOA. Although serum FSH levels reflect the predominant pattern of spermatogenesis, they may not reflect isolated areas of spermatogenesis within the testis and are not related to the more advanced stages of spermatogenesis. The relationship between FSH and the presence of any spermatogenesis is not straightforward in men with NOA. Some men with normal-ejaculate-volume azoospermia have a regular testicular test, normal FSH, and a testicular biopsy that exhibits a spermatogenesis defect (most often maturation arrest). These men have NOA and should not be offered scrotal exploration and reconstruction. Inhibin B has also been found to be slightly more sensitive than FSH as an index of spermatogenic status. However, it was concluded that the inhibin B level alone, or in combination with the serum FSH level, fails to predict successful biopsy for spermatozoa in patients with NOA. By the evaluation of the azoospermic male, the key question is whether spermatogenesis is occurring in the testes and to what degree.

In general, testicular tissue may be sampled for diagnostic purposes via multi-site fine-needle aspiration (or "testicular mapping") and open testicular biopsy. The success of sperm cell retrieval is dependent on the status of spermatogenesis in the testes, rendering it essential to characterize the status [16]. Testicular sperm aspiration (TESA) or testicular fine-needle aspiration (TFNA) are aspirations performed using a butterfly needle of 21 gauge or thinner attached to a 20 ml syringe. The testis is punctured and negative pressure is applied on the syringe primed with nutrient medium. The needle is moved back and forth four to five times in different directions without removing it from the puncture site. The negative pressure is then reduced over 30–60 seconds and the needle is withdrawn. Any protruding tubules from the puncture site are transferred to a small plate or tube containing a sperm nutrient medium. The procedure enables minimally invasive sampling of the tubules from various portions of the testis. An ideal sperm cell retrieval method should allow for retrieval of sufficient spermatozoa with minimal trauma and with a single intervention. Usually, 10–20 needle passes are required to obtain adequate specimens by TESA/TFNA. Sperm cell retrieval rates vary depending upon the type of azoospermia, with success rates of ~100% in OA patients and only about 30% success in NOA cases [17].

Testicular sperm extraction (TESE) differs from TESA in that it requires an incision to reach the testicular tissue. During the TESE method the hemiscrotum is opened and the testis is extruded to the surface of the incision point, the protruding tissue is excised sharply and placed in sperm nutrient medium. The process is repeated several times in other areas of the testis. Obtained testicular tissue is then processed in the laboratory. Two 23–25 gauge insulin needles on 1 ml insulin syringes are bent to 70–80 degrees. These bent needles are used to press and spread the testicular tissue and tubules. Within a few minutes, a delicate suspension with very little particulate matter is obtained. The suspension is drawn up leaving the tissue fragments behind. The suspension is allowed to settle in the tube for 0.5–1 hour at room temperature, and the supernatant is aspirated, without debris, and then centrifuged at 900 × g for 5 minutes, and the formatted pellet is resuspended in a small volume (~50 µl) of sperm medium. Droplets of 5 µl are placed in an ICSI dish. The testicular suspension is kept at <37°C. Storing human testicular tissue at 37°C causes a significant increase in the number of apoptotic cells [18].

For all azoospermia patients, the remaining testicular tissue fragments should be tested by a pathologist for conclusive determination of azoospermia type and for possible early cancer diagnosis. The European Germ Cell Cancer Consensus Group recommends the use of Stieve's or Bouin's solution for the fixation of testicular tissue [19]. Testicular germ cell tumor (TGCT) is the most common cancer in men aged 15–40 years. The incidence of TGCT has more than doubled over the past 50 years; however, the underlying etiology is unknown. Tumors are found in 4% of men who present to the fertility center for infertility evaluation and 50% of men with testis cancer are infertile/subfertile at the time of diagnosis [20–21]. Carcinoma *in situ* (CIS) is challenging to identify in testicular biopsies. Several markers for CIS of the testis have been developed, including placental alkaline phosphatase, AP2-gamma, and stem cell factor receptor c-KIT. OCT3/4 is a highly specific marker for CIS and currently the best marker for noninvasive diagnosis [22].

Today, TESE is the most frequently used technique for sperm cell extraction in azoospermic men with a mean sperm cell recovery rate of ~50% [23]. Repeat TESE has been found to be progressively more difficult and a minimum 6-month period is recommended between repeat procedures [24]. For men with ongoing spermatogenesis, sperm cell banking must be offered as a first-line management, therefore in azoospermic men cryopreservation of a testicular biopsy provides the option of using testicular spermatozoa for fertilization after thawing.

Obstructive Azoospermia (OA)

In the case of an obstruction somewhere along the sperm journey path, spermatozoa can be obtained from the epididymis or the testicular tissue. The epididymis is readily imaged on ultrasound and epididymal pathology can easily be determined. As the typical thickness of a human epididymal head is in the 7–8 mm range, enlargement can be an indication of an obstructive etiology [25]. Missing epididymis segments or total absence of the epididymis on ultrasound suggest an obstructive etiology as well. Solid tumors of the epididymis, though rare, would also suggest an obstructive etiology. As genital tract infection can also cause epididymal obstruction, the ultrasound findings may differentiate between OA and NOA, rather than a singular find.

Percutaneous epididymal sperm cell aspiration (PESA) for ICSI was described in 1994 by Tsirigotis and colleagues [26]. It offers a relatively fast, minimally invasive, and relatively inexpensive method for sperm cell retrieval and is the first choice due to its minimally invasive nature. Epididymal sperm cells offer the advantage of great maturity and motility relative to testicular sperm cells. The PESA technique is similar to that of TESA. The needle is moved back and forth inside the epididymis. Once the fluid is seen just above the needle hub, it is expelled into a tube with a sperm nutrient medium. If PESA does not retrieve sperm cells, microsurgical epididymal sperm cell aspiration (MESA) is suggested in the setting of multiple prior surgeries and extensive scarring. Relative to PESA, MESA offers the advantage of controlled exposure of the epididymal tubule with the ability to extract far more significant quantities of motile sperm cells. Usually, large numbers of sperm cells can be collected from the epididymis. If a sufficient number of epididymal sperm cells are collected, density gradient centrifugation can be used to prepare the spermatozoa for assisted reproductive technology.

In the case of no spermatozoa being obtained from the epididymis, sperm cells can be retrieved from the testes by open biopsy or by percutaneous needle biopsy. TFNA, using a small butterfly needle attached to a syringe, may be used to harvest spermatozoa for ICSI, especially in men with OA. The advantage of TFNA is that it does not require surgical equipment and experience, and can be performed in an outpatient setting under local anesthesia. Testicular samples contain large numbers of non-germ cells, such as erythrocytes, leukocytes, and Sertoli cells, and therefore spermatozoa must be separated from these non-germ cells. Sperm cells collected from the testes are used for ICSI and not for classic in vitro fertilization (IVF) because the samples generally contain only small numbers of spermatozoa, with poor motility. Pentoxifylline and theophylline, phosphodiesterase inhibitors, both inhibit the breakdown of cAMP and are occasionally applied to increase the motility of epididymal and testicular spermatozoa before ICSI [27–28].

Re-evaluation of an ejaculated semen specimen on the day of planned sperm retrieval is critical for the management of men with azoospermia. Approximately 5–10% of men with presumed azoospermia bear rare sperm cells, which can be found on careful evaluation of a semen sample, using an extended sperm preparation technique. Extended sperm examination of additional microdroplets (under oil to prevent evaporation) allows observation of the entire specimen, and not merely a limited part of the sample. Identification of such rare sperm cells can avoid an unnecessary sperm cell retrieval operation.

Nonobstructive Azoospermia (NOA)

Most patients with primary testicular dysfunction resulting in azoospermia show a Sertoli cell-only pattern in their testicular histology. Others have maturation arrest or have sclerosed and/or atrophied seminiferous tubules. A few seminiferous tubules may still show occasional foci of active spermatogenesis. Incomplete Sertoli cell-only syndrome describes cases in which the current histopathology is germ cell aplasia (Sertoli cell-only syndrome), but some tubules do show active spermatogenesis. The same applies to maturation arrest: when full spermatogenesis is present in several tubules, the condition is referred to as incomplete maturation arrest. A biopsy can identify five main histological patterns of spermatogenesis: the absence of seminiferous tubules (tubular sclerosis), no germ cells within the seminiferous tubules (Sertoli cell-only syndrome), incomplete spermatogenesis (spermatogenic arrest), all germ cell stages present with decline in spermatozoa count (hypospermatogenesis), and normal spermatogenesis [22]. The diagnosis of "nonobstructive azoospermia" should be made according to the histopathological findings, rather than based on clinical indicators only, such as FSH levels or testicular size.

Histological diagnosis of NOA revealed Sertoli cell-only syndrome in 60.6% of patients, while 23.8% had hypospermatogenesis and 15.4% of patients had maturation arrest [29]. The sperm cell retrieval rate is higher in patients with hypospermatogenesis compared with patients with Sertoli cell-only syndrome or maturation arrest (88.2% vs. 30.5% and 30.9%, respectively) [29]. The observation that sperm cells could be identified in testis biopsies of men with NOA drove the development of TESE. Indeed, even the most intense forms of NOA, such as Klinefelter syndrome (XXY), were effectively treated with TESE and ICSI, with the successful sperm cell retrieval rate ranging from 27% to 69% [30]. Sperm cell retrieval rates in all cases of NOA range from 16.7% to 44.3% [29]. The use of TFNA was shown to provide limited numbers of sperm cells in men with NOA.

Multiple-biopsy sperm cell retrieval was also shown to be effective, but in some cases, up to 20 biopsies were required to identify sperm cells needed for ICSI [31]. In TESA, the aspirations are usually carried out using a needle attached to a syringe. The needle is introduced through the scrotal skin into the testis (Figure 14.3). The testicular parenchyma is

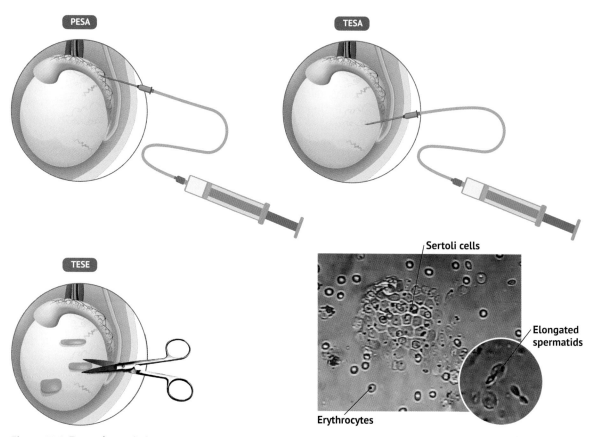

Figure 14.3 Types of testicular biopsy.

aspirated by creating negative pressure. In general, for multiple-biopsy TESE, the tunica albuginea is incised transversely at several locations of the center and upper and lower poles of each testis. The testis is then gently squeezed, and the protruding tissues are excised. The multiple-biopsy TESE results in the interruption of testicular blood supply and even to devascularization of the testis since the vessels supplying the testicular parenchyma migrate under the surface of the tunica albuginea. This operation can lead to a risk of damage to the testis.

Testicular microdissection, micro-TESE (mTESE), as developed by Schlegel and Li in 1998 [32], was a revolutionary innovative technique that has enabled men with the most severe defects in sperm cell production to become biological fathers. mTESE involves a wide transverse opening of the tunica albuginea of the testis, which exposes all areas of

seminiferous tubules for inspection under high power operative microsurgery. The technique relies on the ability of a surgical microscope to identify the individual seminiferous tubules that are engorged with sperm cells. This technique seems to offer the most comprehensive search for sperm cells in the testis of men with NOA [33]. After exposing the seminiferous tubules, a systematic search is performed with a microscope (~×20–40 magnification) (Figure 14.4). Larger tubules thought to contain sperm cells are isolated, placed into the nutrient medium, and examined. Successful mTESE, as a salvage procedure in cases of failed TESE, has been reported [34], while others have reported a limited chance of sperm cell retrieval using mTESE in such men [35]. A surgical procedure such as TESE has possible complications: hematoma, devascularization, inflammation, testicular microlithiasis, and a transient but significant decrease in total testosterone levels, which recover to

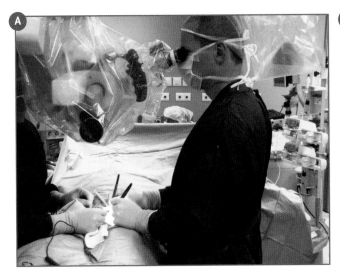

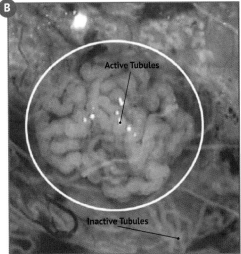

Prognostic Factor	Probability for spermatozoa
Obstructive azoospermia	100%
AZFc deletion	75%
Cryptorchidism	74%
Hypo-Hypo	73%
Klinefelter syndrome	57%
Testicular tumor	45%
Gonadotoxic agents	45%
High FSH	29%
AZF complete deletion (a/b or a+b+c)	0%

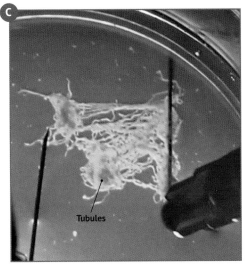

Figure 14.4 mTESE procedure. (A) mTESE under microscope control; (B) visualization of testicular active tubules; (C) spread and tearing of tubules; (D) probability of spermatozoa detection.

baseline levels between 18 and 26 months after TESE preparation [36]. The use of an operating microscope to identify the sites of sperm cell production is a more effective way of finding sperm cells compared with multi-biopsy TESE, and provides for sperm cells with less tissue removed [33]. Using microsurgical inspection, the more distended tubules can be selected for excision. mTESE is considered the standard for sperm cell retrieval among NOA patients, with the highest sperm cell retrieval rates while minimizing tissue loss [37]. Subsequent studies have documented that mTESE is 1.5-fold more effective than random

multiple-biopsy TESE, which was twofold more effective than TESA in controlled trials [38]. The vast majority of seminiferous tubules in men with NOA lack significant numbers of germ cells and demonstrate a collapsed and thin morphology on microscopic appearance. However, rare seminiferous tubules with a full complement of spermatogenesis are larger and more opaque on microscopic appearance and are therefore selected from the surrounding tubules. mTESE succeeded in increasing the sperm cell retrieval rate to the range of 42.9–63% [39]. The sperm cell retrieval was most significant from dilated seminiferous tubules (90%), followed by testes where tubules were slightly dilated (47%), and finally, from testes with no dilated tubules (7%) [40]. Another study with NOA men supported these findings and showed with mTESE a sperm cell retrieval rate of 31% among tubules less than 200 μm in diameter, compared with 44% and 84% among 200–300 μm-diameter and greater than 300 μm-diameter tubules, respectively [41]. Anatomical studies have demonstrated that the highly coiled seminiferous tubules originate and terminate in the center of the testis (in the mediastinum or intratesticular rete region), traveling out to the periphery of the testicle. A typically very fine filamentous septum separates each tubule with blood vessels running parallel to the tubules. This organization allows dissection deep within the testicular parenchyma, which, in turn, enables direct observation of nearly every region of the hundreds of seminiferous tubules within the testis. If the sperm cells are not found on one side of the testis, the other side of the testis is opened.

Stimulation of spermatogenesis with clomiphene citrate before mTESE/TESE for 3–9 months results in more sperm cells produced and a higher probability of finding sperm by mTESE/TESE [42]. Sperm cells were successfully obtained at the second mTESE in 21% of men who had negative initial mTESE and received human chorionic gonadotropin (hCG) and recombinant FSH, whereas no sperm were retrieved from untreated men; success at the second mTESE was more likely when histology at the first mTESE showed hypospermatogenesis [43]. However, others have seen no benefit of neoadjuvant medical therapy before mTESE sperm cell retrieval [44]. The level of evidence supporting the use of adjuvant hormonal therapy is still limited.

Varicocele repair before performing mTESE in men with NOA may be performed if a concurrent varicocele is clinically evident. The mean acceptable interval between varicocele repair and mTESE is 23–24 months [45]. Varicocele repair in men with oligozoospermia and azoospermia was associated with a higher pregnancy rate and with higher sperm cell retrieval rates [46].

When mTESE involves extensive dissection of testicular tissue following the anatomical evaluation of the testis, limited removal of tissue, and careful management of intratesticular structures, there are limited effects on testosterone production and testis loss. Severe damage to the testicle is not a measurable risk of mTESE [47]. An additional intervention that helps to identify rare sperm cells is an aggressive mechanical dispersion of these tissues before an attempt to examine them. A small aliquot of this dispersed tissue suspension is examined under a phase-contrast microscope at magnification (×200–400) for the detection of sperm cells. Sperm cells can be immotile immediately after retrieval, but often acquire at least twitching motility upon incubation in a sperm wash medium.

Testis histology has been found to be the most reliable predictive factor of successful sperm cell retrieval in NOA patients [29; 48]. The overall success rate of sperm cell retrieval for NOA patients stands at ~50% and is highest among men with a histological diagnosis of hypospermatogenesis (~80%) and lowest in those with Sertoli cell-only syndrome (~25%). Sperm cells are successfully retrieved in patients with mosaic Klinefelter syndrome (~65–70%) but not in patients with non-mosaic Klinefelter syndrome. There are statistically lower chances of embryo development if sperm cells have not acquired motility by the time of ICSI. Freezing of residual fresh sperm cells after ICSI is recommended since NOA men have severely limited sperm cell production.

Men with NOA should be offered genetic testing to rule out chromosomal abnormalities and Y chromosome microdeletions. Men with complete deletions involving the azoospermia factor (AZF) regions AZFa, AZFb, or AZFbc of the Y chromosome have minimal chance of sperm cell retrieval. On the other hand, men with AZFc deletions alone often have sperm cells in the ejaculate and even a chance of sperm cell retrieval. Men with NOA and history of cryptorchidism have a good chance of sperm cell retrieval. Similarly, men with Klinefelter syndrome have a good chance of sperm cell retrieval, whereas men with a history of prior chemotherapy and azoospermia have a low chance of retrieval.

Stimulation for Spermatogenesis in the Azoospermic Male

Hypogonadotropic hypogonadism is one of the reasons for NOA. Severe hypogonadotropic hypogonadism results from hypothalamic disorders such as

Kallmann syndrome, or from congenital or acquired pituitary disorders, including both functional and nonfunctional tumors, which may be associated with undetectably low gonadotropins. Also, suppression of the hypothalamic–pituitary–gonadal axis with very low or undetectable gonadotropins resulting in absence of testicular stimulation may be due to feedback inhibition secondary to exogenous testosterone or illicit anabolic androgenic steroid use. Men with bilateral testicular atrophy and hypogonadotropic hypogonadism should, therefore, be asked about previous/current use of testosterone, anabolic androgenic steroids, and workout supplements. Regardless, azoospermic men with hypogonadotropic hypogonadism should have further evaluation, including measurement of serum prolactin and pituitary imaging. Patients with hypogonadotropic hypogonadism require hormonal stimulation by FSH and LH, or pulsatile gonadotropin-releasing hormone (GnRH) to restore their fertility.

FSH is essential for initiation and maintenance of normal spermatogenesis. Lack of FSH results in defective chromatin packaging and reduction in acrosomal glycoprotein content of sperm cells. In addition, FSH may synergize with testosterone by stimulating androgen receptor synthesis. It was suggested that FSH facilitates the transport and localization of testosterone within Sertoli cells [49]. Also, high intratesticular testosterone levels are required for maintenance of spermatogenesis, are responsible for maturation of round spermatids into mature sperm cells, and maintain the adhesion between germ cells and Sertoli cells, as testosterone withdrawal leads to premature release of round spermatids. For normal spermatogenesis, higher levels of testosterone are required for androgen receptors in the testis compared with those in other androgen-dependent tissues. In conclusion, both FSH and testosterone are required for the initiation and maintenance of normal spermatogenesis.

Successful hormonal replacement therapy with hCG and human menopausal gonadotropin (hMG) in NOA or idiopathic azoospermic patients restores the average level of FSH and LH and stimulates Leydig cells in the testis to produce testosterone and initiate spermatogenesis [50]. Alternatively, pulsatile injection of GnRH can restore normal FSH and testosterone levels and lead to the successful production of sperm cells in men with hypogonadotropic hypogonadism [51]. The reason for gonadotropin administration in idiopathic azoospermia is based on its observed efficacy in the treatment of hypogonadotropic hypogonadism. However, its effectiveness in treating normogonadotropic azoospermia is uncertain; the administration of hCG and hMG in men with normal levels of FSH and LH is useless.

Targeting the imbalance between circulating levels of testosterone and estradiol has been investigated as a potential therapeutic tool in men with NOA. Aromatase converts the circulating testosterone and other androgens into estrogen within fat cells, liver, and testes. In markedly obese men, this may lead to the excessive endogenous conversion of testosterone into estrogen, resulting in a reversible imbalance in the testosterone/estradiol ratio. Estradiol suppresses the pituitary secretion of FSH and LH and consequently inhibits testosterone biosynthesis in the testes and impairs sperm cell production. Aromatase inhibitors correct the suppressive effect of estrogen on gonadotropins and testosterone production and have been suggested to improve spermatogenesis in obese men.

The success of endocrine stimulation of spermatogenesis depends mainly on the functional capacity of the testis, which is manifested by the serum levels of FSH and testosterone. High levels of FSH and LH with low or normal testosterone in azoospermic men indicate a primary testicular failure and there is no role of medical treatment. The only option for these cases is mTESE/TESE and ICSI.

It is preferred that the NOA/idiopathic patient continues on endocrine stimulation for 6 months, which is equivalent to two spermatogenic cycles, and semen analysis is advised monthly, starting from the third month of treatment. If the patient remains azoospermic after 6 months of treatment, despite the achievement of the target levels of FSH and serum testosterone, mTESE is recommended, with continued endocrine stimulation treatment up to the day of mTESE.

It was shown that tamoxifen citrate 20 mg/day treatment for 6 months significantly improved sperm parameters [52].

Genetic Counseling for Men with Azoospermia

The sperm cells retrieved from men with NOA are often more frequently cytogenetically abnormal [53]. Testicular sperm samples of NOA patients show a higher incidence of numerical chromosomal abnormalities compared with ejaculated sperm cells of control donors [54]. Genetic diagnosis has a significant impact for men with azoospermia. Genetic evaluations that include karyotype determination, genetic Y chromosome evaluation, and a cystic fibrosis panel are recommended for any man with azoospermia with no apparent underlying cause, such as prior vasectomy or use of exogenous testosterone. The presence of one or another genetic defect determines the diagnosis. Genetic testing brought a significant advance in the evaluation of azoospermia, since sperm cells can always be found in OA patients yet not in NOA patients. Deletions on the Y chromosome have been associated with 15–20% of cases of azoospermia or severe oligozoospermia. Amongst azoospermic men, 10–15% will have an abnormal number of chromosomes. Chromosomal structural anomalies, e.g., translocations, are 10 times more likely in infertile men compared with the general population [55]. Autosomal inversion of chromosome 9 is especially relevant to male infertility and presents in 3–5% of such patients. Congenital absence of the vas deferens is most often associated with mutations within the cystic fibrosis gene.

Men with 47,XXY (Klinefelter syndrome) will be NOA, while men with cystic fibrosis mutations are OA. The presence of a Y chromosome microdeletion indicates NOA.

Any genetic defect in sperm cells can be transmitted to the embryo and couples must be counseled accordingly upon learning about transmissibility. Also, preimplantation genetic testing, testing the embryo for the presence of a specific gene defect, has become routinely available, even in community IVF centers, and, armed with this information, the couple counseled by medical staff can decide which embryo to implant.

Genetic Testing for Men with NOA

The reasons for male infertility are often multifactorial, with approximately 50% of cases involving genetic abnormalities. Chromosomal abnormalities can be identified by the karyotype of peripheral leukocytes in approximately 7% of azoospermic men. Karyotype analysis reveals broad-scale genetic abnormalities, such as deletions of whole chromosomes or substantial portions of a chromosome, as well as translocations. The occurrence of such abnormalities relates inversely to the sperm cell concentration and has been reported to be 10–15% in azoospermic men, approximately 5% in oligozoospermic men, and less than 1% in men having average sperm cell concentrations [56]. Sex chromosome aneuploidy (e.g., Klinefelter syndrome) forms about two-thirds of chromosomal abnormalities observed in infertile men. Men with Klinefelter syndrome are prone to other medical problems besides infertility. Many of these men have low to low-to-normal testosterone levels. The prevalence of structural abnormalities in the autosomes, such as translocations and inversions, is also higher in infertile men than in the general population.

The Y chromosome contains vital components of male differentiation and sperm cell function. Y chromosome microdeletions are too small to detect by karyotyping but can be identified using polymerase chain reaction techniques. Most Y chromosome microdeletions occur in long-arm regions designated as AZFa, AZFb, or AZFc. Deletions in these sites are responsible for varying degrees of spermatogenic dysfunction and are found in 10–15% of men with azoospermia or severe oligozoospermia [57]. Sperm cells can be present in the ejaculate of men with deletions in the AZFc region, while others with deletions in the AZFc region are azoospermic, but still may have sufficient sperm cell production to enable sperm cell extraction by conventional or microsurgical testicular sampling [58]. However, deletions involving the AZFa or AZFb regions are associated with inferior sperm cell retrieval prognosis, and as such, sperm cell retrieval should not be attempted in these patients [59]. Sons of men with AZFc deletions will inherit the abnormality and will likely be severely oligozoospermic or azoospermic [60]. Although Y chromosome microdeletions are not known to be associated with other health problems, data concerning the phenotypes of sons of men with such abnormalities are still quite limited [60].

Therefore, men with NOA should be tested for karyotyping and Y chromosome microdeletions analysis, and receive genetic counseling, if necessary, before their sperm cells are used for ICSI [61].

References

1. Stephen EH, Chandra A. Declining estimates of infertility in the United States: 1982–2002. *Fertil. Steril.* 2006; **86**:516–523.

2. Jarow JP, Espeland MA, Lipshultz LI. Evaluation of the azoospermic patient. *J. Urol.* 1989; **142**:62–65.

3. Dohle GR, Halley DJ, Van Hemel JO et al. Genetic risk factors in infertile men with severe oligozoospermia and azoospermia. *Hum. Reprod.* 2002; **17**:13–16.

4. Desai N, Gill P, Tadros NN, et al. Azoospermia and embryo morphokinetics: testicular sperm-derived embryos exhibit delays in early cell cycle events and increased arrest prior to compaction. *J. Assist. Reprod. Genet.* 2018; **35**:1339–1348.

5. Carpi A, Sabanegh E, Mechanick J. Controversies in the management of nonobstructive azoospermia. *Fertil. Steril.* 2009; **91**:963–970.

6. Singer R, Sagiv M, Barnet M, Levinsky H. Semen volume and fructose content of human semen. Survey of the years 1980–1989. *Acta Eur. Fertil.* 1990; **21**:205–206.

7. Paick J, Kim SH, Kim SW. Ejaculatory duct obstruction in infertile men. *BJU Int.* 2000; **85**:720–724.

8. Roberts M, Jarvi K. Steps in the investigation and management of low semen volume in the infertile man. *Can. Urol. Assoc. J.* 2009; **3**:479–485.

9. Schlegel PN, Shin D, Goldstein M. Urogenital anomalies in men with congenital absence of the vas deferens. *J. Urol.* 1996; **155**:1644–1648.

10. Hall S, Oates RD. Unilateral absence of the scrotal vas deferens associated with contralateral mesonephric duct anomalies resulting in infertility: laboratory, physical and radiographic findings, and therapeutic alternatives. *J. Urol.* 1983; **50**:1161–1164.

11. Chillon M, Casals T, Mercier B, et al. Mutations in the cystic fibrosis gene in patients with congenital absence of the vas deferens. *N. Engl. J. Med.* 1995; **332**:1475–1480.

12. Yu J, Chen Z, Ni Y, Li Z. CFTR mutations in men with congenital bilateral absence of the vas deferens (CBAVD): a systemic review and meta-analysis. *Hum. Reprod.* 2012; **27**:25–35.

13. McCallum T, Milunsky J, Munarriz R, et al. Unilateral renal agenesis associated with congenital bilateral absence of the vas deferens: phenotypic findings and genetic considerations. *Hum. Reprod.* 2001; **16**:282–288.

14. Schwarzer JU, Schwarz M. Significance of CFTR gene mutations in patients with congenital aplasia of vas deferens with special regard to renal aplasia. *Andrologia* 2012; **44**:305–307.

15. Meng MV, Black LD, Cha I, et al. Impaired spermatogenesis in men with congenital absence of the vas deferens. *Hum. Reprod.* 2001; **16**:529–533.

16. Friedler S, Raziel A, Schachter M, et al. Outcome of first and repeated testicular sperm extraction and ICSI in patients with non-obstructive azoospermia. *Hum. Reprod.* 2002; **17**:2356–2361.

17. Matsumiya K, Namiki M, Takahara S, et al. Clinical study of azoospermia. *Int. J. Androl.* 1994; **17**:140–142.

18. Faes K, Goossens E. Short-term storage of human testicular tissue: effect of storage temperature and tissue size. *RBM Online* 2017; **35**:180–188.

19. Krege S, Beyer J, Souchon R, et al. European consensus on diagnosis and treatment of germ cell cancer: a report of the European Germ Cell Cancer Consensus Group (EGCCCG). *Ann. Oncol.* 2004; **15**:1377–1399.

20. Honig SC, Lipshulz LI, Jarow J. Significant medical pathology uncovered by a comprehensive male infertility evaluation. *Fertil. Steril.* 1994; **62**:1028–1034.

21. Shefi S, Turek PJ. Definition and current evaluation of subfertile men. *Int. Braz. J. Urol.* 2006; **32**:385–397.

22. Dohle GR, Elzanaty S, van Casteren NJ. Testicular biopsy: clinical practice and interpretation. *Asian J. Androl.* 2012; **14**:88–93.

23. Donoso P, Tournaye H, Devroey P. Which is the best sperm retrieval technique for nonobstructive azoospermia? A systematic review. *Hum. Reprod. Update* 2007; **13**:539–549.

24. Schlegel PN, Su LM. Physiological consequences of testicular sperm extraction. *Hum. Reprod.* 1997; **12**:1688–1692.

25. Pilatz A, Rusz A, Wagenlehner F, Weidner W, Altinkilic B. Reference values for testicular volume, epididymal head size and peak systolic velocity of the testicular artery in adult males measured by ultrasonography. *Ultraschall Med.* 2013; **34**:349–354.

26. Tsirigotis M, Bennett V, Nicholson N, et al. Experience with subzonal insemination (SUZI) and intracytoplasmic sperm injection (ICSI) on unfertilized aged human oocytes. *J. Assist. Reprod. Genet.* 1994; **11**:389–394.

27. Henkel RR, Schill WB. Sperm preparation for ART. *Reprod. Biol. Endocrinol.* 2003; **1**:108–122.

28. Kovacic B, Vlaisavljevic V, Reljic M. Clinical use of pentoxifylline for activation of immotile testicular sperm before ICSI in patients with azoospermia. *J. Androl.* 2006; **27**:45–52.

29. Caroppo E, Colpi EM, Gazzano G, et al. Testicular histology may predict the successful sperm retrieval in patients with non-obstructive azoospermia undergoing conventional TESE: a diagnostic accuracy study. *J. Assist. Reprod. Genet.* 2017; **34**:149–154.

30. Selice R, Di Mambro A, Garolla A, et al. Spermatogenesis in Klinefelter syndrome. *J. Endocrinol. Invest.* 2010; **33**:789–793.

31. Ostad M, Liotta D, Ye Z, Schlegel PN. Testicular sperm extraction for nonobstructive azoospermia: results of a multibiopsy approach with optimized tissue dispersion. *Urology* 1998; **52**:692–696.

32. Schlegel PN, Li PS. Microdissection TESE: sperm retrieval in non-obstructive azoospermia. *Hum. Reprod. Update* 1998; **4**:439.

33. Schlegel PN. Testicular sperm extraction: microdissection improves sperm yield with minimal tissue excision. *Hum. Reprod.* 1999; **14**:131–135.

34. Turunc T, Gul U, Haydardedeoglu B, et al. Conventional testicular sperm extraction combined with the microdissection technique in nonobstructive azoospermic patients: a prospective comparative study. *Fertil. Steril.* 2010; **94**:2157–2160.

35. Jensen CFS, Ohl DA, Hiner MR, et al. Multiple needle-pass percutaneous testicular sperm aspiration as first line treatment in azoospermic men. *Andrology* 2016; **4**:257–262.

36. Eliveld J, van Wely M, Meibner A, et al. The risk of TESE-induced hypogonadism: a systematic review and meta-analysis. *Hum. Reprod. Update* 2018; **24**:442–454.

37. Kalsi J, Thum MY, Muneer A, Abdullah H, Minhas S. In the era of micro-dissection sperm retrieval (m-TESE) is an isolated testicular biopsy necessary in the management of men with non-obstructive azoospermia? *BJU Int.* 2012; **109**:418–424.

38. Bernie AM, Mata DA, Ramasamy R, Schlegel PN. Comparison of microdissection testicular sperm extraction, conventional testicular sperm extraction, and testicular sperm aspiration for nonobstructive azoospermia: a systematic review and meta-analysis. *Fertil. Steril.* 2015; **104**:1099–1103.

39. Deruyver Y, Vanderschueren D, Van der Aa F. Outcome of microdissection TESE compared with conventional TESE in non-obstructive azoospermia: a systematic review. *Andrology* 2014; **2**:20–24.

40. Caroppo E, Colpi EM, Gazzano G, et al. The seminiferous tubule caliber pattern as evaluated at high magnification during microdissection testicular sperm extraction predicts sperm retrieval in patients with nonobstructive azoospermia. *Andrology* 2019; **7**:8–14.

41. Amer M, Zohdy W, Abd El Naser T, et al. Single tubule biopsy: a new objective microsurgical advancement for testicular sperm retrieval in patients with nonobstructive azoospermia. *Fertil. Steril.* 2008; **89**:592–596.

42. Hussein A, Ozgok Y, Ross L, Niederberger C. Clomiphene administration for cases of nonobstructive azoospermia: a multicenter study. *J. Androl.* 2005; **26**:787–791; discussion 792–793.

43. Shiraishi K, Ohmi C, Shimabukuro T, Matsuyama H. Human chorionic gonadotrophin treatment prior to microdissection testicular sperm extraction in non-obstructive azoospermia. *Hum. Reprod.* 2012; **27**:331–339.

44. Reifsnyder JE, Ramasamy R, Husseini J, Schlegel PN. Role of optimizing testosterone before microdissection testicular sperm extraction in men with nonobstructive azoospermia. *J. Urol.* 2012; **188**:532–536.

45. Esteves SC, Miyaoka R, Roque M, Agarwal A. Outcome of varicocele repair in men with nonobstructive azoospermia: systematic review and meta-analysis. *Asian J. Androl.* 2016; **18**:246–253.

46. Kirby EW, Wiener LE, Rajanahally S, Crowell K, Coward RM. Undergoing varicocele repair before assisted reproduction improves pregnancy rate and live birth rate in azoospermic and oligospermic men with a varicocele: a systematic review and meta-analysis. *Fertil. Steril.* 2016; **106**:1338–1343.

47. Ramasamy R, Yagan N, Schlegel PN. Structural and functional changes to the testis after conventional versus microdissection testicular sperm extraction. *Urology* 2005; **65**:1190–1194.

48. Tournaye H, Verheyen G, Nagy P, et al. Are there any predictive factors for successful testicular sperm recovery in azoospermic patients? *Hum. Reprod.* 1997; **12**:80–86.

49. Verhoeven G, Cailleau J. Follicle-stimulating hormone and androgens increase the concentration of the androgen receptor in Sertoli cells. *Endocrinology* 1988; **122**:1541–1550.

50. Kim ED, Crosnoe L, Bar-Chama N, Khera M, Lipshultz L. The treatment of hypogonadism in men of reproductive age. *Fertil. Steril.* 2013; **99**:718–724.

51. Pitteloud N, Hayes FJ, Dwyer A, et al. Predictors of outcome of long-term GnRH therapy in men with idiopathic hypogonadotropic hypogonadism. *J. Clin. Endocrinol. Metab.* 2002; **87**:4128–4136.

52. Adamopoulos DA, Pappa A, Billa E, et al. Effectiveness of combined tamoxifen citrate and testosterone undecanoate treatment in men with idiopathic oligozoospermia. *Fertil. Steril.* 2003; **80**:914–920.

53. Rodrigo L, Rubio C, Peinado V, et al. Testicular sperm from patients with obstructive and nonobstructive azoospermia: aneuploidy risk and reproductive prognosis using testicular sperm from fertile donors as control samples. *Fertil. Steril.* 2011; **95**:1005–1012.

54. Vozdova M, Heracek J, Sobotka V, Rubes J. Testicular sperm aneuploidy in non-obstructive azoospermic patients. *Hum. Reprod.* 2012; **27**:2233–2239.

55. Schlegel PN. Male infertility: evaluation and sperm retrieval. *Clin. Obstet. Gynecol.* 2006; **49**:55–72.

56. Samli H, Samli MM, Solak M, Imirzalioglu N. Genetic anomalies detected in patients with non-obstructive azoospermia and oligozoospermia. *Arch. Androl.* 2006; **52**:263–267.

57. Pryor JL, Kent-First M, Muallem A, et al. Microdeletions in the Y chromosome of infertile men. *N. Engl. J. Med.* 1997; **336**:534–539.

58. Oates RD, Silber S, Brown LG, Page DC. Clinical characterization of 42 oligospermic or azoospermic men with microdeletion of the AZFc region of the Y chromosome, and of 18 children conceived via ICSI. *Hum. Reprod.* 2002; **17**:2813–2824.

59. Hopps CV, Mielnik A, Goldstein M, et al. Detection of sperm in men with Y chromosome microdeletions of

the AZFa, AZFb and AZFc regions. *Hum. Reprod.* 2003; **18**:1660–1665.

60. Lee SH, Ahn SY, Lee KW, et al. Intracytoplasmic sperm injection may lead to vertical transmission, expansion, and de novo occurrence of Y-chromosome microdeletions in male fetuses. *Fertil. Steril.* 2006; **85**:1512–1515.

61. Practice Committee for the ASRM. Evaluation of the azoospermic male: a committee opinion. *Fertil. Steril.* 2018; **109**:777–782.

Chapter 15

Donation and Surrogacy

For persons who wish to have children but are unable to produce their gametes, assisted reproductive technology (ART) involving donated gametes suggests a means of becoming gestational and social parents (Figure 15.1). Conceiving with a donor gamete ultimately yields a child who lacks genetic relations with one or both of the parents. In order to compensate for this genetic lack, some fertility clinics match the ethnicity of gamete donors and recipient parents, to increase the likelihood that the resulting child will have phenotypic characteristics of the receiving parent despite the absence of a direct genetic link. This matching allows the family to keep secrecy about the use of a donor by ensuring that the child could look as a genetic child. Nonetheless, given that such "ethnic" matching also involves the classification and matching of people based on characteristics that are typically associated with "race," such as skin color and hair color, it raises ethical concerns regarding racism [1].

The ready availability of sperm donors and the ease of artificial insemination have long enabled couples to treat male infertility. The development of in vitro fertilization (IVF) and related techniques has made oocyte and embryo donation another option for infertile couples. Gamete donation is an ethically and legally accepted procedure in most countries. Donation is also associated with the highest pregnancy and live birth rates after IVF (Figures 15.2 and 15.3) [2].

The family and medical history of the donor is established to exclude the presence of major Mendelian disorders, chromosome rearrangements, and multifactorial disorders that have a significant genetic component [3]. In most assisted reproduction clinics, donors of sperm, eggs, or embryos undergo some genetic screening procedures in order to maximize the health of the donor-conceived offspring. Genetic tests may include karyotyping and genetic

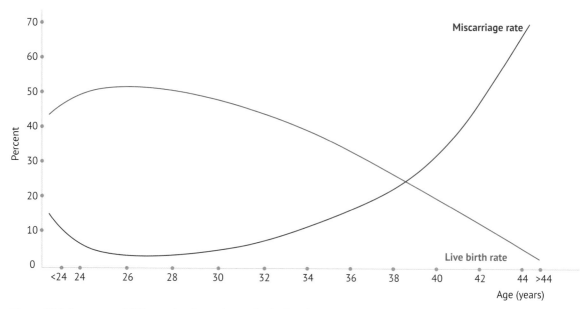

Figure 15.1 Percentage of ART general cycles resulting in live birth and miscarriage by age of women.

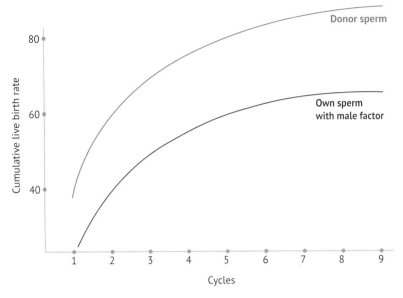

Figure 15.2 Sperm donation impact on IVF success rates.

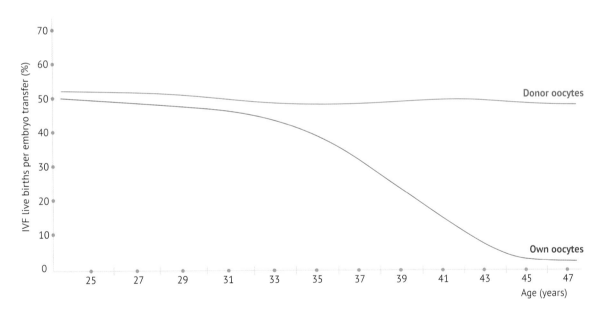

Figure 15.3 Egg donation impact on IVF success rates.

screening for the carrier status of specific conditions such as cystic fibrosis, spinal muscular atrophy, thalassemia, Tay–Sachs disease, and fragile X syndrome. Recent advances in genetic testing technologies now enable more extensive genetic testing of donors than ever before. To date, most attention is directed towards expanded carrier screening for autosomal recessive disorders [4]. New genetic testing technologies could potentially be used to screen for undiagnosed autosomal dominant disorders and even for susceptibility to some multifactorial diseases [5]. Donors and recipients alike acknowledge the importance of genetic information. Recipients are concerned that expanded genetic screening of donors might lead to additional financial costs, but still recognize the potential benefits of performing more extensive genetic screening of donors [6]. Both recipients and donors are apprehensive about extended genomic

183

technologies, with concerns relating to how this information can be used and the ethics of genetic selectivity.

Usually, female and male donors differ in their social status. Over half of the female donors have children of their own when they make a donation. In contrast, male donors are more likely to be single at the time of donation.

The communication and interaction between gamete donors and fertility clinic staff remain to be improved, as donors often feel disrespected and treated as a commodity by clinic staff [7].

Sperm Donation

Sperm donation has been used in the treatment of male infertility for more than 100 years. It is known that pregnancy rates using frozen semen are lower than those with fresh semen [8]. Due to the risk of acquired viral infections, as hepatitis (HBV, HCV), human immunodeficiency (HIV), or cytomegalovirus, frozen sperm for clinical use are quarantined for 6 months until the donor has been retested and found to be seronegative.

Sperm donors. Complete medical, genetic, social, sexual, and family histories must be taken at the time of the initial interview and donors must undergo a physical examination. Usually, men younger than 40 years old are eligible donors. The drawback of using sperm from older men is the increased risk of neurological and chromosomal abnormalities in offspring (autism, schizophrenia, achondroplasia). Before cryopreservation and post-thaw cryo-sensitivity testing, two semen analyses must be performed using criteria established by the semen bank.

The fertility and health of the donor must be immutable, and there should not be a family history of genetic disease. Screening for thalassemia in Mediterranean races, Tay–Sachs heterozygosity in donors of Jewish origin, and sickle cell disease in donors of African origin should be executed. Individuals with a history of herpes, chronic hepatitis, or venereal warts should be excluded. There is no simple method of thoroughly ensuring that infectious agents will not be transmitted by donor sperm, but proper screening should make this a remote possibility. Tests should be performed when the donor is first seen and at repeat donations.

Genetic screening is recommended for all potential donors. Moreover, pairs need to be aware of the fact that in 4–5% of pregnancies using donated sperm,

the child could be born with a congenital anomaly. These anomaly rates are comparable to those seen with spontaneous pregnancies [9].

In a sense, most women want the donor to resemble their partner as much as possible. The resemblance is generally limited to hair color and eye color, ethnic origin, height, and blood type.

Quite a debate continues on the type of gamete donors to be recruited and payment of fees or expenses. Traditionally, sperm donors have received a nominal fee, including reimbursement for their direct and indirect expenses. Most sperm donors are young single students and soldiers who are motivated predominantly by financial incentives. It has been recommended that donors should be paid discomfort fees similar to payment made to healthy volunteers who take part in drug and treatment trials [10].

Positive communication and interaction between donors and fertility clinic staff are of critical importance. Donors conveyed frustration after not receiving information on the expenses they could claim. Donors also negatively commented on aftercare, location and condition of the donation room [11], including the location of the waiting room, and visibility of the donation room to fertility patients, and clinic staff. Hygiene of the donation room is also critical.

Limiting donors. There is concern regarding the risk of exposure among the offspring of the same donor. This is a problem in small towns in which a limited supply of donors is available. It has been recommended that in a population of 800 000, limiting a single donor with no more than 25 pregnancies will avoid inadvertent consanguineous conception [12]. However, only 20–30% of the pregnancies produced through commercial donations are ever reported to the sperm banks [13].

Record management. The nearly universal practice is to maintain the confidentiality of both donors and recipients. In the United Kingdom, the Human Fertilisation and Embryology Authority (HFEA) policy dictates that those who donated sperm, eggs, or embryos after April 1, 2005 are, by law, identifiable. Donor-conceived individuals conceived after April 1, 2005 can apply to the HFEA after the age of 16 years, to receive non-identifying donor information; after reaching the age of 18 years, they can apply to the HFEA to find the information their donor provided, including identifying information.

Records, including those about donor suitability, quality assurance, sample collection, processing, storage, and medical and laboratory data, must be booked for at least 10 years after insemination [14]. This allows donors and recipients to be tracked in the event of a medical problem in the donor or donor's family.

Oocyte Donation

Oocyte donation was first described in the early 1980s. It was thought to be a logical method of achieving pregnancy in women with premature ovarian failure as well as in those who wished to avoid passing on to their children a heritable disease. Since cryopreservation was in its infancy, when a more significant number of oocytes were obtained, one or more could reasonably be donated to a potential recipient [15]. The technique used induced no prohibitive immune reaction. Also, it prepared the recipient's uterus for implantation using exogenous estradiol and progesterone (P_4). Donation appeared to be a viable option for women who needed a donated egg to conceive. Early oocyte donation methods relied on natural ovulation and fertilization in the donor. The developing embryo was then flushed from the uterus of the donor before implantation and then transferred to the uterus of the recipient [16], whose ovulation was monitored and thus known to be synchronous with the ovulation of the donor.

Transvaginal ultrasound-guided follicular aspiration revolutionized oocyte donation. Egg donors no longer needed to undergo insemination with sperm or risk a subsequent retained pregnancy. Controlled ovarian stimulation and standard IVF procedure could be used, thus increasing the yield and efficiency of the process. Since oocyte quality could now be controlled, the effect of the age of the uterus on pregnancy success could be estimated. No decrease in pregnancy rates was observed with increasing recipient age, even beyond the age of 40 years [17]. Obstetrical risks are higher for older women, but pregnancy rates with eggs donated by young women remain high, regardless of the age of the recipient.

In oocyte donation the procedure requires the donor to undergo superovulation, as with conventional IVF. Oocyte retrieval is performed and the donor oocytes are fertilized in vitro with the sperm of the partner of the recipient. The fertilized oocyte (embryo) is transferred to the hormonally synchronized recipient or cryopreserved for transfer at a later date. Although the number of potential recipients is increasing continuously, the shortage of donors is one of the significant difficulties in establishing a donor oocyte program. Anonymous donors were recommended to be under 35 years of age. The disadvantage of using oocytes from older women is the increased risk of chromosomal abnormalities. Another possible problem is that older donors produce fewer oocytes than younger women.

In the early 2000s, techniques of oocyte cryopreservation advanced to the point where reliable results could be obtained with elective oocyte cryopreservation and subsequent thawing. In the context of oocyte donation, oocyte cryopreservation made possible the establishment of oocyte banks, which provided frozen donor oocytes to recipients in a manner analogous to that of frozen sperm in sperm banks.

Ovum sharing raises several ethical and medical concerns. A "shared" ovum donation program is limited by the number of ova available for donation and oocyte quality. Ethical problems might arise in cases where the recipient woman conceives and gives birth to a child while the donor herself does not conceive.

Attempts to reverse the age-related drop in oocyte quality through micro-manipulation of the nucleus and cytoplasm have produced disappointing results and ethical concerns have been expressed. In contrast, the use of oocytes from younger donors is associated with very high rates of conception in menopausal women. The increased obstetrical risks in this population, which bear a higher rate of underlying medical comorbidities, must be considered prior to attempt assisted conception, often in consultation with a multidisciplinary team of physicians.

Oocyte donors. Oocyte donors should have attained their legal majority and preferably be between the ages of 21 and 34 years. Proven fertility is desirable but not required. All prospective oocyte donors should be screened for normal karyotype, and genetic and infectious diseases in order to minimize transmission to the recipient or her offspring. The antral follicular count should be more than 10. The history and physical evaluation should rule out inherited disorders, and the possibility of reproductive dysfunction.

A number of controlled ovarian hyperstimulation protocols have been developed for donors, including the administration of gonadotropins in conjunction with gonadotropin-releasing hormone agonists. When follicles, according to size and number, are ready for aspiration, ultrasound-guided transvaginal oocyte recovery is performed. After a preincubation interval of several hours, the donor oocyte is fertilized with the recipient's partner's sperm.

A side effect of the fertility drugs, used to stimulate the ovaries to release oocytes, is an ovarian hyperstimulation syndrome (OHSS) with symptoms including abdominal swelling, nausea, dehydration, and breathing difficulty. Oocyte donors reported to have OHSS often sensed that clinic staff were not concerned about their physical or emotional well-being but instead focused disproportionately on extracting the oocytes [11].

Recipients. Initially, the primary indication for oocyte donation was a premature ovarian failure, defined as hypergonadotropic hypogonadism occurring before the age of 40 years. Later, oocyte donation became widespread throughout the world to treat a variety of reproductive disorders, some of which are age-related.

Both the oocyte recipient and her partner should be healthy, and there should be no physical contraindication to pregnancy. Screening for infectious diseases in the patient and her partner generally includes tests for HIV, hepatitis, chlamydia and syphilis. Hysterosalpingography should be performed to evaluate any uterine abnormalities.

Many young women are electing to delay childbirth for personal, economic, or professional reasons. However, fertility potential decreases with advancing maternal age and it is expected that older women between the ages of 35 and 45 will be unsuccessful in their effort to reproduce. The introduction of oocyte donation to establish pregnancy in patients with age-related infertility has allowed many older women a new opportunity to conceive. Maximal age of recipients for egg donation in most European countries is 45 years, in England is 50 years, in Israel is 55 years, and in the USA, it is only suggested before the age of 50 years.

Though implantation and clinical pregnancy rates are similar between vitrified donor oocytes and fresh donor oocytes [18], pregnancy presents a high medical risk for the elderly mother and her fetus [19]. It has been shown that most of the complications in pregnancy associated with older age are caused by age-related confounders such as diabetes mellitus, hypertension, and multiparity [20]. Postmenopausal women are considered at a particularly increased risk of vascular complications during pregnancy. There are increased rates of obstetrical and maternal complications with increasing maternal age, including maternal death, fetal and neonatal death, preterm delivery, and low birth weight and efficient delivery

[21–25]. However, these risks are already increased in women over the age of 40; nonetheless, treatment is offered to women between the ages of 40 and 55 without significant debate.

Embryo Donation

Embryo donation is a new procedure and is a well-established and successful form of ART when both partners are infertile. The vast majority of embryo donors are couples who completed IVF procedures and who had the extra embryos cryopreserved. The embryo donors must sign an informed consent document stating their consent to donate their embryos, renouncing all rights to the embryo and any child that may result from the transfer of these embryos. They should be screened for genetic and infectious diseases to prevent transmission to the recipient or the offspring.

Recipient couples should be made aware of the limitations of genetic and infectious disease screening and informed that there is no guarantee that the resulting child will be born free of birth defects or illnesses. Couples who receive embryo donation should be thoroughly evaluated, including medical history, physical examination, and psychological counseling. A pelvic ultrasound evaluation should be performed to assess uterine size and endometrial thickness and to rule out pelvic pathologies such as endometrial polyps, myomas, or ovarian cysts.

Ooplasma Donation (Mitochondria Donation)

At the end of the 1990s, an alternative to oocyte donation termed "cytoplasmic donation" was developed [26–27]. In 1997, Jacques Cohen and coworkers reported on the first human pregnancy following the transfer of cytoplasm from donor oocytes to oocytes of a patient with a history of poor embryo development [26]. In this technique, a fraction of ooplasm from a donor oocyte is co-injected into a recipient oocyte with sperm during intracytoplasmic sperm injection (ICSI). This ooplasm contains mitochondria and other organelles, proteins, and mRNAs. The presence of extraneous cytoplasm appears to increase the quality of the recipient oocyte to the level where the embryo produced is viable. To note, significant improvement in embryo quality does not always occur after cytoplasmic transfer. The donation of ooplasm appeared to result in a reduction in the level of embryo fragmentation and an increase in the number of blastomeres present in the embryo [28]. The mixed (heterologous) ooplasmic transfer has also been reported to lead to successful pregnancies [29]. Donor mitochondrial DNA was identified in the offspring as "three genetic parents." The sufficient benefit of this technology was never fully proved; its safety has been questioned by many specialists and it has raised both ethical and genetic questions. The US Food and Drug Administration banned the procedure in 2001 until a clinical study could be conducted to determine its safety. Although no such study was performed, this technology is still commercially available in IVF clinics in numerous countries worldwide.

Mitochondria are a key component of ooplasm. Mitochondria constitute the powerhouse of cells, as they synthesize ATP by oxidative phosphorylation. They possess their own small genome in the form of mitochondrial DNA (mtDNA). Mitochondrial replication starts in the primordial germ cells (PGCs) and continues during early oogenesis; however, a sharp increase in mitochondria counts is observed during later stages of oogenesis [30]. Thus, whereas PGCs only contain a few hundred copies of mtDNA, mature oocytes contain up to several hundred thousand copies [31]. Since mitochondria in oocytes are ancestral to all somatic mitochondria of the next generation and to all cells of future generations, oocytes must prepare for the high energetic demands of maturation, fertilization, and embryogenesis. Unlike the nuclear genome, which is derived from both the egg and sperm at fertilization, the mtDNA in the embryo is derived almost exclusively from the egg, i.e., it is of maternal origin. Mutations in mtDNA occur at a ≥10-fold rate than in nuclear DNA, possibly due to the high concentration of free oxygen radicals, lack of histones, and limited mtDNA repair mechanisms in the mitochondria [32]. Pathogenic maternally inherited mtDNA mutations are a frequent cause of severe human disease and are found in 0.5% of the population [33], with disease affecting at least 1 in 5000 individuals [34]. Interest in mtDNA mutations has grown due to the increasing number of associated diseases and because they can affect patients throughout life. Also, mtDNA mutations are increasingly implicated in high-energy requirement body systems such as the brain, skeletal muscle, heart, and liver, and are associated with Alzheimer's, Parkinson's, Huntington's diseases and Leigh syndrome [35–37]. ART could eliminate the transmission of mitochondrial diseases in affected families by performing cytoplasmic, germinal vesicle (GV), and pronuclear transfer.

Typically a cell contains only one type of mtDNA (homoplasmy). Mixtures of mtDNA types (heteroplasmy) allow lethal mutations to persist and, most importantly, to pass to the next generation. Many mtDNA diseases are heteroplasmic. Currently, there are no therapies for mitochondrial disorders and available treatments only alleviate symptoms and slow disease progression. Therefore, there is a significant necessity to consider new therapeutic approaches that could prevent the transmission of mtDNA mutations from mother to child.

Another possibility of treatment is transferring nuclear DNA from a mother with mtDNA disease to a cytoplast (or spindle-free oocyte) containing normal mtDNA obtained from a healthy egg donor. The procedure comprises removal of nuclear DNA from an unfertilized oocyte of a patient carrying abnormal mitochondria, followed by its transfer to an enucleated donor oocyte containing assumed healthy mitochondria. ICSI subsequently fertilizes this constructed oocyte. However, such mitochondrial manipulations have come under criticism worldwide [38] as these techniques raise the risks of heteroplasmy, linked to the use of mitochondria or ooplasm from a donor. A pronuclear transfer is essentially the same procedure, except that the nuclear material, both the male and female pronuclei (pN), is removed after fertilization. Spindle–chromosomal apparatus transfer is free of mitochondria [39].

Injection of purified mitochondria instead of ooplasm presents a potential alternative means of delivering more massive amounts of mitochondria into the oocyte [40]. For such procedures, the mitochondria should be obtained from the patient's cells, which, optimally, should be of ovarian or oocyte origin [41–42], and the mtDNA from these cells should be of high quality, without deletions or mutations [43].

Transfer of mitochondria from putative oogonial stem cells (OSCs) into oocytes of low responders [44] led to limited improvement in oocyte functions. In the context of ICSI, the mitochondria were injected into oocytes to augment oocyte performance; healthy live births or ongoing pregnancies have been reported [45]. It was established that the oocyte mtDNA copy numbers per cell and accumulation of mtDNA mutations were not found to be different between older patients with a low ovarian reserve and younger patients [46], so a number of mitochondria per cell should not be a point reason in the reduction of functionality. Furthermore, if OSCs are homologous with PGCs or oogonia, they are expected to have only a few thousand copies of mtDNA compared with the 160 000 copies found in mature oocytes. It remains unclear how mitochondria transfer restores oocyte competence if the aneuploidy is preexisting at metaphase II (MII) in oocytes from aging patients. It is unlikely that mitochondria transfer can boost the embryonic developmental potential of low-quality oocytes obtained from subfertile patients.

So, which of the existing genome replacement approaches available offers the best means of completely eliminating affected mtDNA? While the three options (GV, MII, and pN) are technically similar, they differ significantly from a cell cycle point of view. Mitochondria undergo redistribution along with meiotic progression, a process that has been documented in human oocytes [47]. In GV-stage oocytes, mitochondria are concentrated in the perinuclear space, often associated with lipid vesicles [48]. Thus, there is tremendous potential for transferring a significant amount of patient mtDNA into the donor oocyte following GV transplantation. During meiotic progression, mitochondria scatter in the cytoplasm, where they tend to concentrate in the inner cytoplasm. At the pN stage, mitochondria are again concentrated in a perinuclear position, particularly during pronuclear opposition [49]. Hence, it is likely that there will be less carryover of patient mtDNA in MII karyoplasts compared with pN transfer. The proportion of mtDNA copies carried over has been estimated to be 1% in MII [50], versus 8% [51] in pN transfer, which aligns with the mitochondria distribution dynamics.

Surrogacy

The word "surrogate" is rooted in the Latin "*subrogare*" (to substitute), which means "appointed to act in the place of," and refers to a substitute, especially a person deputizing for another in a specific role. The surrogate mother implies a woman who becomes pregnant, gives birth to a child, and gives away this child to another person or couple, commonly referred to as the "intended" or "commissioning" parent [52]. Law recognizes motherhood on the basis of the biological fact of pregnancy, which leads to a presumption that the mother of a child is the woman who gave birth. Surrogacy requires changes in the legal regulation of parentage and challenges

traditional accounts of motherhood, parenthood, pregnancy, and family. Brazil was one of the first countries to allow surrogacy procedures, as described in Resolution 1358/1992 of the Federal Board of Medicine. Surrogacy is a vital fertility treatment, wherein the advent of IVF has made motherhood possible for women without a uterus, with uterine anomalies preventing pregnancies, with serious medical problems, or with other contraindications for pregnancy. It enables couples to achieve parenthood through the use of an embryo created by themselves or a donor and transferred to the uterus of a gestational carrier. This technique also allows gay couples and single men to achieve paternity by having an embryo created with their sperm and donor oocytes, which is then transferred to the surrogate [53]. Couples seeking equal genetic parenthood can choose to mix their sperm together, or the oocytes of a donor can be fertilized with sperm from both partners and then, multiple embryos can be transferred to the surrogate (referred to as "intentional unknowing") [54]. Other couples may choose to take genetic fatherhood in turns, with one partner providing sperm for the first child and the second partner providing sperm for the subsequent attempts. Gay couples, as lesbian and heterosexual couples, who created their families using ART, are motivated to do so, to establish a genetic relationship with the child.

Surrogacy can be of two types: traditional and gestational. Traditional (genetic/partial/straight) surrogacy is the result of artificial insemination of the surrogate mother with the sperm of the intended father, rendering her a genetic parent along with the intended father. Gestational surrogacy (host/full surrogacy) involves the transfer of an embryo from the intended parents or from a donated oocyte or sperm to the surrogate uterus. In gestational surrogacy, the implanted embryo shares no genetic link with the surrogate mother. Also, surrogacy may be divided into altruistic and commercial surrogacy, depending on whether the surrogate mother is paid a service fee for conceiving, carrying, and giving birth to the child.

Women with a severe Müllerian anomaly or congenital absence of a uterus and/or vagina are typical candidates for surrogacy. An absolute indication for surrogacy is the absence of a uterus. Causes for it can be Mayer–Rokitansky–Kuster–Hauser syndrome [55] or history of obstetric hysterectomy or hysterectomy for gynecological indications such as cervical cancer or endometrial cancer. Also, significant structural abnormalities, such as a small unicornuate uterus, T-shaped uterus, or multiple fibroids with failed attempts to treat fertility, also constitute indications. Women with severe medical conditions (heart or renal diseases), which are contraindications of pregnancy, are also recommended for surrogacy [56]. Further to the above, women suffering from complete androgen insensitivity syndrome, where the uterus and ovaries are absent [56], also elect for surrogacy. Surrogacy can also be considered as a last resort for treating patients with repeated miscarriages and recurrent implantation failures after all possible tools for self-pregnancy have been exhausted [57].

The surrogate woman is generally 23–35 years old and married (for traditional surrogacy) or 23–45 years old (for gestational surrogacy), with at least one child of her own and at minimum 3 years old, with no less than a 2-year interval between two deliveries, and no more than five deliveries or three caesarean sections. The consent of the surrogate's spouse is mandatory. A typical screening process includes an extensive medical and psychological assessment, as well as thorough criminal and financial background checks. The psychological assessment estimates the surrogate's ability to sustain gestation and delivery emotionally. Routine blood tests are performed, along with tests to rule out HIV, HBV surface antigen, and HCV. Also, an electrocardiogram, Pap smear, and mammogram are recommended. The woman will also undergo a thorough pelvic and abdominal ultrasound to rule out anatomical abnormalities.

It is of paramount importance for in-depth counseling of all the parties involved in surrogacy arrangements. They must be confident and comfortable with their decisions and have trust in each other. The surrogate cycle may take account of not only the surrogate mother, but also the oocyte donor, sperm donor, and the commissioning couple or individual.

The surrogate embryo transfer could be fresh or a frozen–thawed transfer and is subject to the availability of the gestational carrier. For a fresh transfer, the surrogate and the intended mother cycle can be synchronized with oral contraceptive pills or P_4 pills, or the surrogate can be put on agonist injection for flexibility of transfer dates.

The surrogate is started on estrogen from the third day of her cycle, for approximately 10 days. On reaching a minimum 8 mm endometrium, she is then put on P_4 supplementation for 3 days or 5 days before a cleavage-stage or blastocyst transfer, respectively.

Once pregnancy is confirmed in the gestational carrier, she either stays in the surrogate house or at her home, depending on the ART clinic facilities. The concept of the surrogate house has recently drawn much attention for various reasons. A surrogate house is a place where the surrogate stays for the entire antenatal period until the date of delivery and where all her medical and personal requirements are taken care of. The obstetric care of the surrogate is extensive due to the preciousness of the pregnancy. Staying at a surrogate house should be optional for surrogate mothers.

Surrogates undergo an obstetric assessment every 20 days until the date of delivery, an obstetric scan at 6–8 weeks, an anomaly scan at 11–13 weeks, an anomaly scan at 20–22 weeks, and a growth scan at 28 weeks and 34–36 weeks. Each additional scan is subject to the obstetric needs of each woman.

The intended couple is sent regular updates regarding the surrogate's pregnancy, including her weight gain and vitals, fetal growth, and antenatal investigation reports and scans (Figure 15.4). Contact with the surrogate can help intended parents feel involved in the pregnancy and emotionally connected to the unborn child. Postdelivery, the surrogate is kept under observation for a minimum of 15 days before discharge.

The significant risk associated with surrogacy is that of obstetric complications, with multiple order pregnancy being the most common. Pregnancy, birth, and the postpartum period include complications such as preeclampsia and eclampsia, stress incontinence, urinary tract infections, gestational diabetes, and rare complications such as amniotic fluid embolism and the possibility of postpartum hemorrhage. However, these risks are associated with pregnancy in general and are not specific to surrogacy. Pregnancies deriving from ART cycles, including surrogacy cycles, may be related to increased risk of perinatal complications compared with natural conception. The perinatal results of gestational surrogacy in comparison to autologous IVF do not show a significant increase in the risks of preterm birth, live birth rate, and congenital anomalies [58].

Surrogacy has raised many ethical debates. Feminist scholars critically queried surrogacy, and saw its commercial variety as an instance of reproductive prostitution, as sex and pregnancy are put on sale, and pleasure and babies are "produced" to please others. The prime ethical concerns raised regarding

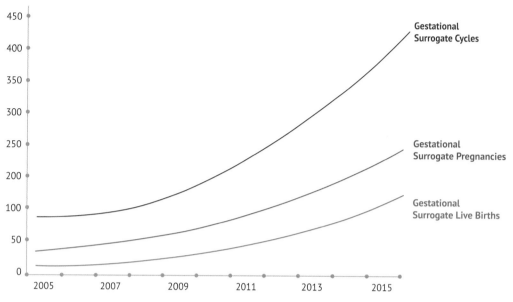

Figure 15.4 Gestational surrogate cycles, pregnancies, and live births.

surrogacy include taking advantage, commodification, and/or coercion when women are paid to be pregnant and deliver babies. However, the counter to it is a woman's right to enter into a contract and make decisions regarding her own body. By becoming commercial surrogates, women enable themselves to improve not only their lives but also the lives of their families. To earn in 9 months of pregnancy, the surrogate mother can give herself and her entire family access to better housing, food, education, and sanitization that would otherwise be difficult. What can be considered fair pay is, of course, notoriously hard to work out. "Equal pay for equal work" is on the face of it attractive. A second thought is how surrogates are treated in other (nonfinancial) ways. Several countries allow for both altruistic and commercial surrogacy. In many countries, the legal status of surrogacy is undefined; it is neither expressly prohibited nor permitted. In many countries, any payment to gestational carriers is legally prohibited by law, solely allowing for some financial aid relating to pregnancy-related expenses only. Are surrogates sufficiently informed at the outset? What conditions must they live under during pregnancy? How is their health care managed? What rights do they have during and after birth, including the rights to make contact with the child? Some Indian surrogates are housed in clinical compounds where all their meals and activities are

supervised, and from which they are not allowed to leave until delivery. The surrogates generally recognized that they have no genetic connection with the baby, but emphasized the strong ties they had with the baby because of shared substances, namely blood and sometimes breast milk.

Surrogacy is a transnational social and legal challenge, as people from countries where the practice is not allowed are forced to travel to other jurisdictions in search of surrogates and intermediary agencies, provided that they have the economic resources to do so.

People who are unable to bear biologically related children should have the same right to access commercial surrogacy as another form of assisted reproductive service, as do those whose infertility can be addressed via commercial IVF or compensated gamete provision. Surrogacy, as an assisted type of reproduction, is conceivable as a type of "third-party reproduction" [59] or "collaborative reproduction" [60]. These definitions draw attention to surrogacy as a reproductive arrangement, understood as an agreement between and joining of different people with the ambition of making new people, i.e., children. Surrogacy results appear to be satisfying and promising, with a reported rate of up to 60% live births, as surrogate women tend to be fertile and young.

Adoption

Adoption is a process in which a person assumes the parenting of another, usually a child, from that person's biological or legal parent(s). Historically, most adoptions occurred within a family, but today also involve unrelated individuals. Intra-family adoption can also occur through surrender, as a result of parental death, or when the child cannot otherwise be cared for and a family member decides to take over. Legal adoptions permanently transfer all rights and responsibilities, along with filiation, from the biological parent(s).

Infertility is the main reason parents seek to adopt unrelated children. Co-adoption by same-sex couples is legal in many countries. Most gay and lesbian adoptive parents choose adoption as their preferred way of parenting, as opposed to heterosexual couples who typically consider adoption only after failed attempts at natural and/or assisted reproduction [61].

References

1. Maung HH. Ethical problems with ethnic matching in gamete donation. *J. Med. Ethics* 2019; **45**:112–116.

2. Sauer M, Paulson R, Lobo R. Pregnancy in women over 50 or more years: outcome of 22 consecutive established pregnancies from oocyte donation. *Fertil. Steril.* 1995; **64**:111–115.

3. Isley L, Falk RE, Shamonki J, Sims CA, Callum P. Management of the risks for inherited disease in donor-conceived offspring. *Fertil. Steril.* 2016;**106**:1479–1484.

4. Henneman L, Borry P, Chokoshvili D, et al. Responsible implementation of expanded carrier screening. *Eur. J. Hum. Genet.* 2016; **24**:e1–e12.

5. Martin J, Asan, Yi Y, et al. Comprehensive carrier genetic test using next-generation deoxyribonucleic acid sequencing in infertile couples wishing to conceive through assisted reproductive technology. *Fertil. Steril.* 2015; **104**:1286–1293.

6. Amor DJ, Kerr A, Somanathan N, et al. Attitudes of sperm, egg and embryo donors and recipients towards genetic information and screening of donors. *Reprod. Health* 2018; **15**:26.

7. Kenney NJ, McGowan ML. Looking back: egg donors' retrospective evaluations of their motivations, expectations, and experiences during their first donation cycle. *Fertil. Steril.* 2008; **93**:455–466.

8. Subak LL, Adamson GD, Boltz NL. Therapeutic donor insemination: a prospective randomized trial of fresh versus frozen sperm. *Am. J. Obstet. Gynecol.* 1992; **166**:1597–1604.

9. Amuzu B, Laxova R, Shapiro SS. Pregnancy outcome, health of children, and family adjustment after donor insemination. *Obstet. Gynecol.* 1990; **75**:899–905.

10. Sauer M. Reproductive prohibition: restricting donor payment will lead to medical tourism. *Hum. Reprod.* 1997; **12**:1844–1845.

11. Williams RA, Machin LL. Rethinking gamete donor care: a satisfaction survey of egg and sperm donors in the UK. *Plos One* 2018; **13**:e0199971. https://doi.org/10.1371/journal.pone.0199971.

12. American Society for Reproductive Medicine. Guidelines for gamete and embryo donation. *Fertil. Steril.* 1998; **70**:1S–4S.

13. Prateek S, Sindhu SG. Ethical and legal aspects in ART. In: Talwar vsm Lt Col P, Sindhu SG, eds., *Step by Step Protocols in Clinical Embryology and ART*. New Dehli: Jaypee Brothers Medical Publishers. 1995; 441–461.

14. Linden JV, Centola G. New American Association of Tissue Banks standards for semen banking. *Fertil. Steril.* 1997; **68**:597–600.

15. Trounson A, Leeton J, Besanko M, Wood C, Conti A. Pregnancy established in an infertile patient after transfer of a donated embryo fertilised in vitro. *Br. Med. J.* 1983; **286**:835–838.

16. Rosenwaks Z. Donor eggs: their application in modern reproductive technologies. *Fertil. Steril.* 1987; **47**:895–909.

17. Sauer MV, Paulson RJ, Lobo RA. A preliminary report on oocyte donation extending reproductive potential to women over 40. *N. Engl. J. Med.* 1990; **232**:1157–1160.

18. Domingues TS, Aquino AP, Barros B, et al. Egg donation of vitrified oocytes bank produces similar pregnancy rates by blastocyst transfer when compared to fresh cycle. *J. Assist. Reprod. Genet.* 2017; **34**:1553–1557.

19. Van Katwijk C, Peeters LL. Clinical aspects of pregnancy after age of 35 years: a review of the literature. *Hum. Reprod. Update* 1998; **4**:185–194.

20. Sauer M, Paulson RJ, Lobo R. Oocyte donation to women of advanced age: pregnancy results and obstetrical outcomes in patients 45 years and older. *Hum. Reprod.* 1996; **11**:2540–2543.

21. Jacobsson B, Ladfors L, Milsom I. Advanced maternal age and adverse perinatal outcome. *Obstet. Gynecol.* 2004; **104**:727–733.

22. Simchen MJ, Yinon Y, Moran O, Schiff E, Sivan E. Pregnancy outcome after age 50. *Obstet. Gynecol.* 2006; **108**:1084–1088.

23. Cleary-Goldman J, Malone FD, Vidaver J, et al. Impact of maternal age on obstetric outcome. *Obstet. Gynecol.* 2005; **105**:983–990.

191

24. Joseph KS, Allen AC, Dodds L, et al. The perinatal effects of delayed childbearing. *Obstet. Gynecol.* 2005; **105**:1410–1418.

25. Schutte JM, Schuitemaker NW, Steegers EA, van Roosmalen J; Dutch Maternal Mortality Committee. Maternal death after oocyte donation at high maternal age: case report. *Reprod. Health* 2008; **5**:12.

26. Cohen J, Scott R, Schimmel T, Levron J, Willadsen S. Birth of infant donor after transfer of anucleate donor oocyte cytoplasm into recipient eggs. *Lancet* 1997; **350**:186–187.

27. Cohen J, Scott R, Alikani M, et al. Ooplasmic transfer in mature human oocytes. *Mol. Hum. Reprod.* 1998; **4**:269–280.

28. Dale B, Wilding M, Botta G, et al. Pregnancy after cytoplasmic transfer in a couple suffering from idiopathic infertility. *Hum. Reprod.* 2001; **16**:1469–1472.

29. Soini S, Ibarreta D, Anastasiadou V, et al. The interface between assisted reproductive technologies and genetics: technical, social, ethical and legal issues. *Eur. J. Hum. Genet.* 2006; **14**:588–645.

30. St John J. The control of mtDNA replication during differentiation and development. *Biochim. Biophys. Acta* 2014; **1840**:1345–1354.

31. Otten AB, Smeets HJ. Evolutionary defined role of the mitochondrial DNA in fertility, disease and ageing. *Hum. Reprod. Update* 2015; **21**:671–689.

32. Scheibye-Knudsen M, Fang EF, Croteau DL, Wilson DM III, Bohr VA. Protecting the mitochondrial powerhouse. *Trends Cell Biol.* 2015; **25**:158–170.

33. Elliott HR, Samuels DC, Eden JA, Relton CL, Chinnery PF. Pathogenic mitochondrial DNA mutations are common in the general population. *Am. J. Hum. Genet.* 2008; **83**:254–260.

34. Schaefer AM, McFarland R, Blakely EL, et al. Prevalence of mitochondrial DNA disease in adults. *Ann. Neurol.* 2008; **63**:35–39.

35. Trushina E, McMurray CT. Oxidative stress and mitochondrial dysfunction in neurodegenerative diseases. *Neuroscience* 2007; **145**:1233–1248.

36. Reeve AK, Krishnan KJ, Turnbull D. Mitochondrial DNA mutations in disease, aging, and neurodegeneration. *Ann. N. Y. Acad. Sci.* 2008; **1147**:21–29.

37. Keating DJ. Mitochondrial dysfunction, oxidative stress, regulation of exocytosis and their relevance to neurodegenerative diseases. *J. Neurochem.* 2008; **104**:298–305.

38. Isasi R, Kleiderman E, Knoppers BM. Genetic technology regulation. Editing policy to fit the genome? *Science* 2016; **351**:337–339.

39. Tachibana M, Sparman M, Sritanaudomchai H, et al. Mitochondrial gene replacement in primate offspring and embryonic stem cells. *Nature* 2009; **461**:367–372.

40. Liu CS, Chang JC, Kuo SJ, et al. Delivering healthy mitochondria for the therapy of mitochondrial diseases and beyond. *Int. J. Biochem. Cell Biol.* 2014; **53**:141–146.

41. Koopman WJ, Willems PH, Smeitink JA. Monogenic mitochondrial disorders. *N. Engl. J. Med.* 2012; **366**:1132–1141.

42. Wolf DP, Mitalipov N, Mitalipov S. Mitochondrial replacement therapy in reproductive medicine. *Trends Mol. Med.* 2015; **21**:68–76.

43. Darbandi S, Darbandi M, Khorshid HRK, et al. Experimental strategies towards increasing intracellular mitochondrial activity in oocytes: a systematic review. *Mitochondrion* 2016; **30**:8–17.

44. Woods DC, Tilly JL. Autologous germline mitochondrial energy transfer (AUGMENT) in human assisted reproduction. *Semin. Reprod. Med.* 2015; **33**:410–421.

45. Fakih MHSM, Szeptycki J, dela Cruz DB, et al. The AUGMENT treatment: physician reported outcomes of the initial global patient experience. *JFIV Reprod. Med. Genet.* 2015; **3**:154.

46. Boucret L, Bris C, Seegers V, et al. Deep sequencing shows that oocytes are not prone to accumulate mtDNA heteroplasmic mutations during ovarian ageing. *Hum. Reprod.* 2017; **32**:2101–2109.

47. Liu S, Li Y, Gao X, Yan JH, Chen ZJ. Changes in the distribution of mitochondria before and after in vitro maturation of human oocytes and the effect of in vitro maturation on mitochondria distribution. *Fertil. Steril.* 2010; **93**:1550–1555.

48. Wilding M, Dale B, Marino M, et al. Mitochondrial aggregation patterns and activity in human oocytes and preimplantation embryos. *Hum. Reprod.* 2001; **16**:909–917.

49. Van Blerkom J, Davis P, Alexander S. Differential mitochondrial distribution in human pronuclear embryos leads to disproportionate inheritance between blastomeres: relationship to microtubular organization, ATP content and competence. *Hum. Reprod.* 2000; **15**:2621–2633.

50. Paull D, Emmanuele V, Weiss KA, et al. Nuclear genome transfer in human oocytes eliminates mitochondrial DNA variants. *Nature* 2013; **493**:632–637.

51. Craven L, Tuppen HA, Greggains GD, et al. Pronuclear transfer in human embryos to prevent transmission of mitochondrial DNA disease. *Nature* 2010; **465**:82–85.

52. Shenfield F, Pennings G, Cohen J, et al. ESHRE Task Force on ethics and law 10: surrogacy. *Hum. Reprod.* 2005; **20**:2705–2707.

53. Blake L, Carone N, Raffanello E, et al. Gay fathers' motivations for and feelings about surrogacy as a path to parenthood. *Hum. Reprod.* 2017; **32**:860–867.

54. Murphy DA. The desire for parenthood: gay men choosing to become parents through surrogacy. *J. Fam. Issues* 2013; **34**:1104–1124.

55. Lindenman E, Shepard MK, Pescovitz OH. Müllerian agenesis: an update. *Obstet. Gynecol.* 1997; **90**:307–312.

56. Beale JM, Creighton SM. Long-term health issues related to disorders or differences in sex development/intersex. *Maturitas* 2016; **94**:143–148.

57. Aflatoonian N, Eftekhar M, Aflatoonian B, Rahmani E, Aflatoonian A. Surrogacy as a good option for treatment of repeated implantation failure: a case series. *Iran. J. Reprod. Med.* 2013; **11**:77–80.

58. Wang AY, Dill SK, Bowman M, Sullivan EA. Gestational surrogacy in Australia 2004–2011: treatment, pregnancy and birth outcomes. *Aust. N. Z. J. Obstet. Gynaecol.* 2016; **56**:255–259.

59. Blyth E, Landau R. (Eds.) *Third Party Assisted Conception Across Cultures: Social, Legal and Ethical Perspectives.* London; New York: Jessica Kingsley Publishers. 2004.

60. Thompson C. *Making Parents: The Ontological Choreography of Reproductive Technologies.* Cambridge; London: MIT Press. 2005.

61. Jennings S, Mellish L, Tasker F, Lamb M, Golombok S. Why adoption? Gay, lesbian, and heterosexual adoptive parents' reproductive experiences and reasons for adoption. *Adopt. Q* 2014; **17**:205–226.

Genetics and Reproduction

Genes and Chromosomes

Our genetic information, sometimes described as the "Book of Life," can be envisaged as a compilation containing two "sets" of information, with one originated from the female and the other from the male. Each set includes 23 "volumes" (chromosomes), and each of these chromosomes contains many "chapters and pages" (clusters of genes). Each gene encodes for a specific message to the cell cytoplasm, where ribosomes translate the codes to specific proteins. The genetic code is made up of combinations of three out of four possible essential nucleotides (A, T, G, and C). These nucleotides are the chemical molecules, components of deoxyribonucleic acid (DNA), creating the genetic information that can be further transcripted and translated by different cell types of machinery to produce the essential cellular proteins. A trinucleotide code (three basic nucleotides), called a codon, encodes a specific amino acid, a basic brick of protein structure. Also, other DNA motifs signal the ribosomes to start or stop producing proteins.

In human, each somatic cell contains 23 pairs of chromosomes (46 in total, 44 autosomes and 2 sex chromosomes, marked as 46,XX for female and 46,XY for male). However, in gametes (oocyte and sperm cell), only one set of chromosomes is present (23 chromosomes). Thus, we describe the chromosome constitution in somatic cells as "diploid," meaning two sets of 23 chromosomes, and as "haploid" in gametes when only one set remains. During the formation of the oocyte or sperm, chromosome pairs exchange homologous regions and separate, therefore only one copy of chromosomes is found in each gamete. Errors occurring in chromosomal pairs and chromatid segregation, during the first and second meiosis, result in very common aberrations in a fertilized cell such as an extra chromosome – trisomy, or loss of a chromosome – monosomy.

The chromosomes are organized in the nucleus of all cells and encode for ~20 000 genes. A small number of genes are included out of the nucleus, in mitochondria, the energy centers of the cell. The function of more than 95% of the DNA is still unclear, while only ~1% of DNA "carries a message" and is often called "coding DNA" (genes coding region). Even in those active regions, only exons are transcribed to mRNA, which exits the nucleus and is finally translated into proteins. Contrary, the introns flanking the exons remain in the nucleus and do not express. Although all cells in individuals have an identical genetic constitution, the genes in each organ and tissue are differently active and expressed. Regulation of gene expression is highly controlled by transcription factors, translation regulation, and epigenetic mechanisms.

Types of Mutations

Recessive mutations. All individuals carry several mutated genes on their chromosomes, which pass on to their offspring. However, usually, family members do not present any clinical symptoms as a result of these changes. "Silence" of the mutation occurs due to the existence of two gene copies, a mutated one and a normal one. When the mutated gene fails to express its coding protein, the other healthy copy gene frequently leads to normal development and function. When both copies of a gene are mutated, there may be no protein production at all or an abnormal production that probably results in a genetic disease.

Dominant mutations. Expression of a mutation that appears only in one of the gene copies hints a dominant pattern of inheritance due to overriding the typical gene sequence or "dominance." Dominant mutation can be inherited from one of the parents; however, in many cases, a dominant mutation occurs during gametogenesis, or when the fertilized oocyte starts the first divisions to produce new cells. These mutations are referred to as *de novo* dominant mutations. In such a case, the affected offspring will be the first individual in the family affected by this condition. There are some genes with a greater tendency for these *de novo* events as in cases of dystrophin, neurofibromatosis, tuberous sclerosis complex genes, etc. This *de novo* mutation occurs probably due to the gene size, genetic structure, or specific hot spots with a predisposition for molecular aberrations.

There are three major types of genetic disorder, which are classified according to the origin of the genetic aberration: **monogenic disorders** (usually due to a point mutation in a single gene), **chromosomal disorders** (structural changes in the chromosomes or the gain or loss of an entire chromosome), and **multifactorial disorders** (due to the interaction of several genes and influence of environmental factors such as diet, chemical exposure, and lifestyle on the expression of genes). Some persons have a higher risk of developing illness than others, due to a specific mutation considered to be "genetically predisposed." Several examples for predisposition include the mutations in mismatch repair genes as in cases such as *BRCA1*, *BRCA2*, *MSH2*, *MSH6*, etc. In mutation carriers of these genes, the risk for cancer is dramatically increased and it tends to appear at an early age and sometimes in several organs.

Some genetic disorders occur more frequently in some populations. For example, cystic fibrosis and hemochromatosis are seen more often in people whose ancestors were European. At the same time, thalassemia is found more frequently in people whose ancestors came from Southern Europe, the Indian subcontinent, the Middle East, Africa and Asian countries.

Monogenic Mutations

The majority of point mutations take place in the coding region and are derived from substitutions of one letter with another in a codon that can result in the production of a different amino acid or in a stop codon that terminates protein synthesis. Other mutations originated from the deletion or insertion of single or several nucleotides that usually leads to a shift in the reading frame of genetic information and termination of translation. Splicing mutations that usually result from the destruction of consensus sequence flanking the exons are also responsible for severe genetic conditions. The genetic expression of point mutations can vary from mild to severe condition and depends on transcription and translation impairment. Examples of disorders that occur due to

monogenic mutations include cystic fibrosis, thalassemia, Tay–Sachs disease, familial dysautonomia, *BRCA* mutation, Gaucher and Bloom diseases, and many others.

Another type of monogenic mutation refers to insertion or deletion of hundreds or thousands of nucleotides, as in cases of hemophilia, Duchenne and Becker types of muscular dystrophy, and neurofibromatosis.

In general, a mutation is usually inherited from one of the parents, but it can also occur *de novo* during gametogenesis or early embryo development.

An additional type of monogenic mutation is the expansion of trinucleotide repeats in specific genes. If the number of repeats increases beyond a critical point, the gene can become "unstable" and may develop further repeats. For example, in fragile X syndrome, CGG repeats are localized in the promoter region of the gene and exceed in repeat numbers over 200 leads to complete inhibition of transcription due to the gene hypermethylation. Other mechanisms characterize different severe disorders, also originated from trinucleotide expansions, as in cases of Huntington's disease and myotonic dystrophy.

Mutations in genes on the X chromosome. Mutations in genes carried on the X chromosome are different in females and males. Females have two copies of the X chromosome, while males have only one X chromosome. Unlike chromosome Y, chromosome X is considered to be "gene-rich," with many genes encoding proteins significant for growth and development. These "gene-rich" genes include genes for the synthesis of muscles' structural protein dystrophin, and several proteins that control blood clotting. When these particular X chromosome genes are mutated, specific genetic disorders, especially in males, result such as Duchenne muscular dystrophy, hemophilia, fragile X syndrome, etc.

Shortly after conception, one of the X chromosomes in each female cell is randomly "switched off" so that (except a few chromosomal regions that are not included in inactivation) males and females both have only one active X chromosome in each cell. Females, who have a mutated gene on one X chromosome, are "carriers" of the gene mutation. The mechanism by which the X chromosome is "switched off" is random. Thus, some cells will have the X chromosome coding for the correct product, while other cells will produce the abnormal product due to the mutation; the correct copy usually protects carrier females from any effects of faulty genes with a recessive inheritance on the X chromosome. Males have no other X chromosome to provide "backup" and will usually be affected due to the mutated X chromosome gene expression, and a disorder may be seen at birth or later in life. Therefore, for disorders caused by recessive mutations on the X chromosome, males in the family are often affected, whereas the females can be unaffected carriers of the mutation.

X Chromosome Inactivation

Inactivation of one copy of the X chromosome in female cells safeguards that both males and females have the same number of X chromosome genes instructing the body to grow, develop, and function. This system of "switching off" of most of the X chromosomes is seen in all mammals and is often called lyonization, named after Mary Lyon, who first clearly described the system in 1962. In humans, it occurs very early in embryonic development. One of the X chromosomes turns out to be very shortened and condensed such that most of its genes cannot be "read" by the cell; the dark body in the cell, called a Barr body, is the inactivated X chromosome. X chromosome inactivation only occurs in the somatic cells of the early embryo (inner cell mass at blastocyst stage), since both X chromosomes need to be active in the oocytes for their normal development. This system of inactivation is usually random, i.e., some cells will have the maternal X chromosome switched off, while other cells will have the paternal X chromosome inactivated. X chromosome inactivation affects most of the genes located on the X chromosome, but not all. Particular genes on the X chromosome have their "partner"; they are active on both chromosomes, such as the gene called ZFK that codes for a protein that is possibly involved in the production of both oocytes and sperm cells.

Mitochondrial DNA

DNA also exists in mitochondria. There are over 80 different genes required to produce the components of the mitochondrial respiratory chain. Defective mitochondrial DNA relates to mitochondrial disorders. The expression and severity of the mitochondrial disorder depend on the ratio between mitochondria with mutation and those free of the mutation.

Chromosomal Structural Rearrangement

Aberrations in chromosome structure may result from the addition or loss of chromosomal material and may occur in many ways, but most commonly by translocation of a part of a chromosome, microdeletion, microduplication, inversion, disomia, or mosaicism.

Translocations. Sometimes, a piece of one autosome or sex chromosome is broken off and attaches to a different autosome or sex chromosome in a process called translocation, occurring in around 1:1000 people. There are two common types of translocation: reciprocal – two chromosomes exchange chromosomal segments in the regions where breakage occurs, and Robertsonian translocation – two acrocentric chromosomes are abnormally sticking one with the other and both are losing their p arms. If all the genetic information is present, but simply rearranged, such a translocation is described as "balanced." If translocation has an uneven distribution of chromosome material, such a translocation is described as "unbalanced." An unbalanced translocation, involving large chromosomal fragments, is usually lethal and aborted during early pregnancy. Unbalanced translocations of smaller DNA regions may result in a viable offspring with possible physical or mental developmental disorders, due to a gain or loss of chromosome material. If a woman is a carrier of a translocation between an autosome and the X chromosome, there is a high chance that she will be infertile.

A Robertsonian translocation (named after an American cytogeneticist) is a particular type of rearrangement mostly involving chromosomes 13, 14, 15, 21, and 22. These structural rearrangements are found in about 1:1000 of the average population. The most common of these (~33% of all Robertsonian translocations) are between chromosomes 13 and 14. Couples, where one partner is the carrier of a Robertsonian translocation, can experience repeated miscarriage and male infertility [1–2].

Deletions. A small part of a chromosome may be lost or deleted during the formation of gametes. If the missing material contains essential information for the body's development and function, a disorder will result. Large deletions are usually lethal. A child with cri du chat syndrome has a small part of the short (p) arm of chromosome 5 deleted, causing a range of disabilities, including a characteristically high-pitched mewing cry in infancy. Deletions are one of the genetic variants causing male infertility [3].

Duplications. A small part of a chromosome may be gained or duplicated along its length. This results in changes to the number of genes present and may result in health, development, or growth problems.

Inversions and rings. Sometimes the chromosomes twist around themselves, become inverted, or joined at the ends to form a ring instead of the usual rod shape. During the formation of these structures, some genetic material may be lost. Inversions and rings may cause problems in physical and/or mental development due to an imbalance of chromosomal material, as well as genetic variants causing male infertility [4].

Uniparental disomy. Uniparental disomy occurs when both members of a pair of chromosomes come from one parent. This phenomenon generally does not cause health problems, except for cases where it is necessary to have one chromosome from each parent due to differential chromosomal imprinting.

Mosaicism. Most people have the same chromosome pattern in all cells in their bodies. People who are chromosomally "normal" would thus have either 46,XX or 46,XY in all their cells. Just as mosaic tiles on a floor have a mixture of patterns, some individuals present a chromosomal mosaic and have a mixture of chromosomal patterns in different cells – usually a mixture of cells with the correct number or structure of chromosomes, together with cells carrying a chromosomal abnormality. The proportions of chromosomally abnormal and normal cells can be quite variable and may also vary between different body tissues. For illustration, people with mosaic for trisomy 21 may have the chromosomal abnormality in 60% of cells in their skin versus only 5% of their blood cells. Some mosaics have a mixture of cells with different abnormal patterns. It is not always known for sure whether an individual is a mosaic. Even in cases where mosaicism is established, the pattern in different parts of the body is not always known, rendering it challenging to predict how severely affected a person may be. An embryo classified as mosaic has a chance of 35% to produce a viable pregnancy, whereas a healthy embryo has a chance of 65% and an abnormal embryo has a chance of less than 4%.

Genetic Testing of Male Infertility

Approximately 2300 genes are involved in the process of spermatogenesis. Spermatogenesis checkpoints are controlled by a multitude of genes and signaling pathways that regulate mitosis, meiosis, and sperm transport. Synaptic defects during meiotic prophase in the male almost always result in spermatocyte death, either at the pachytene stage or at first meiotic metaphase. By contrast, females retain fertility in the face of many mutations that cause complete meiotic arrest and sterility in males. The less stringent pachytene checkpoint mechanisms in the female are likely to underlie the male versus female differences in sex chromosome sensitivity during meiosis. Meiotic sex chromosome inactivation occurs only in males, which explains the difference in male versus female sensitivity to the presence of unsynapsed chromatin. It has been hypothesized that failure to inactivate the sex chromosomes is the leading cause of asynapsis-related male sterility [5–6]. Male infertility accounts for 15–30% of infertility cases, most of them with known genetic factors [7]. Common genetic abnormalities include chromosomal or gene defects and epigenetic alterations. Infertile men may appear with phenotypic abnormalities or with sperm abnormalities. Phenotypic abnormalities include Klinefelter syndrome, congenital absence of vas deferens, Kallmann syndrome, cryptorchidism, hypospadias, ambiguous genitalia, and androgen insensitivity syndrome. Sperm DNA damage has been implicated in both primary infertility and recurrent spontaneous abortions following natural and assisted conception. Sperm DNA damage can be transmitted to offspring and may increase the risk of intergenerational infertility or other serious health problems, such as congenital malformations and childhood cancer. Genetic screening includes cytogenetic analysis to detect numerical and structural chromosomal rearrangements, analysis of single-gene mutations, and assessment of nonspecific DNA damage.

A variety of techniques are necessary for such genetic analyses: gene copy number variations and single-gene mutations/polymorphisms are detected by Sanger DNA sequencing, deletions/microdeletions are detected by polymerase chain reaction (PCR), and cytogenetic tests such as karyotyping detect chromosome aneuploidies. Cytogenetic analysis is the most common diagnostic genetic test used to evaluate men with severe oligozoospermia and azoospermia [8]. The incidence of cytogenetic abnormalities in infertile males ranges from 2.1% to 15.5% [9–10].

Genetic Testing of Female Infertility

In females, genetics plays a role in infertility; these effects are mostly polygenic, rendering it challenging to define a single genetic cause. The difference between spermatogenesis and oogenesis begins after pachytene: male gametes proceed quickly through the rest of meiosis, while oocytes arrest in a late stage of prophase for weeks to months, if not decades. For women with unexplained infertility issues, genetic tests such as karyotyping or DNA sequencing of selected genes are performed. The two most common female factor conditions, ovulatory dysfunction (25%) and endometriosis (15%), have a familial predisposition, suggesting a genetic basis [11]. Also, sex chromosome alterations [12] and several single-gene mutations have been shown to impact female fertility [13], causing conditions such as hypogonadotropic hypogonadism, premature ovarian insufficiency, endometriosis, and polycystic ovary syndrome. Most aneuploidies are due to errors in maternal meiosis and occur in approximately 65% of oocytes when maternal age is 36 and over, with rates increasing with maternal age [14].

There are many ways in which chromosome dynamics can be disturbed in oogenesis and, consequently, there are many routes to human aneuploidy. The impact of maternal age points to multiple mechanisms by which aging affects chromosome segregation. The subsequent loss of sister chromatid cohesion from chromosome arms at anaphase I and from sister centromeres at anaphase II is essential to orchestrate the complex chromosome segregation events necessary to produce haploid gametes. Failure to establish connections between homologs is one of the oldest postulated mechanisms of human aneuploidy [15] and studies of human trisomies suggest that recombination failure is, indeed, an essential mechanism of human nondisjunction. It has also been suggested that the premature separation of sister centromeres is a major mechanism of human aneuploidy [16]. Because cohesion is established during the premeiotic S phase in the fetal ovary, but chromosome segregation occurs years later in the adult, the idea that degradation of cohesion occurs during the protracted meiotic arrest is the basis of the effect of human maternal age on chromosome segregation

abnormalities. Cohesins observed during fetal development are necessary and sufficient to mediate cohesion in the adult fully mature oocyte [17–19]. Meiotic recombination occurs in the fetal ovary and failure to recombine and/or suboptimally located crossovers are prominent contributors to human trisomy. Incidence of chromosome misalignment on the first meiotic spindle and disruptions of the anaphase-promoting complex (regulation of the progression from metaphase to anaphase) result in an increased incidence of aneuploidy [20].

Cytogenetic Analysis and Reproduction

Cytogenetic analysis, e.g., karyotyping, is the most commonly used diagnostic genetic test for the evaluation of men with severe oligozoospermia and azoospermia.

Klinefelter syndrome. Klinefelter syndrome is the most frequent cytogenetic/sex chromosomal/numerical anomaly (aneuploidy) detected in infertile men and leads to nonobstructive azoospermia. Men with Klinefelter syndrome have a 47,XXY chromosomal complement in all cells or are "mosaic" [21–23]. The karyotype arises spontaneously when paired X chromosomes fail to disjoin in the first or second phase of meiosis during oogenesis or when XY chromosomes fail to segregate during spermatogenesis. The presence of two X chromosomes in Klinefelter syndrome leads to seminiferous tubule dysgenesis in approximately one-third of all cases. The failed inactivation of the X chromosome is the most plausible reason for impaired spermatogenesis in these patients. The frequency of Klinefelter syndrome is 0.2% of male newborns and 11% of azoospermic men [24]. The adult Klinefelter syndrome testis shows extensive fibrosis and hyalinization of the seminiferous tubules [25]. However, foci of spermatogenesis can be present in these patients, allowing them to become a genetic father after testicular sperm extraction (TESE) and subsequent intracytoplasmic sperm injection. In its non-mosaic form, Klinefelter syndrome is associated with elevated serum follicle-stimulating hormone (FSH) and luteinizing hormone (LH) levels, as well as low testosterone levels. The sterility in Klinefelter syndrome is due to the high prevalence of azoospermia, seen in 92% of Klinefelter syndrome men capable of providing a semen sample, with the remainder having a median of 0.1 million sperm cells/ml. It has also been reported that there is an advanced decline in spermatogenesis by age in men with Klinefelter syndrome; hence early sperm retrieval or sperm banking (if possible) is advocated in such cases [26–27]. Controversial data show that collecting spermatozoa by TESE at early adolescence does not appear to result in higher sperm retrieval efficiency compared with TESE at adult age [28]. Moreover, histological studies have shown that only small numbers of spermatogonia are present in the testicular biopsies from adolescent boys [29] and germ cells are lost at a very young age, even before the initiation of the fibrotic process. However, focal areas of spermatogenesis may be present within the testis of azoospermic men with Klinefelter syndrome, with sperm successfully extracted in approximately 40–50% of cases after TESE [30]. In most men with nonobstructive azoospermia, clinical parameters do not predict success in sperm retrieval. The majority of offspring born from 47,XXY fathers are genetically normal, although chromosomally abnormal fetuses have also been reported [31–32]. Fluorescence *in situ* hybridization analysis has demonstrated that the frequency of sex chromosome aneuploidy is 1.5–7% in sperm from Klinefelter mosaic patients [21], and ~45% in the sperm of men who appear to have a non-mosaic 47,XXY karyotype [23; 33].

Men with Klinefelter syndrome, with serum testosterone levels of less than 250 ng/dl, treated with aromatase inhibitors, clomiphene citrate, or human chorionic gonadotropin before micro-TESE responded to treatment, leading to an elevation of testosterone to 250 ng/dl or higher, and higher sperm retrieval rates compared with men in whom post-treatment testosterone levels were under 250 ng/dl (77% vs. 55%) [31].

The **46,XX male syndrome**, also known as De la Chapelle syndrome, is a rare aneuploidy, with approximately 90% of these males showing translocation of a sex-determining region on the Y (*SRY*) chromosome to the X chromosome or an autosome [34–35]. *SRY* is a gene responsible for the testicular determination and is essential for initiating testis development and differentiation of the bipotential gonad into Sertoli cells, which then support differentiation and development of the male germline. When the paternal X with the SRY gene combines with a normal X from the mother during fertilization, the result is an XX male. Although 46,XX males exhibit normal internal and external male genitalia, they lack the major spermatogenic regions (basically on the Y chromosome) and are azoospermic [36].

Jacob's syndrome. The genetic cause of this syndrome, 47,XYY, is paternal nondisjunction during meiosis, resulting in YY sperm [37]. These patients exhibit tall stature, and 1–2% of them show aggressive behavioral characteristics. Most are azoospermic or severely oligozoospermic and testis biopsy findings range from Sertoli cells only to maturation arrest patterns. Unlike Klinefelter syndrome, serum testosterone levels are normal.

Triple X syndrome. Trisomy X (47,XXX) is a genetic disorder that affects about 1 in 1000 females and most commonly occurs as a result of nondisjunction during meiosis [38]. Many females with triple X syndrome experience no or only mild symptoms; it is therefore estimated that only 10% of individuals with trisomy X are actually diagnosed. Most females with triple X syndrome experience regular sexual development, presenting with late menarche and menstrual irregularities in some cases, and can become pregnant. A taller than average stature is the most typical physical feature. Symptoms in females with triple X syndrome may include an increased risk of delayed development of motor skills, such as sitting up and walking, as well as speech and language skills, dyslexia, hypotonia, behavioral problems, such as attention-deficit/hyperactivity disorder, and psychological problems, such as anxiety and depression.

X0 (Turner) syndrome. Turner syndrome (described in 1938 by Henry Turner) is a condition that affects only females, resulting when one of the X chromosomes is entirely (monosomy 45,X0) or partially missing. Turner syndrome occurs in 1 in 2500 born females and can cause a variety of medical and developmental problems, including short stature, failure of the ovaries to develop (estrogen deficiency, no menstruation, and infertility), poor breast development, and heart defects [39]. Most women with Turner syndrome are infertile due to oocyte loss that starts during embryonic life: they experience regular migration and mitosis of germ cells, but the oogonia do not undergo meiosis, and rapid loss of oocytes leaves the gonad without follicles early in life, and ovarian tissue appears as a fibrous streak. Most women with Turner syndrome require egg-donation treatment for infertility. Spontaneous pregnancies are seen in 2–5% of Turner syndrome patients and are most likely to occur in women with the mosaic form of this syndrome.

Y0 syndrome. As the X chromosome carries about 800 protein-coding genes, some of which are critical

199

for embryo viability, compared with the 70 genes on the Y chromosome, there is no known Y0 syndrome.

Autosomal translocation. Autosomal translocations are 4–10 times more common in infertile males than in the fertile population [40–41]. Most translocations do not affect other tissues but can severely impair spermatogenesis. This effect may be due to the disruption of genes responsible for spermatogenesis or due to impaired synaptic complex pairing and segregation during meiosis [42–45]. Unbalanced reciprocal translocation carriers have a higher risk of producing unbalanced gametes or offspring with abnormalities. Both the chromosomes involved in translocation and the location of the breakpoints are supposed to be determining factors for the fidelity of synapsis, and thus the carrier's fertility status [45]. Carriers of autosomal translocation always have a reduced number of gametes with an unbalanced karyotype [46].

Sex chromosome translocation. Any part of the sex chromosome can translocate to autosomes like other chromosomal translocations. Sex chromosome translocations have direct consequences on genes required for germ cell differentiation. Translocations between the Y chromosome and autosomes are rare and can involve any part of the Y chromosome, every so often leading to abnormal spermatogenesis and hence infertility [47–48]. The suggested mechanisms for impaired fertility due to sex chromosome translocation are the transformed gene loci or impaired formation of the sex vesicle during meiosis. During the first meiosis of spermatogenesis, pairing between the X and Y chromosomes occurs in primary spermatocytes, resulting in a condensed sex vesicle. Sex chromosome pairing seems to be distinct from autosome pairing, as it is limited to the telomere pseudoautosomal regions (PARs), PAR1 (at Xp/Yp) and PAR2 (at Xq/Yq). Changes of pseudoautosomal sequences result in impaired pairing between the X and Y chromosomes, therefore indicating that there is a recombination event in the DNA homolog segment located in PARs during the first meiosis, which is essential to promote meiotic pairing and ensure sperm production [49].

Defects and mutations of the short stature homeobox gene (*SHOX*) in the PAR1 are related to the short stature of Turner syndrome and idiopathic growth retardation [50–51]. Translocations concerning a sex chromosome and an autosome are more likely to cause infertility than translocations involving autosomes.

Y Chromosome Microdeletions

Y chromosome microdeletions are found in 5–15% of infertile men with azoospermia and are a relatively common cause of male infertility [52]. Such deletions are characterized by azoospermia or severe ($<1 \times 10^6$ sperm cells/ml of semen) to moderate oligozoospermia ($1–5 \times 10^6$ sperm cells/ml of semen), with only rare cases of mild oligozoospermia ($5–15 \times 10^6$ sperm cells/ml of semen). Males with Y chromosome infertility usually do not have obvious symptoms, although physical examination may reveal small testes and/or cryptorchidism, or varicocele. The incidence of Y chromosome microdeletions is estimated to be about 1:2000 to 1:3000 males [53–55]. Y microdeletion analysis is usually carried out by polymerase chain reaction (PCR) amplification of three loci, named the azoospermia factor (AZFa, AZFb, and AZFc loci), in the q arm of the Y chromosome (region Yq11). AZFc is the most commonly found (60%) deletion compared with AZFa (5%), AZFb (16%), or their combination (14%) [56]. This commonly found deletion is in part because AZFc is four times longer than AZFa [56]. Genes within the repeats, called the "amplicons" portion of the male-specific Y region, are expressed exclusively in the testis and are believed to contribute to the development and proliferation of germ cells. Multiplex PCR is a rapid method for the detection of submicroscopic Y chromosome deletions, which are undetectable by conventional cytogenetic analysis and conventional PCR.

The azoospermia factor comprises several genes such as *USP9Y* (ubiquitin-specific protease 9Y), *DBY* (DEAD box Y-linked), *RBMY* (RNA-binding motif Y-linked), *PRY* (PTPN-related gene on Y), *UTY* (ubiquitously transcribed tetratricopeptide repeat containing Y), *CDY* (chromodomain protein Y-linked), *DAZ* (deleted in azoospermia), and *HSFY* (heat shock transcription factor Y-linked). These genes are critical for spermatogenesis at different stages of germ cell development. Deletions of AZFa and AZFb are usually rare and are associated with Sertoli cell-only syndrome and maturation arrest, respectively [57]. Therefore, it has been proposed that patients with a microdeletion involving AZFa and AZFb should not undergo TESE. AZFa is expressed in spermatogonial stem cells and AZFb in premeiotic germ cells (primary spermatocyte). In contrast to AZFa and AZFb, partial or complete AZFc loss is related to a highly variable heterogeneous phenotype, ranging from oligozoospermia to azoospermia. Chromosome Y infertility is inherited in a Y-related manner; however, AZF region deletions in the long arm of the Y chromosome are usually *de novo*.

Monogenic Mutation and Infertility

Fragile X syndrome. Fragile X syndrome is an X-linked, inherited condition caused by a mutation of the fragile X mental retardation 1 (*FMR1*) gene (locus Xq27.3). The *FMR1* gene produces a protein called the FMR-1 protein (or FMRP), which is most commonly found in the brain. FMRP is the primary protein regulator of the translation of many RNAs involved in synaptic plasticity, is necessary for proper brain development, and is essential for healthy cognitive development and female reproductive functions. The most crucial feature of fragile X syndrome is intellectual disability, mental retardation, and autism. The mutation (more than 200 CGG repeats interrupted by AGG in the *FMR1* gene) can result in and occurs primarily in men who carry only one mutated X chromosome. Reduction of AGG interruptions could increase the number of secondary RNA structures (RNA loops) in the *FMR1* mRNA, which bind cell cytosolic proteins and inhibit their biological functions, which could cause cell dysfunction within the ovaries [58]. The average number of CGG repeats on the X chromosome stands at 5–44, while 45–54 repeats belong to the "gray zone." Women who carry the premutation (55–200 repeats), occurring at a frequency of 1:170 in the female population, do not have an increased risk of intellectual disability, but have a 13–26% increased risk of developing premature ovarian insufficiency (POI) [59] and tremor ataxia syndrome. Premutation is also characterized by amenorrhea or oligomenorrhea before the age of 40. POI is expressed in women as a low ovarian reserve, with higher follicle-stimulating hormone (FSH) levels on day 3 of the cycle, lower antral follicle count and anti-Müllerian hormone, and low ovarian response to in vitro fertilization hormonal stimulation. Frequency of the fragile X syndrome (mutation with more than 200 CGG repeats) in males is 1:4000 and in females is 1:6000 [60]. It was suggested that the diminished ovarian function that occurs among carriers of 80–120 repeats is due to increased follicular granulosa cell *FMR1* mRNA accumulation [61]. If diagnosed early, women with premutation and a mid-range number of repeats, and one or no

AGG interruption, can make an informed decision about their fertility and try to conceive earlier in life or to pursue fertility preservation options.

The reproductive effect of fragile X syndrome on men is expressed by low sperm quality and postpubertal macro-orchidism.

BPES. Blepharophimosis (narrowing of the eye-opening), ptosis (droopy eyelids), and epicanthus inversus (upward fold of the skin of the lower eyelid near the inner corner of the eye) syndrome (BPES) affects the development of the eyelids. Mutations in the *FOXL2* gene cause BPES type 1 and type 2. The *FOXL2* gene encodes expression of a protein, which is active in the eyelids and ovaries [62]. The protein controls the growth and development of specific ovarian cells before birth and in adulthood. Mutations that cause partial loss of FOXL2 protein function generally lead to BPES type 2. Mutations that cause complete loss of FOXL2 protein function often lead to BPES type 1. These mutations harm the regulation of eyelid development as well as various activities in the ovaries, resulting in abnormally accelerated maturation of certain ovarian cells and the premature death of oocytes.

Congenital bilateral absence of vas deferens (CBAVD). CBAVD is a syndrome characterized by vasa deferentia agenesis that accounts for approximately 2% of infertility cases and at least 6% of obstructive azoospermia. CBAVD, in at least 95% of affected men, is related to cystic fibrosis transmembrane conductance regulator (*CFTR*) gene mutation [63]. The *CFTR* gene is located on chromosome 7 (locus 7q31.20), and has been associated with over 1500 mutations reported so far [64], with the delta F508 mutation being the most common. The CFTR protein is a glycosylated transmembrane protein that functions as a chloride channel and is expressed in epithelial cells of exocrine tissues, such as the lungs, pancreas, sweat glands, and vas deferens. It was also suggested that azoospermic men with idiopathic obstruction of vas deferens and those who have the triad of chronic sinusitis, bronchiectasis, and obstructive azoospermia (Young syndrome) are at high risk of *CFTR* mutation [65].

Androgen Insensitivity Syndrome

Androgen insensitivity syndrome (AIS) is a disorder that implicates the androgen receptor (AR) function due to mutations in the *AR* gene. AR activity is essential for the development of the male phenotype and spermatogenesis. In normal males, androgens (testosterone/dihydrotestosterone) bind to the AR, and form a complex that activates the transcription of genes responsible for secondary sexual characteristics and spermatogenesis. Unlike other autosomal genes, the *AR* gene is a single-copy gene containing eight exons, located on the X chromosome (Xq11-q12). Because the AR mediates the actions of androgens, mutation of the *AR* gene manifests by various androgen insensitivity phenotypes, ranging from 46,XX infertile females to 46,XY azoospermic males [66]. *AR* gene mutations may severely impair the amount, structure, and function of the AR [67], thus causing AIS, which can express as various phenotypes, such as ambiguous genitalia, partial labioscrotal fusion, hypospadias, bifid scrotum, and gynecomastia [68]. Mutations in this gene include point mutations, insertions or deletions, and altered triplet (CAG)n and (GGC)n repeats. CAG repeats are present in the first exon domain of the *AR* gene and contain an average of 21 ± 2 repeats. In male infertility, an *AR* mutation is believed to affect at least 2% of men [69] and CAG repeats (>28) up to 35% of men [70]. Mutations in *AR* may also result in depressed spermatogenesis without any abnormalities in male secondary sexual characteristics. It is recommended to screen the entire *AR* gene (8 exons) for mutations/deletions using bidirectional sequencing in infertile males with regular 46,XY karyotype [71]. Screening for the CAG repeats in the *AR* gene is usually performed as they have been most often detected in patients with AIS.

Steroid 5-Alpha-Reductase 2 (SRD5A2) Deficiencies

SRD5A2 is an enzyme encoded by the *SRD5A2* gene, which comprises five exons and is located in chromosome 2 (locus 2p23). The primary function of SRD5A2 is the conversion of testosterone into dihydrotestosterone (DHT). In SRD5A2 deficiency, DHT levels are below average with normal levels of testosterone. DHT is essential for the development of the external genitalia (penis, scrotum) and testes descent to the scrotum. At the same time, testosterone plays a vital role during embryogenesis in the normal development and differentiation of male genitalia, including the vas deferens, epididymis, and the seminal vesicles. At adolescence and adulthood both androgens are involved in the development of male secondary sexual characteristics and spermatogenesis. Patients with an *SRD5A2* mutation may

exhibit a female phenotype or a complex phenotype due to partial virilization that includes hypospadias, low sperm quality, bifid scrotum, and micropenis [72–73].

Cryptorchidism

Cryptorchidism is one of the most common congenital abnormalities among infertile males. Cryptorchidism is characterized by failure of testicular migration from an abdominal cavity, through the inguinal canal, into the ipsilateral scrotum at roughly the time of birth under the influence of the androgen hormone. Descent of the testes may be bilateral or unilateral. About 30% of preterm born boys are delivered with at least one undescended testis, making cryptorchidism the most common congenital disability of male genitalia. Men with an anamnesis of cryptorchidism are frequently subfertile in adulthood due to impaired spermatogenesis [74]. Impairment of fertility potential, as tested by abnormal sperm count, is observed in about 50% of individuals in unilateral cases and about 80% of bilateral ex-cryptorchid males [75]. Rare cases of cytogenetic anomalies have been reported in combination with cryptorchidism; however, the exact genetic mechanism and the candidate genes are still unclear. Mutations in the *INSL3* and *LGR8* genes located on chromosomes 19 and 13, respectively, have been linked to cryptorchidism [76].

Other Genetic Male Defects

A substantial proportion of infertile patients are still categorized as an idiopathic disorder. Thus it is important to consider other possible genetic defects associated with male infertility. *FSHR* (FSH receptor, chromosome 2), *DAZL* (deleted in azoospermia-like chromosome 3, locus 3p24), *DMRT1* (doublesex and mab-3 related transcription factor 1, chromosome 9), *LGR8* (Leucine G-protein coupled receptor, chromosome 13), *BLM* (Bloom syndrome, chromosome 15, locus 15q26.1), *Ozf1* (oligozoospermic factor, chromosome 15), *SHBG* (sex hormone binding globulin, chromosome 17), *USP26* (Ubiquitin specific peptidase 26, a gene located on the long arm of X chromosome, expressed throughout the testis in the preliminary stages of spermatogenesis and involved in histone removal during spermatogenesis), *TEX11* (chromosome X, locus Xq13.1), *TAF7L* (TATA-box binding protein associated factor, chromosome X, locus Xq22.1; promotion of synapsis and regulation of crossover), and other genes have been associated with male infertility.

For example, *DAZL* is located on chromosome 3 (locus 3p24) and shares homology (~83% similarity) with the *DAZ* gene on the Y chromosome. *DAZL* is believed to be the regulator of germline gene expression, as it leads to the differentiation of embryonic stem cells into pre- and postmeiotic germ cells [77].

Hypogonadism

Hypogonadism is a disorder characterized by decreased gonadal activity. Androgen deficiency (during the testicular age-related changes) is known as secondary hypogonadism or hypogonadotropic hypogonadism. Primary hypogonadism can be a result of Klinefelter syndrome or impaired testicular development, such as in cryptorchidism. Secondary hypogonadism may result either from decreased gonadotropin-releasing hormone (GnRH) that controls LH and FSH production, or from decreased production of LH or FSH itself. The GnRH gene has seven transmembrane domains, comprising three exons, and is located on chromosome 4 (locus 4q21.2). Mutation in this gene is a rare reason of hypogonadism and screening for mutations is not recommended unless there is a family history of hypogonadism. Mutations in the LH or FSH receptor genes are also rarely seen. LH deficiency causes pseudohermaphroditism, delayed puberty, micropenis, and azoospermia, whereas FSH deficiency is associated with decreased testicular volume and various degrees of impaired spermatogenesis, regardless of normal virilization. Another form of hypogonadism is Kallmann syndrome (abnormal migration of GnRH neurons), which is an X-linked recessive disease with marked genetic heterogeneity. This syndrome is described as the association of hypogonadotropic hypogonadism and anosmia. There are at least six genes, *KAL1*, *FGFR1*, *PROKR2*, *PROK2*, *CHD7*, and *FGF8*, known to be linked to Kallmann syndrome. The *KAL1* gene is located on chromosome X (locus Xp22.3) and encodes a neural cell adhesion molecule, anosmin-1, which is secreted from embryonic olfactory bulb. Mutations involving these genes account for about 30% of all Kallmann syndrome cases. Various *KAL1* mutations have been described in hypogonadotropic hypogonadal males [78–79]. Mutations in *FGFR1* or *FGF8*, encoding fibroblast growth factor receptor-1 and fibroblast growth factor-8 respectively, cause an autosomal dominant form of Kallmann syndrome with incomplete penetrance. Mutations in *PROKR2* and *PROK2*, encoding prokineticin receptor-2 and prokineticin-2 have been described. The mutations in *PROK2* were detected in the heterozygous state, whereas *PROKR2* mutations were found in the heterozygous, homozygous, or compound heterozygous state [80]. *PROKR2* and *PROK2* are likely to be related to both monogenic recessive and digenic/oligogenic Kallmann syndrome transmission.

Genetic Counseling

Genetic testing plays an essential role in the evaluation of infertility, both for diagnosis and prevention of iatrogenic transmission of the genetic defect to the offspring. Numerous organizations have established recommendations concerning genetic tests for couples seeking infertility treatment. Genetic counseling is provided by a team of experts in problems relating to growth, development, and health issues, which may have a genetic basis. This counseling can assist families and individuals in understanding and adjusting to the diagnosis of a genetic disorder. During the consultation, a family health history is collected. A diagnosis of a genetic disorder may be made or confirmed before pregnancy, during pregnancy, after birth, in childhood, or later in life. The diagnosis is performed based on clinical features, biochemical tests, or genetic tests. This diagnosis may mean that other family members are at risk. On the other hand, such tests can be reassuring to individuals who find out that they do not have a particular disorder. Where there is a genetic disorder in a family, the genetic counselor can estimate the chances that other family members, or future children, will be affected. Both verbal and written information about the condition and its impact is provided to assist people in dealing with some of the issues that may arise from a diagnosis of a genetic disorder.

Many genetic disorders can be established before the birth. During genetic counseling, prenatal diagnosis and other reproductive options can be discussed to ensure that any decision is made on an informed basis. Appropriate testing, including carrier, predictive, and presymptomatic testing, can be arranged. Genetic counseling is recommended in various scenarios, including a disorder linked to a family history; a personal risk either to develop the condition or to pass on the condition to his/her children; when a previous child is affected by a serious problem in growth, development, or health, or one or more family members have unusual features, a number of different abnormalities, or a serious health problem; when a woman is in her mid-30s or older and is planning a pregnancy; when intending parents are close relatives; when a fetal abnormality is detected during pregnancy; and when there is concern about exposure to some chemical or environmental agent which might cause birth defects.

References

1. Mau-Holzmann UA. Somatic chromosomal abnormalities in infertile men and women. *Cytogenet. Genome Res.* 2005; 111:317–336.

2. Therman E, Susman B, Denniston C. The nonrandom participation of human acrocentric chromosomes in Robertsonian translocations. *Ann. Hum. Genet.* 1989; 53:49–65.

3. Kuroda-Kawaguchi T, Skaletsky H, Brown LG, et al. The AZFc region of the Y chromosome features massive palindromes and uniform recurrent deletions in infertile men. *Nat. Genet.* 2001; 29:279–286.

4. Sasagawa I, Ishigooka M, Kubota Y, et al. Pericentric inversion of chromosome 9 in infertile men. *Int. Urol. Nephrol.* 1998; 30:203–207.

5. Royo H, Polikiewicz G, Mahadevaiah SK, et al. Evidence that meiotic sex chromosome inactivation is essential for male fertility. *Curr. Biol.* 2010; 20:2117–2123.

6. Homolka D, Jansa P, Forejt J. Genetically enhanced asynapsis of autosomal chromatin promotes transcriptional dysregulation and meiotic failure. *Chromosoma* 2011; 121:91–104.

7. Neto FTL, Bach PV, Najari BB, Li PS, Goldstein M. Genetics of male infertility. *Curr. Urol. Rep.* 2016;17:70–82. https://doi.org/10.1007/s11934-016-0627-x.

8. Lissitsina J, Mikelsaar R, Punab M. Cytogenetic analyses in infertile men. *Arch. Androl.* 2006; 52:91–95.

9. Balkan M, Tekes S, Gedik A. Cytogenetic and Y chromosome microdeletion screening studies in infertile males with oligozoospermia and azoospermia in Southeast Turkey. *J. Assist. Reprod. Genet.* 2008; 25:559–565.

10. Rives N, Joly G, Machy A, et al. Assessment of sex chromosome aneuploidy in sperm nuclei from 47,XXY and 46,XY/47,XXY males: comparison with fertile and infertile males with normal karyotype. *Mol. Hum. Reprod.* 2000; 6:107–112.

11. Mallepaly R, Butler PR, Herati AS, Lamb DJ. Genetic basis of male and female infertility. *Monogr. Hum. Genet.* 2017; 21:1–16.

12. Grynberg M, Bidet M, Benard J, et al. Fertility preservation in Turner syndrome. *Fertil. Steril.* 2016; 105:13–19.

13. Huang H-L, Lv C, Zhao Y-C, et al. Mutant ZP1 in familial infertility. *N. Engl. J. Med.* 2014; 370:1220–1226.

14. Hassold T, Hunt P. To err (meiotically) is human: the genesis of human aneuploidy. *Nat. Rev. Genet.* 2001; 2:280–291.

15. Henderson SA, Edwards RG. Chiasma frequency and maternal age in mammals. *Nature* 1968; 218:22–28.

16. Angell RR. Predivision in human oocytes at meiosis I: a mechanism for trisomy formation in man. *Hum. Genet.* 1991; 86:383–387.

17. Angell RR, Xian J, Keith J, Ledger W, Baird DT. First meiotic division abnormalities in human oocytes: mechanism of trisomy formation. *Cytogenet. Cell Genet.* 1994; 65:194–202.

18. Pellestor F, Andreo B, Arnal F, Humeau C, Demaille J. Maternal aging and chromosomal abnormalities: new data drawn from in vitro unfertilized human oocytes. *Hum. Genet.* 2003; 112:195–203.

19. Revenkova E, Herrmann K, Adelfalk C, Jessberger R. Oocyte cohesin expression restricted to predict stages provides full fertility and prevents aneuploidy. *Curr. Biol.* 2010; 20:1529–1533.

20. Reis A, Madgwick S, Chang HY, et al. Prometaphase APC cdh1 activity prevents non-disjunction in mammalian oocytes. *Nat. Cell Biol.* 2007; 9:1192–1198.

21. Lim AS, Fong Y, Yu SL. Estimates of sperm sex chromosome disomy and diploidy rates in a 47,XXY/46,XY mosaic Klinefelter patient. *Hum. Genet.* 1999; 104:405–409.

22. Thomas NS, Hassold TJ. Aberrant recombination and the origin of Klinefelter syndrome. *Hum. Reprod. Update* 2003; 9:309–317.

23. Lenz P, Luetjens CM, Kamischke A, et al. Mosaic status in lymphocytes of infertile men with or without Klinefelter syndrome. *Hum. Reprod.* 2005; 20:1248–1255.

24. Schiff JD, Palermo GD, Veeck LL, et al. Success of testicular sperm extraction and intracytoplasmic sperm injection in men with Klinefelter syndrome. *J. Clin. Endocrinol. Metab.* 2005; 90:6263–6267.

25. Aksglaede L. Natural history of seminiferous tubule degeneration in Klinefelter syndrome. *Hum. Reprod. Update* 2005; 12:39–48.

26. Ichioka K, Utsunomiya N, Kohei N, et al. Adult onset of declining spermatogenesis in a man with nonmosaic Klinefelter's syndrome. *Fertil. Steril.* 2006; 85:1511.e1–1511.e2.

27. Plotton I, Giscard d'Estaing S, Cuzin B, et al. Preliminary results of a prospective study of testicular sperm extraction in young versus adult patients with

nonmosaic 47,XXY Klinefelter syndrome. *J. Clin. Endocrinol. Metab.* 2015; 100:961–967.

28. Van Saen D, Vloeberghs V, Gies I, et al. When does germ cell loss and fibrosis occur in patients with Klinefelter syndrome? *Hum. Reprod.* 2018; 33:1009–1022.

29. Van Saen D, Pino Sánchez J, Ferster A, et al. Is the protein expression window during testicular development affected in patients at risk for stem cell loss? *Hum. Reprod.* 2015; 30:2859–2870.

30. Corona G, Pizzocaro A, Lanfranco F, et al. Sperm recovery and ICSI outcomes in Klinefelter syndrome: a systematic review and meta-analysis. *Hum. Reprod. Update* 2017; 23:265–275.

31. Ron-El R, Raziel A, Strassburger D, et al. Birth of healthy male twins after intracytoplasmic sperm injection of frozen-thawed testicular spermatozoa from a patient with nonmosaic Klinefelter syndrome. *Fertil. Steril.* 2000; 74:832–833.

32. Friedler S, Raziel A, Strassburger D, et al. Outcome of ICSI using fresh and cryopreserved-thawed testicular spermatozoa in patients with non-mosaic Klinefelter's syndrome. *Hum. Reprod.* 2001; 16:2616–2620.

33. Estop AM, Munne S, Cieply KM, et al. Meiotic products of a Klinefelter 47,XXY male as determined by sperm fluorescence in-situ hybridization analysis. *Hum. Reprod.* 1998; 13:124–127.

34. Maduro MR, Lamb DJ. Understanding new genetics of male infertility. *J. Urol.* 2002; 168:2197–2205.

35. Quinn A, Koopman P. The molecular genetics of sex determination and sex reversal in mammals. *Semin. Reprod. Med.* 2012; 30:351–363.

36. Oates RD. The genetic basis of male reproductive failure. *Urol. Clin. North Am.* 2008; 35:257–270, ix.

37. Davis JL, Kurek JA, Morgan JC, Sethi KD. Tremor and dystonia in Jacob's syndrome (47,XYY). *Mov. Disord. Clin. Pract.* 2019; 7:107–108.

38. Otter M, Schrander-Stumpel CT, Curfs LM. Triple X syndrome: a review of the literature. *Eur. J. Hum. Genet.* 2010; 18:265–271.

39. Kosteria I, Kanaka-Gantenbein C. Turner syndrome: transition from childhood to adolescence. *Metabolism* 2018; 86:145–153.

40. Chandley AC, Seuanez H, Fletcher JM. Meiotic behavior of five human reciprocal translocations. *Cytogenet. Cell Genet.* 1976; 17:98–111.

41. Elliott DJ, Cooke HJ. The molecular genetics of male infertility. *Bioessays* 1997; 19:801–809.

42. Estop AM, Van Kirk V, Cieply K. Segregation analysis of four translocations, t(2;18), t(3;15), t(5;7), and t(10;12), by sperm chromosome studies and a review of the literature. *Cytogenet. Cell Genet.* 1995; 70:80–87.

43. Cifuentes P, Navarro J, Blanco J, et al. Cytogenetic analysis of sperm chromosomes and sperm nuclei in a male heterozygous for a reciprocal translocation t(5;7)(q21;q32) by in situ hybridisation. *Eur. J. Hum. Genet.* 1999; 7:231–238.

44. Alves C, Carvalho F, Cremades N, Sousa M, Barros A. Unique (Y;13) translocation in a male with oligozoospermia: cytogenetic and molecular studies. *Eur. J. Hum. Genet.* 2002; 10:467–474.

45. Ferguson KA, Chow V, Ma S. Silencing of unpaired meiotic chromosomes and altered recombination patterns in an azoospermic carrier of a t(8;13) reciprocal translocation. *Hum. Reprod.* 2008; 23:988–995.

46. Guo JH, Zhu PY, Huang YF, Yu L. Autosomal aberrations associated with testicular dysgenesis or spermatogenic arrest in Chinese patients. *Asian J. Androl.* 2002; 4:3–7.

47. Gunel M, Cavkaytar S, Ceylaner G, Batioglu S. Azoospermia and cryptorchidism in a male with a de novo reciprocal t(Y;16) translocation. *Genet. Couns.* 2008; 19:277–280.

48. Pabst B, Glaubitz R, Schalk T, et al. Reciprocal translocation between Y chromosome long arm euchromatin and the short arm of chromosome 1. *Ann. Genet.* 2002; 45:5–8.

49. Mohandas TK, Speed RM, Passage MB, et al. Role of the pseudo-autosomal region in sex chromosome pairing during male meiosis: meiotic studies in a man with a deletion of distal Xp. *Am. J. Hum. Genet.* 1992; 51:526–533.

50. Ellison JW, Wardak Z, Young MF, et al. PHOG, a candidate gene for involvement in the short stature of Turner syndrome. *Hum. Mol. Genet.* 1997; 6:1341–1347.

51. Rao E, Weiss B, Fukami M, et al. Pseudoautosomal deletions encompassing a novel homeobox gene cause growth failure in idiopathic short stature and Turner syndrome. *Nat. Genet.* 1997; 16:54–63.

52. Poongothai J, Gopenath TS, Manonayaki S. Genetics of human male infertility. *Singapore Med. J.* 2009; 50:336–347.

53. Kamp C, Huellen K, Fernandes S, et al. High deletion frequency of the complete AZFa sequence in men with Sertoli-cell-only syndrome. *Mol. Hum. Reprod.* 2001; 7:987–994.

54. Krausz C, Forti G, McElreavey K. The Y chromosome and male fertility and infertility. *Int. J. Androl.* 2003; 26:70–75.

55. Dada R, Gupta NP, Kucheria K. Yq microdeletions-- azoospermia factor candidate genes and spermatogenic arrest. *J. Biomol. Tech.* 2004; 15:176–183.

56. Walsh TJ, Pera RR, Turek PJ. The genetics of male infertility. *Semin. Reprod. Med.* 2009; 27:124–136.

57. Krausz C, Quintana-Murci L, McElreavey K. Prognostic value of Y deletion analysis: what is the clinical prognostic value of Y chromosome microdeletion analysis? *Hum. Reprod.* 2000; 15:1431–1434.

58. Lekovich J, Man L, Xu K, et al. CGG repeat length and AGG interruptions as indicators of fragile X-associated diminished ovarian reserve. *Genet. Med.* 2017; 20:957–964.

59. Karimov CB, Moragianni VA, Cronister A, et al. Increased frequency of occult fragile X-associated primary ovarian insufficiency in infertile women with evidence of impaired ovarian function. *Hum. Reprod.* 2011; 26:2077–2083.

60. Crawford DC, Acuña JM, Sherman SL. FMR1 and the fragile X syndrome: human genome epidemiology review. *Genet. Med.* 2001; 3:359–371.

61. Elizur SE, Lebovitz O, Derech-Haim S, et al. Elevated levels of FMR1 mRNA in granulosa cells are associated with low ovarian reserve in FMR1 premutation carriers. *PLoS One* 2014; 9:e105121.

62. Gustin SE, Hogg K, Stringer JM, et al. WNT/β-catenin and p27/FOXL2 differentially regulate supporting cell proliferation in the developing ovary. *Dev. Biol.* 2016; 412:250–260.

63. Carrell DT, De Jonge C, Lamb DJ. The genetics of male infertility: a field of study whose time is now. *Arch. Androl.* 2006; 52: 269–274.

64. Radpour R, Gourabi H, Gilani MA, Dizaj AV. Molecular study of (TG)m(T)n polymorphisms in Iranian males with congenital bilateral absence of the vas deferens. *J. Androl.* 2007; 28:541–547.

65. Practice Committee of American Society for Reproductive Medicine in collaboration with Society for Male Reproduction and Urology. Evaluation of the azoospermic male. *Fertil. Steril.* 2008; 90:S74–S77.

66. Arnedo N, Nogues C, Bosch M, Templado C. Mitotic and meiotic behaviour of a naturally transmitted ring Y chromosome: reproductive risk evaluation. *Hum. Reprod.* 2005; 20:462–468.

67. Stouffs K, Tournaye H, Liebaers I, Lissens W. Male infertility and the involvement of the X chromosome. *Hum. Reprod. Update* 2009; 15:623–637.

68. Galani A, Kitsiou-Tzeli S, Sofokleous C, Kanavakis E, Kalpini-Mavrou A. Androgen insensitivity syndrome: clinical features and molecular defects. *Hormones (Athens)* 2008; 7:217–229.

69. Hiort O, Holterhus PM, Horter T, et al. Significance of mutations in the androgen receptor gene in males with idiopathic infertility. *J. Clin. Endocrinol. Metab.* 2000; 85:2810–2815.

70. Mifsud A, Sim CK, Boettger-Tong H, et al. Trinucleotide (CAG) repeat polymorphisms in the androgen receptor gene: molecular markers of risk for male infertility. *Fertil. Steril.* 2001; 75:275–281.

71. Sharma V, Singh R, Thangaraj K, Jyothy A. A novel Arg615Ser mutation of androgen receptor DNA-binding domain in three 46,XY sisters with complete androgen insensitivity syndrome and bilateral inguinal hernia. *Fertil. Steril.* 2011; 95:804. e19–804.e21.

72. Yuan S, Meng L, Zhang Y, et al. Genotype-phenotype correlation and identification of two novel SRD5A2 mutations in 33 Chinese patients with hypospadias. *Steroids* 2017; 125:61–66.

73. Li SP, Li LW, Sun MX, et al. Identification of a novel mutation in the *SRD5A2* gene of one patient with 46, XY disorder of sex development. *Asian J. Androl.* 2018; 20:518–519.

74. La Vignera S, Calogero AE, Condorelli R, et al. Cryptorchidism and its long-term complications. *Eur. Rev. Med. Pharmacol. Sci.* 2009; 13:351–356.

75. Caroppo E, Niederberger C, Elhanbly S, et al. Effect of cryptorchidism and retractile testes on male factor infertility: a multicenter, retrospective, chart review. *Fertil. Steril.* 2005; 83:1581–1584.

76. Ferlin A, Zuccarello D, Garolla A, Selice R, Foresta C. Hormonal and genetic control of testicular descent. *RBM Online* 2007; 15:659–665.

77. Kerr CL, Cheng L. The dazzle in germ cell differentiation. *J. Mol. Cell. Biol.* 2010; 2:26–29.

78. Albuisson J, Pecheux C, Carel JC, et al. Kallmann syndrome: 14 novel mutations in KAL1 and FGFR1 (KAL2). *Hum. Mutat.* 2005; 25:98–99.

79. Trarbach EB, Baptista MT, Garmes HM, Hackel C. Molecular analysis of KAL-1, GnRH-R, NELF and EBF2 genes in a series of Kallmann syndrome and normosmic hypogonadotropic hypogonadism patients. *J. Endocrinol.* 2005; 187:361–368.

80. Dodé C, Teixeira L, Levilliers J, et al. Kallmann syndrome: mutations in the genes encoding prokineticin-2 and prokineticin receptor-2. *PLoS Genet.* 2006; 2(10):e175. doi:10.1371/journal. pgen.0020175.

Chapter 1

Preimplantation Genetic Testing (PGT)

Eliezer Girsh and Mira Malcov

Introduction to Preimplantation Genetic Testing

The risk for transmission of genetic disorders to off-spring has been a critical obstacle for couples known to be carriers for severe genetic disorders. To prevent the birth of an affected child, prenatal testing by amniocentesis or chorionic villus sampling (CVS) is offered. An alternative approach, available with assisted reproductive technology (ART), is preimplantation genetic testing – PGT – enabling testing of the embryo for the familial disorder before the corresponding embryo is transferred to the uterus of the mother.

The concept of PGT (until recently termed "preimplantation genetic diagnosis – PGD") emerged in the early 1960s when sexing of rabbit embryos at the blastocyst stage was attempted [1]. The first clinical applications of PGT were reported in 1990, with the first pregnancies obtained following blastomere biopsy and sex determination by polymerase chain reaction (PCR) in couples at risk of having children with X-linked disorder [2]. Since then, the list of diseases for which PGT has been used is rapidly growing, and thousands of children have been born following intracytoplasmic sperm injection (ICSI)-PGT cycles, with no identified adverse neonatal, obstetrical, or cognitive risks. Blastomere biopsy for PGT has no added adverse effects compared with ICSI pregnancies [3–5].

Initially, the indication for PGT focused on preventing the birth of a child affected with a severe familial disorder associated with a monogenic mutation or chromosomal rearrangement, carried by the parents, e.g., cystic fibrosis (CF), thalassemia, fragile X, spinal muscular atrophy (SMA) [6–7], as well as structural chromosomal aberrations, mainly translocations that can be diagnosed by the use of different technologies [8–10]. Theoretically, PGT can be performed for any genetic condition for which the gene sequence is

available, and the familial causative mutation has been identified. However, in the past decade, PGT has been widely performed for chromosomal screening during in vitro fertilization (IVF) cycles to enhance pregnancy and take-home baby rates. In these cases, an aneuploidy screening is performed without any specific parental genetic indication but with the hope that since chromosomal abnormalities represent one of the significant causes of implantation failures and spontaneous abortions, a selective transfer of a euploid embryo will increase implantation rate and reduce spontaneous abortion, due to the enhanced viability of the euploid embryo. Theoretically, an embryo diagnosed as euploid has a higher chance to be implanted, likely reducing the number of attempts until a viable pregnancy and healthy offspring is achieved [11].

The increasing use of chromosomal screening during IVF treatments has recently promoted a modern classification and subdivision of PGT into three major branches: PGT for monogenic disorders (PGT-M), PGT for structural chromosomal rearrangements (PGT-SR), and PGT for chromosomal screening for aneuploidy (PGT-A).

Steps in Preimplantation Genetic Testing

Method of Fertilization for PGT

As PGT is performed using a very limited amount of genetic material, aspirated oocytes should be denuded from the surrounding maternal cumulus cells in order to prevent maternal contamination. The fertilization is regularly performed by ICSI instead of insemination, in order to avoid paternal contamination of sperm cells remaining attached to the zona pellucida (ZP). During the biopsy procedure, it is most important to make sure that perforated ZPs are free of parental cells that might lead to misdiagnosis [12].

Biopsy

Biopsy of preimplantation embryos consists of two main steps: the creation of an opening in the ZP and removal of polar bodies (PBs) or embryonic cells. For PGT, embryos are subjected to biopsy in the IVF laboratory using an inverted microscope and micro-manipulator with holding and biopsy pipettes on hydraulic arms. The ZP is perforated using an in-contact laser beam and the genetic origin is aspirated by gently pulling the biopsy pipette [13–15]. When blastomeres are biopsied from a cleavage-stage embryo, it is highly recommended to make sure that the cell contains genetic material, i.e., a nucleus, which is fundamental for DNA analyses. However, nuclei are not always visible due to rapid mitotic divisions of early embryonic stages and blastomeres are characterized by a rapidly dissolving and regenerating nuclear membrane. Several methods have been described for ZP opening and genetic material removal, depending on the stage and morphology of the oocyte/embryo biopsied. Removal of genetic material (PB or blastomere) by aspiration into the biopsy micropipette is the most widely used method and is applicable for all stages of biopsy (mature oocytes and embryos at cleavage or blastocyst stages). Blastomere removal by extrusion or flow displacement can also be applied at any stage of the embryo. While cleavage-stage biopsy was the most widely practiced form of embryo biopsy for over a decade [16], its clinical use has now been reduced compared with the blastocyst-stage biopsy. Nevertheless, the preferred stage for biopsy remains under substantial debate. For blastocyst biopsy, aspiration and excision with a laser can be used as well as an aspiration in combination with the mechanical cutting of the trophectoderm (TE) cells. It is critical to be extremely accurate in matching between the numerical mark of the embryo and numerical mark of a corresponding isolated biopsied cell, in order to prevent mismatch at diagnosis of different embryos. Double-checking by two embryologists is highly recommended at this stage. After a biopsy, the embryo is carefully washed, returned to the culture medium and incubated or cryopreserved until embryo transfer.

Zona Pellucida Opening

A sampling of any genetic material from the embryo (the first and second PBs, blastomere, or TE) is only possible following oocyte/embryo ZP-envelope perforation. Three methods have been developed for this purpose: mechanical, chemical, and laser-aided.

Mechanical opening. The mechanical method was the first method used to open the ZP and is still applied clinically, although in a very limited number of centers. The method involves creating slits in the ZP, using a sharp micropipette, and scratching the strung ZP by a sharp micropipette onto the holding one. In this way, a V-shaped triangular or square flap opening for biopsy in the ZP is created [17].

Chemical opening. This type of biopsy is practically no longer in use. It used to utilize acidic Tyrode's solution (pH = 2.3), which is aspirated into the biopsy pipette. The pipette is lowered to close proximity to the embryo to dissolve the ZP locally. When the breach is opened, the excess of acidic solution in the medium, close to the embryo, is aspirated by the same biopsy pipette. The method was mainly used for cleavage-stage embryo biopsies up to two decades ago and was replaced by other methods due to the potential toxicity of the acid Tyrode's on embryo viability [18].

Contact laser opening. In 1990, a laser (ultraviolet [UV] contact) neodymium:yttrium–aluminium–garnet (Nd:YAG) with a potassium titanyl phosphate crystal (the working wavelength to 532 nm) was introduced, and used to drill the ZP of oocytes and embryos [13]. The introduction of the erbium: yttrium–aluminium–garnet (Er:YAG) laser occurred in 1992; this worked at a wavelength of 2900 nm and consequently avoided potential damage to the embryos' genetic structure [19]. The subsequent years saw the emergence of noncontact lasers working in the infrared or near-infrared range (800–1500 nm), further away from the DNA absorption peak of 260 nm. The first laser with a significant impact on the advancement of ART was the indium–gallium–arsenic–phosphorous (InGaAsP) semiconductor diode laser, operating at 1480–2100 nm (infrared) [14; 20], which is still commonly used today. This laser avoided the mutagenicity and contamination that had previously been related to UV contact lasers, and has become a valuable tool for ART. At present, the laser is the most popular method of ZP opening for PB, cleavage-stage, and blastocyst biopsy. The method involves the use of a guided noncontact laser beam, which can be adjusted to create a ZP opening of the desired size, accurately and rapidly. Exposure to the laser should be minimal and efforts should be made to avoid damage of embryonic cells and impairment of embryo development. In the case of PB or cleavage-stage biopsy, the size of the ZP opening should be adapted to the size of the biopsied material. The hole must be extensive and allow the safe pulling and collection of PB or blastomere, while also avoiding the significant rupture of embryo envelope or remaining cells.

Genetic Material Aspiration

During the opening procedure of the ZP, the position of the embryo is selected such that a blastomere intended for nucleation is at the biopsy-opening side "3 o'clock position." For sample aspiration, a 30–40 µm-diameter biopsy pipette is used (larger diameters are used for blastomeres and TE and smaller ones for PB biopsy). The biopsy pipette is carried close to the opening in the ZP. The outer edge of the blastomere/PBs and the tip of the aspiration pipette are kept in focus. Using very gentle aspiration, the blastomere/PB is slowly drawn into the pipette and then released into the medium. Extreme care is required to avoid cell membrane rupture and damage to the biopsied cell or the surrounding blastomeres within the embryo. Aspiration of the blastomere with a visible nucleus and proximal to the hole of the ZP is preferred.

The efficient transfer of biopsied cells to reaction tubes, i.e., "tubing," is a critical step and a determining factor for a successful PGT cycle. In principle, tubing requires careful and accurate handling of embryonic cells to ensure the placement of the genetic material in the tube and to prevent contamination with DNA from exogenous cells.

A sampling of the embryo for genetic testing can be performed using three follow methodologies:

1. Polar body biopsy. During oocyte maturation and meiosis completion, the oocyte extrudes two PBs one after another. Follicle-stimulating hormone and luteinizing hormone surges promote random segregation of homologs from each of the chromosomal pairs to the first PB and the oocyte, while the sister chromatids of the remaining chromosomes are segregated to the second PB following fertilization [21–22].

Biopsy of first and second PB is performed immediately following fertilization and after the appearance of the pronuclei, respectively, and serves as an alternative to blastomere biopsy. The oocyte is secured by the holding pipette at the "9 o'clock" position, with the PB at the "6 or 12 o'clock" position. The opening of the ZP is made at the "3 o'clock" position and the PB is aspirated with an aspiration/biopsy micropipette. PB biopsy does not adversely affect either fertilization or cleavage. The second PB is removed by introducing the biopsy micropipette through the slit previously made to remove the first PB. This step is delicate, as connections may still exist between the second PB and the oocyte membrane [23–24].

This biopsy strategy was initially suggested in order to determine the genetic status of the embryo by sampling genetic material which is not a part of the developing embryo. Later, due to regulations that prohibited embryo biopsy due to religious or moral laws in some countries (Switzerland, Austria, Germany, and Italy), PB biopsy became common, as it only tests the unfertilized oocytes and fertilized oocytes at the stage before they are considered a zygote.

The advantages of PB biopsy include both minimal impairment of the embryonic cellular array, allowance of two additional days for genetic analysis, and enablement of fresh embryo transfer. However, the use of a meiosis oocyte derivate as a source of genetic material is now less practiced due to the following disadvantages: the need for two sequential biopsies and sometimes, when the first PB is homozygous and resulting data are insufficient, a third biopsy is required. Such repetitive and prolonged exposures of the embryo to unmonitored conditions may be harmful to development. Also, the biopsied genetic material is extremely small and sticky, rendering it challenging to be sampled and collected. The most critical limitation of this technique is the absence of paternal genetic material, thereby rendering it irrelevant for testing for paternal-dominant disorders. For this reason, for recessive mutations, 50% of the embryos, instead of 25%, will have to be discarded. For PGT-A, this biopsy technique also lacks information on postmeiotic chromosomal errors that occur in the first mitotic embryonic divisions. Another disadvantage lies in the fact that the embryo is diagnosed by the elimination of the observed three alleles, diagnosed both in the first and second PBs, out of all four maternal known alleles. This is highly inferior when compared with the direct embryo testing of blastomeres and TE biopsies [25].

2. Blastomere biopsy. Biopsy of a single cell from a cleavage-stage embryo, usually performed 72 hours after fertilization, is still a technique commonly used for the diagnosis of monogenic disorders. This stage is particularly essential for those of paternal origin and recessive disorders that cannot be diagnosed by PB analysis. For blastomere biopsy, quality cleavage-stage embryos composed of at least six cells and at the pre-compaction stage are exposed to a bivalent cation-deficient medium (Ca^{2+}/Mg^{2+} free) in order to attenuate tight junctions and disrupt cell adhesions [26]. Following a biopsy, the Ca^{2+}/Mg^{2+}-free medium is rinsed off the embryo with culture medium, at least once, and the embryo is cultured according to standard IVF culture conditions [16; 18]. Embryos with fragmentation exceeding 25% are generally not biopsied and may be cultured to the blastocyst stage for biopsy.

The advantage of this biopsy approach is the direct testing of the embryo (in contrast to "elimination diagnosis" when PBs are tested). The biopsy schedule on day 3 of development allows fresh embryo transfer and, also, in case of amplification failure or inconclusive results, it is still possible to re-biopsy the embryo on day 5 if development to blastocyst stage is accomplished.

The disadvantage of this type of biopsy lies in the limited amount of DNA, resulting in enhanced allele dropout (ADO) rates and amplification failures. For a reliable and accurate analysis, a diagnostic system should be calibrated for single-cell multiplex nested PCR protocols. Besides, blastomere biopsy at this embryo-development stage is not suitable for PGT-A, mainly because of the insufficient amount of DNA required for full chromosomal constitution representation following whole genome amplification. Also, this embryonic stage is characterized by higher rates of mosaicism, compared with the blastocyst stage; as a result, biopsy at this stage may lead to rejection of a euploid embryo due to trisomy or monosomy of the blastomere that represents only the biopsied cell and not the whole embryo [27].

3. Trophectoderm biopsy. This type of biopsy is the most commonly used for PGT-A cycles and the most suitable means of chromosomal diagnosis using advanced molecular methods such as chromosomal microarray (CMA) and next-generation sequencing (NGS). It is also considered to be safer for the embryos, since biopsied cells are carefully taken from the TE lineage cells, without affecting the inner cell mass (ICM), which is destined for fetal development.

Determination of the fate of embryos based on TE sampling is rooted in the assumption that cells from the blastocyst TE represent the comprehensive chromosomal status of the embryo compared with embryonic cells biopsied from day 3 embryos. Also, due to significantly higher amounts of DNA, TE biopsy is considered to be more reliable and successful than blastomere biopsy for PGT-A [27–30]. Therefore, the estimated rate of inconclusive diagnoses is expected to be below 5%. Moreover, whole-genome amplification (WGA) products of blastocyst biopsies enable running multiple analyses for different indications from the same biopsied cells. Such analyses are essential when both a chromosomal aberration and a monogenic disorder should be diagnosed [31].

For biopsy of TE, one of the following procedures can be performed: slitting a hole in the ZP of good-quality embryos by a laser beam on day 3, and 2 days later, slashing of the tail end of the TE of an expanded blastocyst, which hatched from the perforated ZP, using the laser beam. Alternatively, the ZP opening may be performed early on the day of blastocyst formation, followed by a period of culture to allow herniation of TE cells from the ZP and TE cell removal. The third option is to simultaneously perform ZP opening and TE cell excision on the day of full blastocyst expansion [32]. The biopsy procedure can vary, depending on the morphology and quality of the blastocyst, expansion grade, and the position of the ICM. A biopsy is performed in a HEPES-buffered medium. The Ca^{2+}/Mg^{2+}-free medium should not be used. TE cells are aspirated into the biopsy pipette with gentle suction. Laser pulses are directed at the junctions between cells, to either excise the aspirated cells from the blastocyst or to minimize cell damage while detaching. Biopsied TE cells are mechanically released from the pipette, by making a quick flicking movement of the biopsy pipette against the holding pipette. To avoid cross-contamination during biopsy, it is highly recommended to change the biopsy pipette for each blastocyst. Blastocysts are cryopreserved immediately after the biopsy.

The advantage of blastocyst biopsy is a collection of multiple TE cells for analysis, allowing more reliable results, without invading the ICM (Figure 17.1). However, this type of biopsy suffers from several disadvantages, the most prominent one being the need to freeze the embryos immediately after biopsy before the results of diagnosis are obtained. Also, while feasible, the prolonged culture required for blastocyst

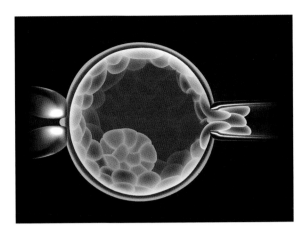

Figure 17.1 Biopsy of a blastocyst.

formation (day 5, 6, and even 7) has been implicated in lower implantation rates. Although reaching the stage of expanded blastocyst formation serves as a selective parameter and as an excellent positive predictor for pregnancy, prolonged culture also might be harmful to embryos at the genetic and epigenetic levels [33–35]. Another essential drawback is if, for some reason, diagnosis is failed or inconclusive, re-biopsy of thawed embryos is exceptionally complicated. In that case, the embryo should be thaw, re-biopsied and frozen again, and all these procedures impair further embryo survival.

General Recommendations on Labeling and Witnessing throughout the Biopsy

Double witnessing is recommended during the following stages: (a) immediately after biopsy, to confirm the embryo and sample number match by two embryologists; (b) during spreading or tubing, to confirm that the sample identification matches the labeling on the relevant slide or tube; (c) further embryo culture, when placing the embryo into the labeled culture dish, and (d) in case of cryopreservation, after the biopsy and before acquiring the genetic analysis results, label the cryopreservation device with specific identification of the embryo.

In general, biopsied oocytes and embryos must be cultured or cryopreserved individually, with an identification system to ensure tracking of the biopsy sample and unambiguous post-diagnostic identification.

Principles of PGT Analyses

In general, for PGT analyses, all blastomeres or TE samples biopsied from tested embryos and intended for PGT-M, PGT-SR, or PGT-A are rinsed in a fresh culture medium. The isolated blastomere or TE is then rinsed twice in phosphate-buffered saline supplemented with 10% polyvinylpyrrolidone to prevent the stickiness of the samples and attachment to the aspirating capillary. After the last rinse, the genetic material representing the embryo is gently transferred to the bottom of a PCR tube under sterile conditions. The tubes, with a single embryonic cell in each of them, are immediately incubated at +70°C for 10 minutes to allow DNase inactivation. This stage is pivotal for the integrity of the DNA sample. The samples are then transferred to -80°C, for at least 1 hour. This step is aimed to facilitate the exposure of covered and condensed DNA molecules to the subsequent ingredients and enzymes of the amplification reactions [36].

In the biopsy work area and the first PCR room, protective clothing (preventing genetic contamination of the sample) should be worn, including a full one-time surgical dress, hair cover, face mask covering both the nose and mouth, and shoe covers. Gloves should be worn at all times and changed frequently, whenever coming in contact with a nonsterile object. The tubing (preamplification) area should be in a DNA-free environment. However, due to IVF good laboratory practices, DNA decontamination protocols cannot be applied, and benches, binocular area, and other surfaces are thoroughly cleaned with water and ethanol 70%. Since such DNA decontamination is suboptimal, it is recommended to design a particular area dedicated to embryo biopsy, in proximity to or within the IVF laboratory.

PGT-M

PGT-M refers to the analysis of a possible monogenic mutation in a single cell biopsied from a preimplanted embryo. The tested mutation has an autosomal dominant, autosomal recessive, or X-linked transmission pattern. The justification for conducting IVF with PGT-M (usually for fertile couples) is determined according to the risk for affected offspring, the severity of the disease, the therapeutic options to treat it, the penetration and variable expression, and the time of onset.

211

In general, PGT-M can diagnose any severe genetic disorder that has already been identified in the family/carrier patient and can also be diagnosed in prenatal samples such as amniocentesis and CVS.

PGT-M, in contrast to PGT-A and PGT-SR, is a tailor-made diagnostic system based on the amplification and characterization of the familial mutation parallel to several polymorphic markers flanking the tested mutation. A qualified molecular laboratory can test as many as several dozen DNA loci in a single biopsied blastomere. This flexibility enables the diagnosis of several genetic conditions simultaneously if needed. For example, to select an immunologically suitable bone marrow donor for an affected sibling, by analyzing the human leukocyte antigen (HLA) typing loci with or without concurrent testing for an additional monogenic disorder [37].

When PGT-M was first introduced, two molecular diagnostic approaches were suggested in order to analyze mutation in a single cell biopsied from a cleavage-stage embryo: WGA and single-cell multiplex nested PCR. In WGA, the DNA of a single cell is randomly amplified (as described later), followed by a second amplification of selected DNA loci, including the mutation of interest and flanking polymorphic markers, custom-designed for each family. For single-cell multiplex nested PCR, only desired DNA loci, including the familial mutation and flanking markers, in contrast to the random amplification in the WGA method, are amplified from DNA originating from the single cell [38]. The second amplification in this method is the nested PCR, in which each of the genetic loci is separately re-amplified, using the same primers of the first reaction or nested primers. The WGA procedure is considered to be less accurate than multiplex PCR and is characterized by higher rates of ADO and total amplification failures. ADO is a phenomenon in which only one of the alleles, maternal or paternal, is amplified, while the other allele is dropped out, likely in the very first PCR cycles. Also, for WGA, a TE biopsy is required, followed by the pre-diagnosed biopsied embryos being frozen separately. The main advantage of WGA is a circumvention of the need for meticulous protocol calibration for single-cell PCR amplification. Nevertheless, most molecular PGT laboratories opt for PGT-M in the single-cell multiplex PCR procedure, which is performed on a single blastomere biopsied from cleavage-stage embryos. Using this highly flexible "home-made" protocol, specific adjustments for each family can be made, enabling the detection of several genetic conditions, all in the DNA from a single blastomere [39–40].

Analysis of a specific DNA locus from a single cell, which contains a single maternal and a single paternal DNA copy, is usually accompanied by amplification failure and relatively high rates of ADO. ADO is a common phenomenon and is the main obstacle in single-cell PCRs and the major cause of misdiagnosis in PGT-M. Such events are especially significant when dominant mutations or recessive disorders, caused by two different mutations, are analyzed. In these cases, ADO of the mutated allele, leading to the demonstration of the normal allele only, may lead to the not desirable transfer of an affected embryo. The main problem with this method is that due to the extremely high sensitivity of the PCR required to amplify a single DNA copy, the yield of the amplicons does not reflect the original amount of DNA in the biopsied blastomere and, therefore, the existence of a single or double normal allele cannot be extrapolated. When ADO of the mutated allele occurs, there is no way to differentiate between normal cells and affected cells carrying the mutated allele that was accidently dropped out [41–42]. When amplifying and analyzing the mutation sequence only, the mutated allele may be dropped out, leading to misdiagnosis since biopsied cells from the affected embryo may be diagnosed as the cells from a normal embryo. In order to prevent such devastating results, monogenic disorders are usually tested by simultaneous amplification of the specific familial mutation, together with several informative polymorphic markers usually represented by short tandem repeats (STRs). The polymorphic markers with STRs are usually long repeats of the C and A nucleotides dispersed throughout the genome. Due to their repetitive nature, cellular DNA polymerase fails to amplify them correctly and deletion or insertion of repeats is frequently observed. Therefore, within generations, variability of these markers increases until it is possible to distinguish both one person from another and also between maternal and paternal alleles in each individual. The diagnosis of a familial mutation by analysis of STR markers flanking the tested mutation decreases the risk for misdiagnosis almost entirely. This immense variability is of value not only for PGT-M but also for other genetic applications, including paternity/maternity determination tests, forensic biology, and others [43–45].

The collection of polymorphic markers closely flanking the mutation of interest (no more than 1.5 million bases upstream and downstream of the mutation) constitutes a stable genomic cluster that, due to the minimal distances between them, is not subject to crossing-over events and is called a "haplotype." It is technically feasible to differentiate between the maternal and paternal haplotypes and, consequently, between mutated and healthy alleles. Informativity of haplotypes depends on the differences in the numbers of CA repeats between the maternal and paternal alleles and the distances between informative markers and the tested mutation. The chances that a calibrated diagnostic system will drop out an entire haplotype are close to zero. The careful design of each molecular PGT-M diagnostic system for each family ensures a negligible risk for misdiagnosis, alongside high reliability and accuracy.

In cases when the causative mutation is localized on the X chromosome and the disease is expressed in a gender-dependent manner, the gender of the embryo is also determined. For this purpose, the sex chromosomes are analyzed using at least three informative STRs, localized on X and Y chromosomes [39].

Following tailoring the diagnostic system for each family, accuracy and reliability should be validated before the clinical PGT-M cycle. For this purpose, single leukocytes are isolated from the peripheral blood of healthy and affected family members in order to simulate the single-blastomere analysis. Only when all single tested leukocytes are correctly diagnosed, with amplification rates above 95% and an ADO rate for each locus below 10%, is the analytic system considered accurate and reliable. After that, hormonal induction for the IVF treatment cycle for PGT is initiated.

In brief, for the PGT-M, single blastomeres are removed from -80°C in a clean room dedicated to the first PCR amplification (multiplex PCR for PGT-M or WGA for PGT-A). The most critical steps of a single-gene molecular analysis are the first ones and faults, errors, or contaminations in these initial stages are frequently fatal and irreversible. The first step of PGT-M analysis is the exposure of DNA, which is naturally condensed within the protecting nucleus and covered with histones, to the PCR reaction components. The DNA is accessed by treating the cell with an alkaline lysis buffer before the PCR amplification [12]. For the first multiplex PCR amplification, all primers, designed to amplify the mutation, flanking

polymorphic markers, and markers located on sex chromosomes (when an X-linked disease is analyzed), are mixed in the tube containing the single blastomere. The tube also contains other ingredients required for single-cell PCR, e.g., the extremely robust DNA polymerase, special additives that stabilize the DNA, suitable buffer, and other reagents. Meticulous calibration of the PCR program, starting with a prolonged denaturation stage and careful designation and purification of relatively long primers, allows for efficient and accurate amplification of many DNA loci from an extremely limited amount of DNA [39]. At the end of the first PCR amplification, the PCR tube content containing a significant but still insufficient amount of DNA of each of the desired loci is subjected to a second PCR reaction, in which each locus is further amplified [46]. To this end, aliquots of each analyzed blastomere (representing each of the analyzed embryos) are prepared. In each tube, each locus amplified in the first PCR reaction is amplified separately. At the end of the second PCR, the amount of DNA is highly amplified and subjected to fragment analysis for haplotype determination and mutation testing, or incubated with specific restriction enzymes which discriminate between normal and mutated alleles. Collecting, editing, and analyzing all data of direct mutation testing, together with haplotype results for each sample, enable accurate genotyping of each of the biopsied embryos. The final results are then shared with the IVF laboratory; after which, the healthy and transferrable embryos are selected.

PGT-SR

PGT-SR refers to the analysis of an unbalanced chromosomal constitution arising from a pathogenic aberration already identified in the family of the patient. Most PGT-SR tests analyze the chromosomal constitution of embryos derived from a couple in which one of them is a carrier of a balanced translocation. Due to meiotic chromosomal segregations, those couples have about 60% risk for unbalanced offspring. In individuals with an unbalanced chromosomal constitution, partial chromosomal deletion and/or addition is observed, and viability and severity of the syndrome will depend on the numbers and functions of genes localized on DNA regions involved in the aberration.

At the very beginning, only fluorescence *in situ* hybridization (FISH) was available. However, in the past decade, advanced molecular methods, such as array-based comparative genomic hybridization (aCGH), single nucleotide polymorphism (SNP) array, and NGS were introduced and serve as the gold standard for PGT-SR as well as for PGT-A [47]. Although these advanced technologies enable detection of all expected unbalanced forms of the chromosomal rearrangement, they do not distinguish between embryos with a normal karyotype and embryos with an abnormal but balanced aberration.

Fluorescence *In Situ* Hybridization (FISH)

When PGT-SR was first introduced, FISH was the standard diagnostic method applied to detect numerical and structural chromosomal aberrations. FISH-based PGT was mainly applied for detection of inherited chromosomal rearrangements but also for embryo sexing, and for the analysis of X-linked diseases, such as Duchenne muscular dystrophy. FISH enables the labeling of specific chromosomal regions that are involved in structural rearrangements or indicative of sex chromosomes. By using specific DNA fragments designed to hybridize with known chromosomal regions and labeled with fluorescent tags in different colors, the number of chromosomal signals can be counted. In the analysis of autosomal chromosomes, two signals represent a balanced embryo and other numerical combinations hint to an unbalanced chromosomal constitution. Fluorochrome probes are specifically designed to hybridize the centromere region, the telomere region, or the entire chromosome (chromosome painting). The specific probes and fluorescent tags are carefully selected according to the chromosomal aberration in question and are usually ordered from a commercial supplier.

For the FISH analysis, two blastomeres are usually aspirated from a cleavage-stage embryo and carefully lysed with a spreading buffer placed over a positively charged glass slide [48], and left until the nucleus is separated from other cell components and is clearly observed. The area on the slide where each nucleus is localized should be immediately bordered with a diamond pencil (mark the opposite side of the slide) and the serial number of the biopsied embryo should be indicated [48]. The slides embedded with embryonic interphase nuclei are treated with proteinase, to remove cytoplasmic remnants and to achieve better exposure of DNA and enhance its accessibility to the probes. Nuclear and probe DNA are simultaneously denatured

and generally incubated with three probes that can differentiate between the balanced and unbalanced chromosomal constitution of the tested aberration. After overnight incubation, excess probes are rinsed and signals are observed using a fluorescence microscope [49–51].

To analyze reciprocal translocations, a combination of three informative probes with three different fluorescent colors (one color per probe), targeting both chromosomes involved in the translocation, are used. In order to detect all unbalanced segregation products of a reciprocal translocation and to reliably discriminate between normal/balanced and unbalanced chromosomal constitution, the three probes should be designed in correlation to the translocation breakpoints, with either two distal and one proximal, or two proximal and one distal. For Robertsonian translocations and inversions, two fluorescent probes are sufficient. For deletions and duplications, locus-specific probes for the deleted or duplicated region should be used, and a control probe (usually on the same chromosome) should be included.

In contrast to conventional cytogenetic analysis, FISH does not require cells at the metaphase stage and can analyze interphase nuclei as well. Compared with other advanced molecular methods, FISH is relatively cheap, rapid, and simple, and does not require dedicated or costly equipment. Also, the biopsy for FISH can be performed on day 3, so diagnosed unaffected embryos can be transferred in fresh cycles. However, this early stage of embryo development is characterized by high mosaic rates. Biopsy of a blastocyst for a FISH-based diagnosis is not recommended because both separation of different nuclei from the same biopsied TE cells and avoidance of overlapping of the nuclei and their signals are difficult. While biopsy of more cells usually increases reliability in this case, it increases the uncertainty of results suffering anyhow from relatively low accuracy and reliability, compared with PCR and CMA/NGS techniques.

Drawbacks of FISH analysis include the delicateness required to spread blastomeres on a slide, requiring high proficiency, and often met with obstacles. Also, the diagnosis is based on a visual and subjective inspection of fluorescent signals, which are often misinterpreted due to overlapping signals, where two different signals may be considered as one and two chromosomes are interpreted as only one. Similarly, when the signal is split, one signal may be considered as two different signals and one chromosome is interpreted as two. These two types of misinterpretations account for the relatively high rates of misdiagnosis. Another significant disadvantage is that, in comparison to other molecular cytogenetic methods, which provide comprehensive details of the chromosomal constitution, FISH results are limited to the loci targeted by the specifically selected probes. The FISH analysis is also limited by the small variety of available fluorescently colored (wavelength) probes. A maximum of three to nine chromosomes from each embryo biopsy specimen (when two separated hybridizations are performed with striping of probes between the first set of DNA probes and the second set) can be analyzed in a single cell. Therefore, FISH-based PGT is currently only used for chromosomal rearrangements involving small fragments or subtelomeric regions of chromosomes that are difficult or impossible to detect using other advanced molecular diagnostic methods, e.g., NGS and DNA array. For sex determination, the use of multiplex single-cell PCR of specific CA repeats localized on X and Y chromosomes is much more accurate, reliable, and cost-effective than FISH analysis, with only one probe for each of the sex chromosomes [32].

Chromosomal Microarray (CMA) and Next-Generation Sequencing (NGS)

Over the last decade, molecular genome-wide technologies, such as aCGH and NGS, have proven to provide a comprehensive means of chromosomal screening, and have gradually replaced the FISH method. In general, for PGT-SR (and for PGT-A as well), advanced molecular methods and significantly higher amounts of DNA are needed to perform both aCGH and NGS. Therefore, TE biopsy should be performed at day 5 or 6 and then subjected to WGA. During this initial and most critical stage of the analysis, the embryonic DNA is randomly and uniformly amplified using random primers. The WGA product can be further analyzed by CMA or NGS techniques, to obtain the complete constitution of all 23 chromosome pairs.

Whole-Genome Amplification (WGA)

When DNA quantity in a tested sample is limited and not sufficient to allow diagnosis by molecular and cytogenetic analysis, WGA can be used to amplify a DNA template of interest. This approach is used when preimplantation embryos are biopsied and comprehensive chromosomal analysis is required. WGA can amplify the original amount of DNA from a small number of single TE cells, enabling further analyses. Technically, it is possible to use the same method for single blastomere amplification. However, in a single cell, the amplified product is often of poor quality, with significant variances in the representation of different genomic regions. While several WGA protocols, using different types of primers or different DNA polymerization enzymes, are available, they are all based on the same principle of random amplification, using complete or partially random primers. Three basic strategies were developed and are still commonly used for WGA. In the primer extension preamplification (PEP) method, the primers utilized for the amplification are entirely random and complementarity between primers and the DNA template is very low. To achieve amplification under these conditions, a relatively low temperature is used during PCR cycles to allow the random primers to anneal to the DNA template. In the degenerate oligonucleotide polymerization (DOP) protocol, only the six nucleotides in the center of each primer are random, while the rest of the nucleotides are constant in all used primers. This structure allows the use of a higher annealing temperature, which increases productivity and uniformity compared with the PEP method. DOP-PCR is the method of choice for the detection of copy number variations (CNV). The third and commonly used method is the multiple displacement amplification (MDA) method. This approach is based on the annealing of random short primers (hexamers) to the DNA template, followed by strand displacement polymerization, which results in many amplification branches on the same strand. This amplification is performed under isothermal conditions instead of the regular PCR program, which is based on repetitive cycles of temperature changes for DNA denaturation, annealing, and elongation. The branching and continuity of amplified amplicons yield PCR products that are much longer than following PEP or DOP amplification. This unique amplification method is enabled by a special DNA polymerase – Phi29, which exhibits very high enzymatic activity compared with the commonly used Taq polymerase. The amplicons in MDA can reach to thousands of base pairs in length, while the average fragment sizes achieved in PEP and DOP are 400–500 bp. It has been claimed that this method of amplification increases fidelity, and prevents slippage, stoppage, and dissociation of the polymerase from the template, resulting in higher uniform amplification of the genome. Commercial kits, based on the PEP, DOP, or MDA technologies or a combination of these methods, are available and frequently compared. Some differences and advantages of the range of commercial products have been described, mainly concerning fidelity, as tested by exome sequencing. Before choosing the method of preference, all the WGA methods should be evaluated with regards to uniformity of genomic coverage, high fidelity of the sequence, reliability of CNV quantification, and technical ADO-rooted errors. For CMA, it seems that the differences between strategies and commercial kits are insignificant [52–53]. A suboptimal WGA product, with regards to the relative and absolute DNA amounts and most importantly, genomic amplification uniformity, will negatively influence test reliability and accuracy. Poor WGA quality may lead to total amplification failure and even to misdiagnosis.

For the WGA procedure, the biopsied TE sample is handled as in PGT-M and is performed precisely according to the manufacturer's protocol. Usually, the WGA protocol includes cell lysis, preamplification preparations, such as fragmentation or ligation, and final amplification. In some of the commercial kits, the quantity and quality of DNA amplification can be estimated by agarose gel separation, before advanced genetic analyses.

Chromosomal Microarray (CMA) – Comparative Genomic Hybridization (CGH)

Comprehensive chromosomal analysis is based on the hybridization of the WGA product of the biopsied embryo sample, with a glass slide microchip embedded with thousands of DNA fragments representing the entire chromosomal constitution. For PGT-SR or PGT-A, CMA hybridization of the WGA product is performed on arrays embedded with DNA probes or oligonucleotides, usually representing each chromosomal locus several times. This system significantly increases the reliability and accuracy of the test. When probes are used, the number of analyzed representative chromosomal regions is usually smaller compared with the dozens of thousands of hybridization loci that can be analyzed when oligonucleotides are imprinted on the glass. The CGH method is based on competitive

hybridization between the analyzed sample and reference DNA, prelabeled with different fluorescent tags. Following the co-hybridization of the test sample and reference DNA on the same array, each hybridized spot displays a color that results from the ratio between two different chromosomal constitutions labeled with different fluorescence. The difference in fluorescence ratio is detected by the scanner and analyzed by software, with variants identified by the addition or deletion of a chromosomal fragment or entire chromosome. These deviations from the 1:1 ratio are translated by the system's software to a visual chromosomal map representing gain or loss of DNA fragments/chromosomes in the analyzed embryo sample. When the analyzed sample is chromosomally balanced, the hybridization ratio in all loci of the array will be 1:1 and the system software will translate this status of fluorescence as "normal." However, when a chromosomal fragment is gained or lost, the fluorescence ratio at the specific aberrant locus will be either lower than the reference sample, indicating loss of chromosomal content, or higher than the reference, indicating a gain of a chromosomal region. The chromosomal gain will increase the ratio of test to control, while a chromosomal loss will decrease the ratio of test to control. The CMA-CGH procedure is relatively rapid and simple, and provides detailed and accurate information concerning chromosomal gain or loss and segmental anomalies, with a resolution of ~10 Mb.

There are a few cases when the detection of translocation segments is limited by the resolution of the CMA platform, due to the absence of probes or oligonucleotides in the specific regions of interest. If the size of more than one of the four translocated segments is below this resolution limit and probe coverage in these regions is very low, CGH-based PGT is not feasible. Detection of small, unbalanced translocation segregations with telomeric or subtelomeric breakpoints is usually performed by FISH, despite the previously described limitations and disadvantages of the method. An additional disadvantage of the CMA method is a requirement of an amount of DNA that is much larger than that found in a single cell. Therefore cleavage-stage embryos are not suitable for the analysis and should be grown to blastocyst stage for the biopsy of TE. It also means that the embryo must be cryopreserved until results are obtained. Also, this analysis is quantitative and cannot distinguish between balanced structural abnormalities and healthy embryos. In such cases, there is a high risk of transmitting an unbalanced constitution to the following generations.

Next-Generation Sequencing (NGS)

NGS, or what was originally called massively parallel sequencing (MPS), was developed from the Sanger chain-termination method of sequencing designed by Frederick Sanger and his colleagues in 1977. Sanger sequencing made it possible to read a single ~300 bp DNA fragment using sequencing by termination [54]. The MPS/NGS revolution greatly enhanced Sanger sequencing and enabled the simultaneous reading of millions of DNA fragments [55–56]. The new platform, for example, enables the sequencing of an entire human genome within a single day.

There are several methods for massive sequencing, based on the enzymatic incorporation of deoxyribonucleotide triphosphates into a DNA template, during sequential cycles of DNA synthesis. Depending on the sequencing platform, each cycle of nucleotide incorporation is followed by the release of fluorophores or hydrogen ions, which are detected by the system and translated by software to a certain nucleotide in a specific position. In all NGS platforms, paralleled sequencing of millions of small DNA fragments is followed by advanced bioinformatics analyses that align all fragments and compare sample reads to the human reference genome. To increase accuracy and reliability, each genomic region is sequenced multiple times, providing the "depth" of the reaction.

In general, NGS involves four necessary steps: library preparation, performed by random fragmentation of the desired DNA source, followed by ligation, normalization, and tagmentation of small DNA oligonucleotides with "DNA barcodes" for further efficient clonal amplification and identification of sequenced DNA fragments by standard PCR. The normalized DNA library is than clonally amplified by the binding of the library adapters to the complementary oligonucleotides in the flow cell, resulting in cluster generation of each DNA fragment. Each cluster is then sequenced by the detection of single bases incorporated into the DNA strand. Nucleotide incorporation is directly monitored by luminescence detection or by changes in electrical charge or pH during the sequencing procedure. The sequenced reads are analyzed by the alignment of the newly identified sequence to a reference genome. Data analysis enables detection of a broad spectrum of genome variations through microdeletion and microduplication of chromosomal aberrations, such as monosomy and trisomy, as used for PGT-SR and PGT-A.

These technologies are extensively used for whole-exome sequencing (WES) and cover more than 95% of human exons for the identification of coding variants involved in human diseases and disorders. In cases when variation cannot be identified in WES, whole-genome sequencing can provide further information concerning introns and other regulatory elements absent in WES. Other studies with NGS technology for the investigation of RNA transcription and sequencing have been performed to assess the differential expression of genes epigenetically regulated by methylation sequencing and following developmental events, differentiation, diseases, and other conditions also reflect transient and environmental factors.

PGT-SR and PGT-A by NGS

While both PGT-A and PGT-SR aim to analyze all 24 chromosome pairs in early developing embryos, the main focus of PGT-A is the diagnosis of whole-chromosome additions or deletions, while in PGT-SR, the analysis identifies specific, relatively small regions of chromosomal aberrations. Recently, a growing number of PGT laboratories analyzing translocation and inversion and providing comprehensive chromosomal screening exchanged CMA technology with NGS. NGS provides for high throughput and higher accuracy and resolution compared with former methods. As the number of samples increases due to the use of genetic barcodes, enabling the analysis of multiple embryos in a single run, the cost per test dramatically decreases. The various NGS platforms for PGT-A/SR demonstrate different levels of accuracy, with all platforms being capable of assessing aneuploidy of full chromosomes with very low error rates. However, only some reliably detect small unbalanced translocations, segmental aneuploidy, polyploidy, and mosaicism [57–58]. NGS technology is usually used as a means of sequencing and fails to identify microdeletion and microduplication smaller than 5 Mb.

The issue of mosaicism is mainly critical in PGT-A analyses, where aneuploidy is acquired during early embryonic mitotic divisions. In PGT-SR, these events are irrelevant. Since unbalanced rearrangements originate in and are carried by one of the parental gametes, the chromosomal aberration will appear in all embryo cells, in contrast to mosaicism acquired during random mitotic chromosomal errors.

PGT-A and Mosaicism

Mosaicism, likely a widespread phenomenon in early developing embryos, is a status when the embryo contains two or more populations of cells, each of which represents different chromosomal constitutions. Some of the embryonic cells present a normal chromosomal constitution, while others are aneuploid or even chromosomally chaotic. These random chromosomal aberrations are a result of postmeiotic errors occurring during massive mitotic divisions after fertilization. Such genetic errors may be of clinical relevance, manifested by impaired embryo viability and decreased potential for live birth. Until recently, it was well accepted that even at low levels of mosaicism, mosaic embryos are not suitable for transfer. However, thanks to new molecular technologies, such as comprehensive chromosomal analysis for PGT-A or PGT-SR by NGS, recent studies have suggested a relatively high frequency of such events in normal implanted embryos as well [59–62], raising debates over the value of comprehensive chromosomal screening [63–64]. The Committees of the American Society for Reproductive Medicine and the Society for Assisted Reproductive Technology stated in 2018 that "there is insufficient evidence to recommend the routine use of blastocyst biopsy with aneuploidy testing in all infertile patients" [65]. There is also a deep debate over the degree to which the biopsied sample from TE truthfully represents the ICM. Some studies claim that chromosomal aberrations appear in higher frequencies in TE compared with the developing embryo [66]. These higher frequencies are specially related to segmental chromosomal anomalies and it seems that their clinical effect is limited and rather reflects the TE quality [67].

Uniquely Challenging PGT Cases

Combined PGT-M and PGT-A Diagnosis

Since prenatal and postnatal CMA examinations have become very common, a growing number of monogenic diseases should be diagnosed in parallel to the detection of chromosomal microduplication, microdeletions, and chromosomal rearrangements. In the past, to test for a monogenic mutation with chromosomal aberration, two consecutive biopsies were required: one blastomere for monogenic diagnosis and another blastomere for FISH analysis (instead of two blastomeres generally used for FISH analysis due

to the relatively low accuracy and reliability of this method). The remarkable improvement in the reliability and uniformity of WGA allowed for the combined diagnosis of PGT-A and PGT-M, with the same WGA source material derived from a single TE biopsy. The amplified DNA is sufficient for several dozens of tests, including PCR and CMA analyses [68]. However, when NGS is applied, it allows for the detection of single nucleotide variations and small insertions and deletions, common in monogenic disorders, in parallel to aneuploidies by target sequencing. In this procedure, primers aimed to amplify the mutation region and flanking haplotype are included in a single NGS reaction. This approach potentially enables the analysis of multiple mutations in many genes alongside aneuploidy screening, in contrast to other PGT-A techniques, such as CMA, which allow for chromosomal evaluation only [69].

"Karyomapping" is a platform based on SNP array technology, developed for simultaneous monogenic and chromosomal analysis [70]. SNPs are very abundant in the human genome (one SNP per 300–1000 bp), and analysis can be easily interpreted. SNP arrays containing several millions of probes allow for SNP genotyping of entire chromosomes in a single reaction. More specifically, as with NGS, it enables the simultaneous analysis of single gene defects and aneuploidies. The advantage of this platform is that the built-in millions of SNPs are distributed throughout the genome, with high density and coverage of all coding regions. This enables the immediate testing of any monogenic disease, without requiring the meticulous bioinformatic and molecular preparations, taking into consideration specific familial genotype variables. The main disadvantage of "karyomapping" is the high cost relative to other platforms; PGT laboratories with accurate and reliable single-cell PCR amplification capacities will usually opt for single-cell multiplex nested PCRs instead of "karyomapping." This is the preferred route, especially for the diagnosis of common diseases, such as those tested in national screening programs (fragile X, CF, TS, SMA, etc.). However, this technology can still be cost-effective when the diagnosis of several new or private mutations is required [71]. A similar, "home-made" diagnostic system, also based on SNPs, was developed [72]. This approach demonstrated very high accuracy and reliability for PGT-A, PGT-SR, and PGT-M testing. In addition to the three known types of PGT, this platform also tested, for the first time, the prediction risk of polygenic disorders, such as hypothyroidism and type 1 diabetes.

PGT-M for Late-Onset Neurodegenerative Disorders

When a couple has a significant risk for an offspring affected by a severe, incurable late-onset disease, such as Huntington's disease, several diagnostic and reproduction options can be considered. Since biochemical and physical screening tests cannot prevent the onset of disease, many potential carriers with unknown definitive status prefer to remain undiagnosed due to social and financial (e.g., insurance, occupation) negative impact of such knowledge. There are two different ways to ensure that the next generation will be free of the familial devastating disease while leaving the genetic status unknown. The first and less common option is the "nondisclosure" in which a regular PGT, including direct testing of carrier status, is performed, but results are not transferred to the patient. Such a situation in which the medical staff is aware of a "secret" is prone to produce uncomfortable medicolegal situations. The second and more common procedure is called the "exclusion test." In this approach, the mutation is never tested; embryos are diagnosed by haplotype analyses only. This method is based on the discrimination of all embryos that inherited from the suspected carrier parent one of both alleles from the affected grandmother or grandfather. This is determined only by haplotype and cannot define whether the suspected inherited allele carried by the parent is the mutated or normal gene. Transfer of embryos that inherited the allele from the unaffected grandmother or grandfather eliminates the risk for the familial late onset disease. This method eliminates the risk for affected offspring without revealing carrier status. However, the disadvantage of this procedure is the possible waste of healthy embryos and the need to perform IVF in cases when the suspected parent is actually healthy [73].

HLA Typing

Prenatal and preimplantation testing aims to enable the selection of embryos free of a severe familial mutation. However, when a couple has a child affected by an inheritable disease, such as thalassemia, adrenoleukodystrophy, Fanconi anemia, or other life-threatening malignant diseases, unresponsive to standard treatments, bone marrow transplantation from a suitable donor is lifesaving. In these cases, PGT-M for HLA matching, with or without a diagnosis of a familial mutation, serves as the only solution for treatment. For this purpose, an HLA region located on the short arm of chromosome 6 is completely and precisely haplotyped in order to distinguish between all four possible genotypes in this region. The embryo achieved following ART is biopsied and the same HLA region is characterized. For transfer, only embryos with an HLA haplotype identical to that of the affected sibling is transferred. In most cases, a genetic disorder is also involved, and the analysis of the biopsied single cell requires both HLA typing and a PGT-M for autosomal dominant, recessive or X-linked disorders. Such analyses are highly complex, due to a large number of tested genetic loci and the relatively high crossover tendency within the HLA region. If HLA is the only selection criterion, 25% of the embryos will be suitable for transfer. However, when a genetic disorder must also be excluded, the chances for a suitable embryo are even lower: 18.75% for recessive or X-linked disorders (25% chance for HLA match times the 75% chance for a healthy embryo) and 12.5% for dominant disorders (25% chance for HLA match times the 50% chance for a healthy embryo). When the desired embryo is eventually selected, transferred, and develops into a healthy pregnancy, umbilical cord stem cells with the sibling HLA match are collected following labor and serve for future transplantation.

De Novo Mutations

Accurate PGT-M is based on direct testing of the familial mutation, with the additional characterization of the informative haplotype. Genotyping the carrier parent is not adequate for the phase resolve, i.e., resolving which haplotype represents the normal allele and which represents the mutated one. For this purpose, haplotyping of a close family member with a known genotype, such as one of the parents of the carrier patient, siblings, or an offspring, is performed. However, there are cases when the mutation first arose in the carrier patient, and haplotype phasing by analysis of another family member is irrelevant. To overcome this limitation, a meticulous analysis of single haploid genetic material of the *de novo* carrier, containing only one allele, i.e., mutated or healthy, is performed. Parallel examination of the mutation and haplotype of the same haploid cell enables the linkage

219

of each haplotype to the normal or mutated allele. When the carrier patient is male, single haploid sperm cells are isolated under an inverted microscope, each of the single sperm cells is placed in a different PCR tube and further subjected to multiplex nested single-cell PCR using primers aimed to amplify the mutation sequence together with a panel of informative markers constituting the tested haplotype. When the carrier patient is a female, the first and second PBs are biopsied right after ICSI fertilization and the following day, respectively. The second PB, extruded following fertilization, is haploid (contains only one chromatid of each chromosome pair) and therefore, can be individually collected and diagnosed similarly to the diagnosis of single sperm cells. Once haplotypes are affiliated to normal or mutated alleles, the rest of the diagnostic analysis is performed according to the routine protocol [74–75].

Mitochondrial DNA Disorders

Maternally inherited mitochondrial DNA (mtDNA) mutations, the frequent cause of mitochondrial disorders, are the cause of severe disorders with a variety of manifestations, usually without treatment options. The mtDNA mutations are not localized to the nuclear DNA but are randomly carried, in different proportions, by mitochondria from the cytoplasm of the maternal oocyte. Due to the heteroplasmic nature of mtDNA mutations, the female cells simultaneously carry mutated and healthy mtDNA and will transmit a variable and unpredictable amount of affected mitochondria to embryos. Therefore, it is essential to determine for each mtDNA disease the specific heteroplasmy threshold, beyond which the disease is expressed. This mission is the major limitation of prenatal diagnosis (PND) and PGT of mtDNA mutations [76–77]. PND is generally inadequate for such maternally inherited mutations due to variation in clinical expression and mutation load. When genetic and fertility options are considered, PGT is preferred over PND due to a large number of embryos available for the analysis, following hormonal stimulation. PGT-M for mtDNA is currently performed by only a few centers, due to the complexity of the genetic analysis, based on quantitative real-time PCR and then quantified by fluorescent last-cycle restriction fragment length polymorphism analysis. For the analysis, a biopsy of two blastomeres is usually performed to enable the accurate evaluation of mutation load for the entire embryo. It was demonstrated that for the majority of mtDNA

mutations, the load in individual blastomeres is representative of the load in the entire embryo. Blastomeres proving free of maternal mutation or harboring a heteroplasmy mutation load below the phenotypic expression threshold indicate a transferable embryo and are associated with a significantly reduced risk for affected offspring [78–80].

An alternative potential fertility option is the mitochondrial replacement techniques that were recently developed but which are still under regulation inspections and clinical investigations [81–82].

Noninvasive PGT

Biopsy of a single blastomere or several TE cells has been shown to be relatively safe and might only slightly decrease implantation rate relative to ICSI [83]. Noninvasive PGT (NI-PGT) is a relatively new approach that analyzes the embryo without the need to aspirate embryonic cells. Two NI-PGT techniques have been suggested as an alternative to embryo biopsy. The first was to collect the fluid from the expanded blastocyst cavity (blastocoele), which is enriched with cells or fragments which dropped out from the ICM or TE during dynamic mitoses. Another source of embryonic DNA is the medium in which the embryo is incubated. However, this approach requires a prolonged incubation time, up until day 6 of development, and has the risk of contamination by sampling the culture medium and cell contaminants, mainly of sperm, corona radiata, and other cells, as well as foreign DNA sources. In general, although these methods have been under examination for several years, outcomes are still unsatisfactory. When PGT-M is performed, matching between results from an analysis of blastomere or TE biopsies and the results of NI-PGT is lower than 80%. This can be explained by the hypothesis that the source of NI-PGT DNA is from apoptotic cells, which includes degraded DNA and less chromosomally normal cells. To date, the accuracy and reliability of this method are still inadequate and it should not yet be broadly applied in PGT cycles [84].

PGT Cycle Follow-Up

PGT is an alternative to PND, with several advantages, alongside a remarkable disadvantage concerning the invasive biopsy of the developing embryo. The question of whether the aspiration of single or several cells interferes with embryo development, future health, and cognitive parameters remains unanswered and unsettling.

Several studies compared the outcome of pregnancies achieved following invasive biopsy during PGT cycles with outcomes of singleton and twin pregnancies following ICSI. Pregnancies following biopsy presented healthy intrauterine growth and development similar to spontaneous and ART-ICSI pregnancies. Perinatal outcomes were similar between PGT and ICSI pregnancies. No association was found between PGT pregnancies and risks of adverse neonatal or obstetrical outcomes, e.g., mean birth weight, gestational age at birth, and pre-term deliveries (<37 weeks). Perinatal mortality and hospital admissions were also found to be similar to those of naturally conceived children. Tracking of incident malformations demonstrated a similar frequency to that observed in ART-ICSI pregnancies as well as in the general spontaneously conceived population. It seems that blastomere biopsy itself has no significant impact on pregnancy outcomes and no correlation with increased risk for adverse perinatal outcomes [4; 85]. When PGT children were further evaluated for blood pressure, anthropometrics, socio-neurodevelopment, emotional development and intellectual abilities, no significant differences or evidence for an adverse effect of biopsy compared with control children were observed. The verbal performance of PGT children was very similar to that of the general population, but IQ scores of PGT children were slightly above the average. This phenomenon is explained by the relatively high educational level of PGT parents [85–87].

PGT Accreditation

For quality purposes, it is recommended to confirm the PGT diagnosis of embryos not transferred or cryopreserved following diagnosis, in line with local regulations. Such confirmation aims to provide quality assurance (QA) as well as accurate and up-to-date misdiagnosis rates to prospective PGT patients. It is recommended to perform these checks on as many embryos as is practicable. In order to validate the diagnosis system, single leukocytes isolated from the peripheral blood of the carrier and affected member of the tested family are analyzed to confirm the feasibility, reliability, and accuracy of the reaction.

When a pregnancy ensues PGT testing, it is recommended that parents are made aware of the chance and risks of misdiagnosis and be informed of prenatal testing possibilities. PGT and IVF centers should make special efforts to follow up with the parents after prenatal testing or birth, especially if confirmatory testing is not possible. Follow-up data should be used for internal quality control/QA purposes. It is recommended that laboratories follow local regulations or accreditation schemes on storage of clinical samples and patient records.

Accreditation, along with proficiency testing through internal and external QA, provides a means to achieve and maintain the highest quality standards. Accreditation is the formal recognition that an authoritative body gives to a laboratory/department/center when it demonstrates competence in carrying out defined tasks, and encompasses all aspects of management, along with technical requirements. Where possible, IVF/PGT centers should be accredited or certified, even when it is not legally required.

Since PGT is multidisciplinary in nature, the various units participating in the process should be accredited/certified for their defined tasks and according to the most appropriate quality standards [16; 51; 88–89]. For each unit, responsibilities should be clearly outlined and transfer of responsibility from one unit to the other during the PGT process should be well defined and guaranteed.

References

1. Gardner RL, Edwards RG. Control of the sex ratio at full term in the rabbit by transferring sexed blastocyst. *Nature* 1968; **218**:346–348.

2. Handyside AH, Kontogianni EH, Hardy K, Winston RM. Pregnancies from biopsied human preimplantation embryos sexed by Y-specific DNA amplification. *Nature* 1990; **344**:768–770.

3. International Working Group on Preimplantation Genetics. 10th anniversary of preimplantation genetic diagnosis. *J. Assist. Reprod. Genet.* 2001; **18**:66–72.

4. Hasson J, Limoni D, Malcov M, et al. Obstetric and neonatal outcomes of pregnancies conceived after preimplantation genetic diagnosis: cohort study and meta-analysis. *RBM Online* 2017; **35**:208–218.

5. Heijligers M, Verheijden LMM, Jonkman LM, et al. The cognitive and socio-emotional development of 5-year-old children born after PGD. *Hum. Reprod.* 2018; **33**:2150–2157.

6. Sermon K, Van Steirteghem A, Liebaers I. Preimplantation genetic diagnosis. *Lancet* 2004; **363**:1633–1641.

7. Dreesen JC, Jacobs LJ, Bras M, et al. Multiplex PCR of polymorphic markers flanking the CFTR gene; a general

approach for preimplantation genetic diagnosis of cystic fibrosis. *Mol. Hum. Reprod.* 2000; **6**:391–396.

8. Harper JC, Harton G. The use of arrays in preimplantation genetic diagnosis and screening. *Fertil. Steril.* 2010; **94**:1173–1177.

9. Sermon K, Capalbo A, Cohen J, et al. The why, the how and the when of PGS 2.0: current practices and expert opinions of fertility specialists, molecular biologists, and embryologists. *Mol. Hum. Reprod.* 2016; **22**:845–857.

10. Frumkin T, Peleg S, Gold V, et al. Complex chromosomal rearrangement—a lesson learned from PGS. *J. Assist. Reprod. Genet.* 2017; **34**:1095–1100.

11. Munné S. Status of preimplantation genetic testing and embryo selection. *RBM Online* 2018; **37**:393–396.

12. Malcov M, Schwartz T, Mei-Raz N, et al. Multiplex nested PCR for preimplantation genetic diagnosis of spinal muscular atrophy. *Fetal. Diagn. Ther.* 2004; **19**:199–206.

13. Tadir Y, Wright WH, Vafa O, et al. Review: micromanipulation of gametes using laser microbeams. *Hum. Reprod.* 1991; **6**:1011–1016.

14. Rink K, Delacrétaz G, Salathé RP, et al. Non-contact microdrilling of mouse zona pellucida with an objective-delivered 1.48-μm diode laser. *Lasers Surg. Med.* 1996; **18**:52–62.

15. Kalma Y, Bar-El L, Asaf-Tisser S, et al. Optimal timing for blastomere biopsy of 8-cell embryos for preimplantation genetic diagnosis. *Hum. Reprod.* 2018; **33**:32–38.

16. Harton GL, Magli MC, Lundin K, et al. ESHRE PGD Consortium/Embryology Special Interest Group--best practice guidelines for polar body and embryo biopsy for preimplantation genetic diagnosis/screening (PGD/PGS). *Hum. Reprod.* 2011; **26**:41–46.

17. Verlinsky Y, Kuliev A. *An Atlas of Preimplantation Genetic Diagnosis.* London: The Parthenon Publishing Group. 2000.

18. De Vos A, Van Steirteghem A. Aspects of biopsy procedures prior to preimplantation genetic diagnosis. *Prenat. Diagn.* 2001; **21**:767–780.

19. Feichtinger W, Strohmer H, Fuhrberg P, et al. Photoablation of oocyte zona pellucida by erbium-YAG laser for in-vitro fertilisation in severe male infertility. *Lancet* 1992; **339**:811.

20. Neev J, Schiewe M, Sung V, et al. Assisted hatching in mouse embryos using a noncontact Ho:YSGG laser system. *J. Assist. Reprod. Genet.* 1995; **12**:288–293.

21. MacLennan M, Crichton JH, Playfoot CJ, Adams IR. Oocyte development, meiosis and aneuploidy. *Semin. Cell Dev. Biol.* 2015; **45**:68–76.

22. Capalbo A, Hoffmann ER, Cimadomo D, Ubaldi FM, Rienzi L. Human female meiosis revised: new insights into the mechanisms of chromosome segregation and aneuploidies from advanced genomics and time-lapse imaging. *Hum. Reprod. Update* 2017; **23**:706–722.

23. Montag M, van der Ven K, Rösing B, van der Ven H. Polar body biopsy: a viable alternative to preimplantation genetic diagnosis and screening. *RBM Online* 2009; **18**(Suppl. 1):6–11.

24. Verlinsky Y, Kuliev A. Preimplantation polar body diagnosis. *Biochem. Mol. Med.* 1996; **58**:13–17.

25. Levin I, Almog B, Shwartz T, et al. Effects of laser polar-body biopsy on embryo quality. *Fertil. Steril.* 2012; **97**:1085–1088.

26. Dumoulin JC, Bras M, Coonen E, et al. Effect of Ca^{2+}/Mg^{2+}-free medium on the biopsy procedure for preimplantation genetic diagnosis and further development of human embryos. *Hum. Reprod.* 1998; **13**:2880–2883.

27. McCoy RC, Demko ZP, Ryan A, et al. Evidence of selection against complex mitotic-origin aneuploidy during preimplantation development. *PLoS Genet.* 2015; **11**:e1005601.

28. Adler A, Lee HL, McCulloh DH, et al. Blastocyst culture selects for euploid embryos: comparison of blastomere and trophectoderm biopsies. *RBM Online* 2014; **28**:485–491.

29. Weissman A, Shoham G, Shoham Z, et al. Chromosomal mosaicism detected during preimplantation genetic screening: results of a worldwide web-based survey. *Fertil. Steril.* 2017; **107**:1092–1097.

30. Liñán A, Lawrenz B, El Khatib I, et al. Clinical reassessment of human embryo ploidy status between cleavage and blastocyst stage by next generation sequencing. *PLoS One* 2018; **13**:e0201652.

31. Del Rey J, Vidal F, Ramírez L, et al. Novel double factor PGT strategy analyzing blastocyst stage embryos in a single NGS procedure. *PLoS One* 2018; **13**:e0205692.

32. Fragouli E, Alfarawati S, Daphnis DD, et al. Cytogenetic analysis of human blastocysts with the use of FISH, CGH and aCGH: scientific data and technical evaluation. *Hum. Reprod.* 2011; **26**:480–490.

33. Ventura-Juncá P, Irarrázaval I, Rolle AJ, et al. In vitro fertilization (IVF) in mammals: epigenetic and developmental alterations. Scientific and bioethical implications for IVF in humans. *Biol. Res.* 2015; **48**:68.

34. Laskowski D, Humblot P, Sirard MA, et al. DNA methylation pattern of bovine blastocysts associated with hyperinsulinemia in vitro. *Mol. Reprod. Dev.* 2018; **85**:599–611.

35. De Rycke M, Goossens V, Kokkali G, et al. ESHRE PGD Consortium data collection XIV-XV: cycles from January 2011 to December 2012 with pregnancy

follow-up to October 2013. *Hum. Reprod.* 2017; **32**:1974–1994.

36. Yaron Y, Schwartz T, Mey-Raz N, et al. Preimplantation genetic diagnosis of Canavan disease. *Fetal Diagn. Ther.* 2005; **20**:465–468.

37. Rechitsky S, Pakhalchuk T, San Ramos G, et al. First systematic experience of preimplantation genetic diagnosis for single-gene disorder, and/or preimplantation human leukocyte antigen typing, combined with 24-chromosome aneuploidy testing. *Fertil. Steril.* 2015; **103**:503–512.

38. Harper JC, Wells D. Recent advances and future developments in PGD. *Prenat. Diagn.* 1999; **19**:1193–1199.

39. Malcov M, Naiman T, Yosef DB, et al. Preimplantation genetic diagnosis for fragile X syndrome using multiplex nested PCR. *RBM Online* 2007; **14**:515–521.

40. Zhao M, Lian M, Cheah FSH, et al. Identification of novel microsatellite markers flanking the SMN1 and SMN2 duplicated region and inclusion into a single-tube tridecaplex panel for haplotype-based preimplantation genetic testing of spinal muscular atrophy. *Front. Genet.* 2019; **10**:1105.

41. Ray PF, Handyside AH. Increasing the denaturation temperature during the first cycles of amplification reduces allele dropout from single cells for preimplantation genetic diagnosis. *Mol. Hum. Reprod.* 1996; **2**:213–218.

42. Rechitsky S, Verlinsky O, Amet T, et al. Reliability of preimplantation diagnosis for single gene disorder. *Mol. Cell Endocrinol.* 2001; **183** (Suppl. 1):S65–S68.

43. Jovanovich S, Bogdan G, Belcinski R, et al. Developmental validation of a fully integrated sample-to-profile rapid human identification system for processing single-source reference buccal samples. *Forensic Sci. Int. Genet.* 2015; **16**:181–194.

44. He G, Zou X, Wang M, et al. Population genetics, diversity, forensic characteristics of four Chinese populations inferred from X-chromosomal short tandem repeats. *Leg. Med. (Tokyo)* 2020; **43**:101677.

45. Liu Y, Sun Y, Wu J, et al. Polymorphisms in IL-1A are associated with endometrial cancer susceptibility among Chinese Han population: a case-control study. *Int. J. Immunogenet.* 2020; **47**:169–174. doi:10.1111/iji.12463.

46. Malcov M, Ben-Yosef D, Schwartz T, et al. Preimplantation genetic diagnosis (PGD) for Duchenne muscular dystrophy (DMD) by triplex-nested PCR. *Prenat. Diagn.* 2005; **25**:1200–1205.

47. Sciorio R, Tramontano L, Catt J. Preimplantation genetic diagnosis (PGD) and genetic testing for aneuploidy (PGT-A): status and future challenges. *Gynecol. Endocrinol.* 2020; **36**:6–11.

48. Frumkin T, Malcov M, Yaron Y, Ben-Yosef D. Elucidating the origin of chromosomal aberrations in IVF embryos by preimplantation genetic analysis. *Mol. Cell Endocrinol.* 2008; **282**:112–119.

49. Coonen E, Dumoulin JC, Ramaekers FC, Hopman AH. Optimal preparation of preimplantation embryo interphase nuclei for analysis by fluorescence in-situ hybridization. *Hum. Reprod.* 1994; **9**:533–537.

50. Barbash-Hazan S, Frumkin T, Malcov M, et al. Preimplantation aneuploid embryos undergo self-correction in correlation with their developmental potential. *Fertil. Steril.* 2009; **92**:890–896.

51. Harton GL, Harper JC, Coonen E, et al. ESHRE PGD consortium best practice guidelines for fluorescence in situ hybridization-based PGD. *Hum. Reprod.* 2011; **26**:25–32.

52. Borgstrom E, Paterlini M, Mold JE, Frisen J, Lundeberg J. Comparison of whole genome amplification techniques for human single cell exome sequencing. *PLoS One* 2017; **12**:e0171566.

53. Deleye L, Gansemans Y, De Coninck D, Van Nieuwerburgh F, Deforce D. Massively parallel sequencing of micro-manipulated cells targeting a comprehensive panel of disease-causing genes: $ comparative evaluation of upstream whole-genome amplification methods. *PLoS One* 2018; **13**:e0196334.

54. França LT, Carrilho E, Kist TB. A review of DNA sequencing techniques. *Q. Rev. Biophys.* 2002; **35**:169–200.

55. Anderson MW, Schrijver I. Next generation DNA sequencing and the future of genomic medicine. *Genes* 2010; **1**:38–69.

56. Muzzey D, Kash S, Johnson JI, et al. Software-assisted manual review of clinical next-generation sequencing data: an alternative to routine Sanger sequencing confirmation with equivalent results in >15,000 germline DNA screens. *J. Mol. Diagn.* 2019; **21**:296–306.

57. Fiorentino F, Biricik A, Bono S, et al. Development and validation of a next-generation sequencing-based protocol for 24-chromosome aneuploidy screening of embryos. *Fertil. Steril.* 2014; **101**:1375–1382.

58. Friedenthal J, Maxwell SM, Munné S, et al. Next generation sequencing for preimplantation genetic screening improves pregnancy outcomes compared with array comparative genomic hybridization in single thawed euploid embryo transfer cycles. *Fertil. Steril.* 2018; **109**:627–632.

59. Popovic M, Dhaenens L, Taelman J, et al. Extended in vitro culture of human embryos demonstrates the complex nature of diagnosing chromosomal

mosaicism from a single trophectoderm biopsy. *Hum. Reprod.* 2019; **34**:758–769.

60. Victor AR, Tyndall JC, Brake AJ, et al. One hundred mosaic embryos transferred prospectively in a single clinic: exploring when and why they result in healthy pregnancies. *Fertil. Steril.* 2019; **111**:280–293.

61. Munné S, Spinella F, Grifo J, et al. Clinical outcomes after the transfer of blastocysts characterized as mosaic by high resolution next generation sequencing – further insights. *Eur. J. Med. Genet.* 2020; **63**:103741.

62. Orvieto R, Gleicher N. Preimplantation genetic testing for aneuploidy (PGT-A)-finally revealed. *J. Assist. Reprod. Genet.* 2020; **37**:669–672. doi:10.1007/s10815-020-01705-w.

63. Magli MC, Jones GM, Gras L, et al. Chromosome mosaicism in day 3 aneuploid embryos that develop to morphologically normal blastocysts in vitro. *Hum. Reprod.* 2000; **15**:1781–1786.

64. Orvieto R, Gleicher N. Should preimplantation genetic screening (PGS) be implemented to routine IVF practice? *J. Assist. Reprod. Genet.* 2016; **33**:1445–1448.

65. Practice Committee of the American Society for Reproductive Medicine, Practice Committee of the Society for Assisted Reproductive Technology. Blastocyst culture and transfer in clinically assisted reproduction: a committee opinion. *Fertil. Steril.* 2018; **110**:1246–1252.

66. Lawrenz B, El Khatib I, Liñán A, et al. The clinicians' dilemma with mosaicism-an insight from inner cell mass biopsies. *Hum. Reprod.* 2019; **34**:998–1010.

67. Escribà MJ, Vendrell X, Peinado V. Segmental aneuploidy in human blastocysts: a qualitative and quantitative overview. *Reprod. Biol. Endocrinol.* 2019; **17**:76.

68. Banker JM, Arora P, Khajuria R, Banker M. India's first child using PGT-M, PGT-A and HLA matching for helping a sibling having β-thalassemia major. *J. Hum. Reprod. Sci.* 2019; **12**:341–344.

69. Backenroth D, Zahdeh F, Kling Y, et al. Haploseek: a 24-hour all-in-one method for preimplantation genetic diagnosis (PGD) of monogenic disease and aneuploidy. *Genet. Med.* 2019; **21**:1390–1399.

70. Natesan SA, Bladon AJ, Coskun S, et al. Genome-wide karyomapping accurately identifies the inheritance of single-gene defects in human preimplantation embryos in vitro. *Genet. Med.* 2014; **16**:838–845.

71. Prates R, Konstantinidis M, Goodall NN, et al. Clinical experience with karyomapping for preimplantation genetic diagnosis (PGD) of single gene disorders. *Fertil. Steril.* 2014; **102**:e25–e26.

72. Treff NR, Zimmerman R, Bechor E, et al. Validation of concurrent preimplantation genetic testing for polygenic and monogenic disorders, structural rearrangements, and whole and segmental chromosome aneuploidy with a single universal platform. *Eur. J. Med. Genet.* 2019; **62**:103647.

73. Van Rij MC, De Rademaeker M, Moutou C, et al. BruMaStra PGD working group preimplantation genetic diagnosis (PGD) for Huntington's disease: the experience of three European centers. *Eur. J. Hum. Genet.* 2012; **20**:368–375.

74. Rechitsky S, Pomerantseva E, Pakhalchuk T, et al. First systematic experience of preimplantation genetic diagnosis for de-novo mutations. *RBM Online* 2011; **22**:350–361.

75. Altarescu G, Brooks B, Kaplan Y, et al. Single-sperm analysis for haplotype construction of de-novo paternal mutations: application to PGD for neurofibromatosis type 1. *Hum. Reprod.* 2006; **21**:2047–2051.

76. Hellebrekers DM, Wolfe R, Hendrickx AT, et al. PGD and heteroplasmic mitochondrial DNA point mutations: a systematic review estimating the chance of healthy offspring. *Hum. Reprod. Update* 2012; **18**:341–349.

77. Johnston IG, Burgstaller JP, Havlicek V, et al. Stochastic modelling, bayesian inference, and new in vivo measurements elucidate the debated mtDNA bottleneck mechanism. *eLife* 2015; **4**:e07464.

78. Sallevelt SC, Dreesen JC, Coonen E, et al. Preimplantation genetic diagnosis for mitochondrial DNA mutations: analysis of one blastomere suffices. *J. Med. Genet.* 2017; **54**:693–697.

79. Sallevelt SC, Dreesen JC, Drüsedau M, et al. PGD for the m.14487 T>C mitochondrial DNA mutation resulted in the birth of a healthy boy. *Hum. Reprod.* 2017; **32**:698–703.

80. Treff NR, Campos J, Tao X, et al. Blastocyst preimplantation genetic diagnosis (PGD) of a mitochondrial DNA disorder. *Fertil. Steril.* 2012; **98**:1236–1240.

81. Wolf DP, Mitalipov N, Mitalipov S. Mitochondrial replacement therapy in reproductive medicine. *Trends Mol. Med.* 2015; **21**:68–76.

82. Tang M, Guggilla RR, Gansemans Y, et al. Comparative analysis of different nuclear transfer techniques to prevent the transmission of mitochondrial DNA variants. *Mol. Hum. Reprod.* 2019; **25**:797–810.

83. Scott KL, Hong KH, Scott RT. Selecting the optimal time to perform biopsy for preimplantation genetic testing. *Fertil. Steril.* 2013; **100**:608–614.

84. Leaver M, Wells D. Non-invasive preimplantation genetic testing (niPGT): the next revolution in reproductive genetics? *Hum. Reprod. Update* 2020; **26**:16–42.

85. Heijligers M, van Montfoort A, Meijer-Hoogeveen M, et al. Perinatal follow-up of children born after preimplantation genetic diagnosis between 1995 and 2014. *J. Assist. Reprod. Genet.* 2018; **35**:1995–2002.

86. Heijligers M, Verheijden LMM, Jonkman LM, et al. The cognitive and socio-emotional development of 5-year-old children born after PGD. *Hum. Reprod.* 2018; **33**:2150–2157.

87. Kuiper D, Bennema A, Bastide-van Gemert S, et al. Developmental outcome of 9-year-old children born after PGS: follow-up of a randomized trial. *Hum. Reprod.* 2018; **33**:147–155.

88. Thornhill AR, deDie-Smulders CE, Geraedts JP, et al. ESHRE PGD Consortium. 'Best practice guidelines for clinical preimplantation genetic diagnosis (PGD) and preimplantation genetic screening (PGS)'. *Hum. Reprod.* 2005; **20**:35–48.

89. Harton GL, De Rycke M, Fiorentino F, et al. ESHRE PGD consortium best practice guidelines for amplification-based PGD. *Hum. Reprod.* 2011; **26**:33–40.

Structure and Management of IVF Laboratory

Structure of IVF Laboratory

Before in vitro fertilization (IVF) was established as a standard treatment for infertility, there was no concern about the laboratory structure and its environment, and how it should be organized. Today, specific standards and legislations exist and the laboratory should also meet international legislations, if cross-border treatments are to be performed. In order to establish a high-quality assisted reproductive technology (ART) clinic, a multidisciplinary skilled task force needs to be formed, to guarantee that all aspects concerning the design of the clinic, selection of equipment and disposables, as well as logistic treatment procedures are taken into consideration.

The IVF laboratory should be adjacent to the operating room where the clinical procedures are performed. Careful attention should be paid to the location of the building in which the IVF laboratory is to be constructed. Also possible sources of particulate and chemical pollution, e.g., parking garages, dry cleaners, foundries, and petroleum processing facilities, should be taken into account [1]. If known pollution sources are identified, this might warrant additional measures to reduce those pollutants within the laboratory environment. In addition, the clinic must actively prevent the exposure of oocytes and embryos to environmental embryotoxic contaminants from within the clinic, building materials, ventilation, laboratory furniture, light and gas sources, disposables, detergents and cleaning agents, and clothing materials; therefore restricted access should be enforced [2–8]. Moreover, the laboratory should provide optimal conditions for gamete and embryo development with high implantation and low miscarriage rates. The workstations should be of the highest quality, preferably antibacterial, easy to clean, resistant to cleaning detergents and disinfectants, and non-embryotoxic. The physical factors of temperature and relative humidity must be maintained within defined limits, and the osmolality, pH, and composition of culture media must be controlled. Critical equipment,

including incubators and cryotanks, should be continuously monitored and equipped with alarm systems. An automatic emergency backup power system must be in place for all such equipment. Nicknamed "dirty" rooms should be separated from the ART suite and include gas cylinder rooms, storage rooms for bulk supplies, fixation and staining rooms, office space for laboratory staff, changing rooms, and janitorial closets. The cryobank itself should also be separate from the ART suite, due to the requirement for continuous extraction ventilation. Maintenance of a clean environment in the ART suite is paramount and requires strategies to reduce outside infiltration.

Local fire protection regulations often apply to gas and cryobank rooms, as they contain significant volumes of volatile liquids. As a result, architects might request the presence of firebreak dampers in ventilation ducts. However, this must be avoided to prevent the risk of anoxia or carbon dioxide intoxication in case of accidental closure of ventilation dampers without an alternative fresh air supply.

Staff must use protective laboratory clothing, preferably with low particle shedding. Hairnets and non-toxic, non-powdered gloves and masks should be used, where appropriate. Needles, glassware, and other sharps should be handled with extreme caution and discarded into sharps containers. Equipment should be repaired and annual services must be registered. The most sensitive and vital equipment must be connected to an uninterrupted power supply to avoid disruption of work, recalibration, and damage to the equipment or gametes and embryos.

All laboratory staff must be trained to use standard operational procedures (SOPs) and quality controls (QCs) [9]. Their competency must be routinely tested. Vaccination of all personnel against hepatitis B or other viral diseases, for which a vaccine is available, is recommended. All body fluids (blood, follicular fluid, semen, etc.) should be treated as potentially contaminated.

A wide range of factors can affect the outcome of IVF. We should keep in mind that no two laboratories practice identically [10]; therefore, within the laboratory, the gametes and embryos can be affected by factors associated with the laboratory environment, equipment, contact materials, methodology, and the staff. The patients themselves represent a source of influence, as their own biology affects the potential of their gametes and resultant embryos. Clinical factors, such as the stimulation, oocyte retrieval, and embryo transfer procedures and luteal phase support, also influence outcomes.

Air and Ventilation

Air supply vents should be located in the ceiling and return ducts should draw from close to floor level. The effectiveness of the clinic's heating, ventilation, and air conditioning (HVAC) system (air change effectiveness, contamination reduction effectiveness, controlling particulates, microorganisms, and volatile organic compounds [VOCs] within the critical areas) should be evaluated; perforated diffusers ensure effective mixing of the inlet air and a cleaner environment. An effective air filtration system is essential for achieving optimal laboratory performance, and can bring a significant decrease in VOC and aldehyde concentrations. Not all VOCs are toxic to gametes and/or embryos; examples of nontoxic VOCs include silicones, which are used in all incubator gaskets and tubing, and high-molecular-weight alkanes, such as paraffinic oil, which is stable and nonreactive, and is in use to cover medium with gametes/embryos. A range of organic compounds are typically found in ART laboratories, including d-limonene and α-pinene, common ingredients in colognes and cleaning products, which are highly oil-soluble and hence should not be used, but because they are unreactive under the conditions of culture, they do not seem to be biologically significant contaminants. Ethanol, however, which is one of the two most common contaminants in ART facilities, can be metabolized into acetaldehyde, and isopropyl alcohol can be metabolized into formaldehyde, both of which are biologically detrimental. According to the Hazardous Substance Data Bank, many of the aldehydes commonly found in ART laboratories, e.g., formaldehyde, acetaldehyde, propionaldehyde, butyraldehyde, benzaldehyde, and n-hexaldehyde, are known carcinogens and mutagens. Thus, among modern ART laboratories, i.e., those built using clean-room concepts, the mean and upper 95% confidence limit for total VOC levels are 339.5 µg/m^3 and 1213.9 µg/m^3, respectively [11]. Medium density fiberboard (MDF) is a significant source of formaldehyde and should not be used in ART laboratory cabinetry. The fixation solution for pathology biopsy samples (10% formalin) can also be a source of formaldehyde. Styrene, the monomer used in the production of polystyrene, can also be found in ART laboratories because of incomplete polymerization during the manufacturing process. Release of styrene molecules occurs when new packages of plasticware are opened.

The olfactory method, i.e., sense of smell, is not a reliable analytical method to detect organic compounds. The smell of odor is susceptible to inter-individual differences in sensitivity, it is highly dependent on the substance and the amount in the environment, and the odor threshold for some substances exceeds the potential level of toxicity in an ART environment. Methods to clean air and reduce VOC levels include centralized units or free-standing towers with activated carbon, potassium permanganate, photocatalytic oxidation (system that works with titanium oxide), high-efficiency particulate air (HEPA) filter, and positive air pressure. Installation of an independent active ventilation system is recommended.

Old IVF laboratories which moved to new clean-room facilities benefited from an increased proportion of high-quality embryos [12]. Laboratories with a carbon air filter and HVAC central filter system showed decreased VOCs and improvements in laboratory performance [13–14].

Generally accepted standards for air quality are fewer than 352 000 particles larger than 0.5–10 µm per m^3 (equivalent to <10 000 such particles per cubic foot), fewer than 10 cfu/m^3, and fewer than two spores/m^3 "at rest." Total VOCs should be lower than 500 µg/m^3 (~400–800 ppb total VOC, depending on molecular species) and lower than 5 µg/m^3 aldehydes [11].

Air change of a minimum of 15 total air changes per hour are necessary for IVF laboratories, including 3 fresh air changes per hour, i.e., 20% outside air. Recommended air movement out of the room is at minimum positive pressure of 15 Pascal, with an ideal target of 30–50 Pascal. This can be attained through a cascade of overpressure across several rooms, e.g., external space to access vestibule to IVF laboratory, or recovery area to access vestibule to procedure room to IVF laboratory, to avoid too great a differential pressure between immediately adjacent rooms. A double-door pass-through between the IVF laboratory and the procedures room (if the procedures room is not as clean as the IVF laboratory) must be air-tight to preserve room air pressure differentials and reduce the number of new materials being brought directly into the laboratory.

Most benches come with thick, high-efficiency particulate air – HEPA (99.99% efficiency in removing 0.3 μm particles) – or ultra-low particulate air – ULPA (99.999% efficiency in removing 0.1–0.3 μm particles) – filters of a high quality that do not easily block and can therefore be used for a very long time before the filter must be replaced. HEPA, carbon, and VOC filters improve air quality [15] and provide the workstation with a clean-room environment, which improves IVF success [16]. The prefilters on top of the benches and the large HEPA/ULPA filters should be easily exchangeable. When a new bench is installed, the distributor must ensure that the filters have not been damaged during the transportation. Some benches can also be fitted with activated carbon filters for partial removal of VOCs.

Laminar Flow Workstation

The vertical laminar flow is the most commonly used workstation within the ART laboratory. The biological safety laminar flow (Class II) protects both the product and operator. Ventilation speed should be controlled for optimal efficiency. If not controlled, there is no guarantee that the work area meets the standards necessary for ensuring culture sterility during the various procedures.

The laminar flow cabinet should run continuously, to ensure the cleanliness of the laboratory. If a bench is switched off and started up again, it initially (15–20 minutes) releases a substantial amount of debris that contaminates everything within the bench. Moreover, turbulence is induced behind each object, which increases the risk of contamination. All this can be avoided with programmable benches, where turn off and on times can be programmed so that all parameters (temperature and ventilation control) are at optimum when work begins in the morning.

A high-quality stereomicroscope (binocular), built-in in a laminar flow cabinet, is commonly used to identify and handle cumulus–oocyte complexes, and for evaluation and selection of embryos for embryo transfer and cryopreservation. The binocular

should be fitted with an adjustable ergonomic triocular tube, so that a camera can also be connected to a TV monitor, within or outside the cabinet. The space between the light source and the objective should allow easy handling of dishes with gametes, zygotes, and embryos; a start point of 0.7–0.8 magnification objective is recommended. The combination of a high-quality stereomicroscope, a camera, and a light source with angled and adjusted mirrors allows a quality picture displayed on a high-resolution screen to be obtained, enabling evaluation of organelles as small as pronuclei and vacuoles. It is very important that the laminar flow cabinet has dampers, to avoid vibrations. Positioning of the high-resolution screen on the outside of the cabinet allows for dual control and evaluation, and is useful for teaching purposes.

Integrated built-in mini-incubators, with individual small doors and a gas inflow purge, for quicker recovery and better maintenance of the culture conditions, are recommended.

The heated surface should provide an equal temperature over the entire surface area. The temperature of all heated surfaces of the laminar flow cabinet must be calibrated with a sensitive temperature probe measuring the most commonly used dish, and not the surface of the bench. In some cabinets, the surface is coated with a silver-ion-impregnated antibacterial/antimicrobial coating, which prevents growth of bacteria and reduces the risk of contaminations.

Cleaning is performed at the end of the day, with special embryo-tested cleaning detergents. However, in between patients and if spillage occurs, the surface is wiped and then rinsed with water for injection and finally cleaned with a detergent. If the surface becomes sticky or greasy from the detergent, it should be cleaned again with water for injection.

ICSI Workstation

A micromanipulator should be installed on an anti-vibration table. During handling and injection of oocytes, it is advisable to use MOPS- or HEPES-buffered media, with an oil overlay. Exposure of oocytes to microscope light of the micromanipulator should be minimized during intracytoplasmic sperm injection (ICSI) or other procedures.

Incubators

Traditional "big-box" incubators, whether they are carbon dioxide-only or tri-gas, for reduced oxygen, regulate the gas levels by the addition of carbon dioxide and nitrogen. Most laboratories average an oxygen calibrate between 4.5% and 5.5%; as for carbon dioxide, between 5.5% and 6.5% [10]. Clearly, this type of incubator is susceptible to the inclusion of VOCs that are circulating in the laboratory. In contrast, modern benchtop incubators include smaller individualized chambers to help maintain stability of the culture environment, and generally function by flushing the incubator chambers with gases, either premixed in outsourced cylinders or mixed inside the benchtop incubator [17]. As the incubator flushes the chambers with the mixed gas, any ambient room air is flushed out of the chamber, thereby leaving the tanks and in-line filters as the only source of contaminants inside the incubation chamber [11].

The connecting gas tube must be of nontoxic and VOC-free material, leak proof, and easily fitted to the gas reduction inlet valve. The concentration of carbon dioxide must be calibrated (~5–6%) to that of the clinic's choice of culture media and the concentration of oxygen should be low, between 4.5% and less than 5.5% [10], although 5–6% oxygen is also tolerated [18]. This low oxygen concentration, compared with that of natural air oxygen (~21%), has been shown to ensure the development of high-quality embryos [19–20], and high implantation rates, clinical rates, and live birth rates [21–22]. Since the incubator door (in traditional, large incubators) is frequently opened, the culture conditions are never optimal, which affects the outcomes of the treatments. Such external disturbances have been reduced by table-top incubators which have individual chambers for each patient.

Minimal handling and removal of dishes from the confines of the incubator results in more stable gas levels (culture pH) and temperature. Furthermore, reduced handling helps avoid potential sheer stress caused by pipetting, and other risks associated with transporting embryos across the laboratory or between dishes.

Many of these new-generation incubators lack humidity. The aim of removing humidity in modern embryo culture incubators, including most time-lapse systems, is to reduce contamination associated with moisture in the incubator. However, if conditions are not optimized to avoid loss of humidity, evaporation of culture media may occur [23]. Embryo culture for 5 days in a single-step medium with no replacement demonstrated that use of dry chambers yielded lower day 3 embryo development, lower blastocyst formation, and reduced clinical pregnancy and implantation rates compared with use of humidified chambers [24–25]. Non-humidified conditions could be prevented by adding a plate with sterile water to each chamber with achievement of humidity levels around 40–45% [26]. The amount of oil that sits above the medium may prevent evaporation; it has been shown that 3 ml of oil results in more evaporation compared with 5–7 ml in the same sized dish [27]. The type of oil also affects the evaporation rate, with heavier and denser oil more effectively reducing evaporation than lighter oil; a difference in density of 0.04 g/ml was shown to have a significant effect on evaporation [28]. Nomenclature of many commercial IVF oils is unclear, and it is therefore difficult to determine the densities of commercial embryo culture oils for comparison. Therefore, when media evaporation occurs, the embryos are not exposed to the same components or concentrations of media solvents as originally designed. For example, recommended starting osmolality should be in the range of 255–265 mOsm/kg [29]. Osmolality exceeding 300 mOsm/kg inhibits embryo development. Evaporation of media during culture in dry incubators varies with media drop size. Media evaporation can also occur in modern embryo culture dishes made for time-lapse culture incubators. Use of different dishes yields differing amounts of evaporation.

Incubators are the main source of magnetic fields in a laboratory. Most people do not differentiate between static magnetic fields (those coming from earth) and dynamic magnetic fields (those induced by electric currents going through wires). Works which studied the effect of both types are limited, with conditions either extremely low or high (high expression of magnetic field in Gauss is small when it is expressed in Tesla) compared with those naturally encountered in the laboratory. The statement that reproductive cells are more sensitive to electro pollution remains therefore more a concern than a proven fact.

Time-Lapse Imaging Incubators

Embryo morphology is not always a robust and absolute indicator for implantation potential as, sometimes, the best looking blastocyst fails to produce pregnancy, while a morphologically suboptimal embryo can develop into a healthy baby. Finally, on average, only one-third of all cycles results in a pregnancy [30].

Morphological evaluation of the embryos at specific time points has been the method of choice for embryo selection for decades [31] and remains the primary line of embryo assessment during IVF cycles. Historically, morphological evaluation included the measurement of features, such as pronuclear size [32], multinucleation in early cleavage stages [33], blastomere fragmentation [34], or blastocyst morphology [35]. However, this evaluation method poses limitations, not only arising from the subjectivity of the embryologist, but also because of the evaluation system itself, which views embryo development statically. Moreover, this approach usually requires the physical removal of the embryos from the incubator, and exposes them to fluctuations in temperature, pH, and oxygen levels. Embryo evaluation is typically based on a few discrete time points, leaving the events occurring in between the observations largely unknown; the status of an embryo can change markedly within just a few hours [36]. While multiple observations increase the robustness of embryo evaluation, they impose multiple disturbances to the culture environment, possibly stressing the embryo and reducing its potential to develop and implant. These limitations can be overcome with time-lapse systems, which enable assessment of dynamic changes of embryo morphology occurring during the preimplantation period of a 5-day culture. The key advantages of time-lapse technology include the provision of an improved culture environment based on embryo evaluation without removal from the incubator, and collection of objective and accurate algorithm information about the kinetic and morphological changes and abnormalities an embryo undergoes in vitro [37]. Use of a time-lapse system has led to a 20% improvement in pregnancy rates [38–39].

Analysis of initial events of embryo development revealed that pronuclei breakdown occurred significantly later in embryos that resulted in a live birth, and never earlier than 20 hours 45 minutes after fertilization [40]. It was observed that ability to reach the blastocyst stage could be predicted by the timing of early developmental stages: first cytokinesis 0–33 minutes, a time interval between first and second mitoses of 7.8–14.3 hours, and a time interval between second and third mitoses of 0–5.8 hours [41]. Two- to five-cell cleavage timing and intervals during two cleavages (t5 – the timing of the cleavage to five cells, and s2 – duration of the transition from a two-cell to a four-cell embryo, cc2 – duration of

the second cell cycle) were shown to be the most predictive parameters for embryo viability and implantation [36; 38]. An association between aneuploidy and irregular division, start time of cavitation (tSB), expansion (tEB), tEB-tSB interval was reported [42–43]. Furthermore, presence of at least two abnormal cleavage features was associated with a poor prognosis for embryo chromosomal status [42]. Using morphokinetics, it has been possible to demonstrate associations between various cleavage-stage kinetic parameters and the ability of the embryos to reach the blastocyst stage [44]. Blastocyst transfer yields higher implantation rates than transfers at the cleavage stage, but this outcome must be balanced against the possible disadvantages of longer culture, such as the risk of canceled cycles and concerns over the possible epigenetic effects of prolonged in vitro culture [45].

The Eeva (early embryo viability assessment) test is facilitated by dark-field microscopy and cell-tracking software algorithms (based on P2 [t3-t2] and P3 [t4-t3], which categorize embryos into groups with either high or low likelihood of forming "usable blastocysts"). Eeva significantly improved the specificity and the positive predictive value of usable blastocyst predictions compared with morphology evaluation alone [46].

Observation by time-lapse imaging showed that embryos with complex aneuploidies presented delays on the first two cleavages as well as prolonged transitions between the two- and four-cell stages [47]. In some countries where preimplantation genetic testing for aneuploidy (PGT-A) is not permitted, usage of time-lapse systems provides key information on embryo development supplying a cheaper, faster, and less invasive means of evaluating embryo ploidy status compared with PGT-A [48].

Significance of the time-lapse system as a benefit regarding embryo ploidy and live birth is still a contentious issue. When no differences in the ploidy at early stages of embryo development are determined, the initiation of cavitation and the timing of the formation of a full blastocyst have been defined as parameters relevant to ploidy [48]. While most studies found significant morphokinetic differences between euploid and aneuploid embryos, none of them provided sufficient evidence to recommend the clinical use of time-lapse technology for embryo ploidy assessment [49]. It was also suggested that investing in time-lapse systems and changing the daily routine would not lead to clinical benefits [50–51], and there are currently no high-quality data to support the clinical use of this technology for selection of preimplantation embryos [52–53]. Existing data do not yet provide any certainty on the improvement in live birth rates using embryo selection by time-lapse monitoring. However, studies based on large sample sizes, which include several centers from different countries, strongly support time-lapse monitoring as a strategy for embryo selection. Nevertheless, general conclusions cannot be made at the moment, as the studies were carried out in selected populations and the quality of some studies included can be questioned [54]. To augment general concerns, time-lapse incubation and conventional incubation have shown similar cumulative live birth rates [55]. The use of techniques designed to maximize the number of live births and minimize the suffering of women who undergo failed embryo transfers is a moral obligation.

Time-lapse technology has significant relevance for other laboratory activities. For example, differences in embryo morphokinetics, detected by time-lapse technology, may be valuable endpoints for determining the compatibility of consumables, cryopreservation protocols, and devices introduced in the IVF laboratory [56].

Gas Supply

Gas cylinders should be located outside the laboratory. There should be an automatic change-over system and sufficient cylinders stocked for immediate replacement. High-purity gas and in-line HEPA and VOC filters are highly recommended [57]. It might be helpful to insist that IVF laboratories purchase new cylinders from the gas supplier, for their exclusive use, thereby assuring that they are relatively clean. When refilling, the supplier should confirm that the same cylinder was not used for acetylene, for example, before it was filled with carbon dioxide. The compressed gases may contain high levels of organic contamination. It is therefore essential that the gas quality be of the highest purity (medical grade for both nitrogen and carbon dioxide) and has the lowest concentration of contaminants [58]. For many gas companies, "medical grade" only means that the cylinders have only been used for medical gases at medical facilities, and never used for industrial gases or at industrial locations. Many clinics also pre-clean the inlet gas via an in-line HEPA, charcoal, and potassium permanganate filter, which can minimize levels of

contaminants that reach the incubator before it is heated and humidified. Evidence is lacking regarding the effectiveness of the different types of in-line filters or the frequency of change-out (monthly, quarterly, or even less frequent changes being recommended). Polyvinyl chloride (PVC) was found to be the most detrimental material to gametes and embryos [59]. However, polytetrafluoroethylene (PTFE)-Teflon gas tubes and phthalate-free manufactured products (e.g., Tygon) are not detrimental to gametes and embryos. Gas supply lines can be made of stainless steel, copper (braised, not soldered), or Tygon.

The gas rooms for compressed gases and liquid nitrogen (LN_2) should be separate from, but ideally adjacent to, the ART laboratory suite. All gas lines into the IVF laboratory suite must be sealed at the piping–wall interface. Adequate ventilation and low oxygen alarms should be installed. Protection devices (e.g., glasses, face shield, cryo-gloves, apron, footwear) should be used during LN_2 handling. All staff dealing with LN_2 should be trained in safety aspects of its use.

Oil Overlay

Oil overlay is commonly used to reduce loss of carbon dioxide and evaporation of medium drops, and to minimize humidity and temperature deviations of cultures when removed from the incubator for procedures. Although shown to be effective for the latter two points, oil overlay has been shown to have only a negligible impact on preservation of carbon dioxide levels, as it has been shown to cause substantial slowing of medium re-gassing [60].

Once VOCs penetrate the culture, it is difficult to remove them, but it is possible to reduce their concentration. VOCs can be either hydrophobic, e.g., benzene, styrene, or hydrophilic, such as ethanol, acrolein, formaldehyde, and glutaraldehyde. Hydrophobic VOCs can partition into the embryos' membranes as they are also oil-like phases. Overlaying the culture medium with oil results in the preferential partitioning of hydrophobic VOCs into the oil phases, thereby reducing their concentration in the aqueous medium [11]. In regular culture dishes, the surface area of the exposed oil is large compared with the depth of the oil, favoring rapid dissolution of air VOCs into the oil. Dissolution of carbon dioxide through the oil into the medium could be affected in a similar manner, likely explaining the need for preincubation to achieve medium pH equilibration [60].

Virus Contamination via LN$_2$

Virus transmission from one sample to another via LN$_2$ containers is one of the most disputed risks, the potential hazard of contamination and disease transmission through cryopreservation. Viruses cannot "jump out" of the solidified drop of a frozen sample (sperm, oocytes, or embryo) to the liquid phase during storage in LN$_2$. No virus transmissions were reported in over 600 000 cryopreserved samples of IVF cases in 40 countries over the last 20 years. Not a single report of infection supposedly caused by LN$_2$-mediated disease transfer has been reported in human. Only one report of disease transmission in bovine has been documented [61]; however, this finding cannot be clearly attributed to the applied cryopreservation and storage conditions. Under experimental settings, such possibility of infection transmission exists [62]. As an alternative to the LN$_2$ phase, the vapor phase of LN$_2$ has been suggested as a safer method for the storage of gametes and embryos.

Laboratory Walls

The walls of the IVF laboratory must run from the concrete floor up to the underside of the concrete of the floor above (often described as "slab-to-slab"), and all perforations must be completely sealed. Suitable materials for walls are true clean-room modular panels with powder-coated antiseptic (with silver ions), metal, gasketed interfaces, or plasterboard coated with VOC-free paint. Standard paints used to seal the wall and ceiling surfaces in laboratories may be a significant source of VOCs. Low-VOC or VOC-free paints are now available [63].

Laboratory Floors

Sheet vinyl with impervious sealed joints must be used for floors. PVC with a metal grid for antistatic floorings is designed for premises where an electrostatically conductive design is required. They have high chemical resistance, suitable for underfloor heating, ease of maintenance, and resistance to the effects of chairs. In areas in which large volumes of LN$_2$ are used, a non-thermally fragile floor covering, such as a stainless-steel tread plate, should be considered. Polished concrete and epoxy (VOC-free) floor coating are also flooring options. They are low maintenance and very durable (in terms of LN$_2$).

Countertops

Nonporous materials that do not release VOC should be used for countertops. Suitable materials include epoxy, Corian, and Trespa. Use of manufactured wood products, such as MDF, linoleum, or oil-based paints is not recommended, as they have all been demonstrated to be embryotoxic [11].

Desktop computers in operation are known to emit VOCs and formaldehyde. A minimum number of computers should be used in the ART suite and they should be switched off when not in use [11].

Laboratory Lighting

All light fittings are recommended to be of yellow light. Warm white light has a yellow-white color, which is less damaging to embryos than cool white light. Light emitted at 400–500 nm (blue light) appears to be more harmful than longer wavelengths (green, orange, or red light) of visible light, and results in oxidative stress [64]. The time-lapse systems with 625–636 nm (using a red LED) combined with very short exposure times reduce stress on the embryo. More than 90% of the light on the embryo is from microscopes. The light tube should be positioned so it can easily and safely be replaced when needed.

Temperature

Working temperature in the laboratories should be stable and maintained in a range comfortable to the staff, typically within the range of 20–24°C (68–73°F), depending on the region. Keeping the temperature within a narrow range facilitates equipment calibration and operation. The total heat output of the laboratory equipment and staff must be considered. Adequate provision must be made for heating and cooling of the incoming fresh air according to local climatic requirements.

While a static (rather than dynamic) core temperature of 37°C in the incubators and on work station surfaces is not optimal, it has become mainstream. In vivo temperature of the reproductive system is biphasic, increasing in the luteal phase; with the caudal region of the oviduct 1–2 degrees cooler than the cranial portion [65]; i.e., in vivo the embryo is subjected to fluctuation of temperature. That would obviously still require close monitoring of equipment temperature. It is known that differences exist in microscope stage warmers and incubators. It is possible that some heat retention devices or practices in successful clinics are performing more optimally than others. It is also known that display temperatures should not be relied upon and incubators should be measured by an external standard [17]. All traditional disposable plastic dishes do not allow the base of the dish to come into direct contact with the microscope stage, so there is always an air gap. Because air is a poor conductor of heat, this air gap greatly reduces the efficacy of heating stages, allowing the medium in dishes to cool below the temperature at which the heated surface is set.

Humidity

Laboratory relative humidity should be between 35% and 50%. Higher levels will promote growth of molds and fungi. A lower humidity is uncomfortable, and can cause eye irritation, as well as evaporative loss during dish preparation and from cultures. Low humidity increases static electricity, which will affect osmolarity of the culture medium, which may be deleterious to embryos in culture [29; 66].

Hand-Washing Facilities

Hand-washing facilities should typically be located in vestibules rather than in laboratories.

Management of Semen Treatment

Patients should be given clear instructions regarding the collection of the sperm sample (hygiene, sexual abstinence, timing, etc.). The use of spermicidal condoms, creams, or lubricants must be avoided. Semen samples should be collected into sterile containers (tissue-grade, sperm-toxicity tested). The container should be clearly labelled and correct identification should be confirmed by the patient [57]. Results from at least two, but preferably three separate seminal analyses must be obtained before a definitive clinical conclusion can be drawn. The interval between the analyses is arbitrary and is generally recommended to be 1–2 weeks. Both sperm analysis and preparation for fertilization should start within 1 hour of sperm collection. Prolonged sperm exposure to seminal plasma is not recommended. Semen, as all other body fluids, (blood, follicular fluid, etc.) should be treated as potentially contaminated.

Partial thawing of a vial with cryopreserved sperm (shaving) is sometimes applied as a measure to preserve sperm for further use, particularly in cases of very restricted sperm quantity. Experimental analysis of partial thaw revealed significantly reduced motility in sperm samples that were previously partially thawed versus fully thawed [67]. While no differences were observed in the rates of oocyte fertilization, the mean number of top-quality embryos was significantly lower in the shaved group than in the complete sperm thawing group [67]. The process of freezing and thawing, by itself, may detrimentally affect chromatin structure [68], potentially risking the decondensation of the sperm nucleus following ICSI [69]. Repeated cycle of freezing and thawing increases fragmentation of sperm DNA [70].

ID Control

Identification of patients and traceability of their reproductive cells are crucial aspects of ART treatments. Each IVF laboratory must have an effective and accurate system to uniquely identify, trace, and locate reproductive cells during each procedural step. A proper identification system should ensure that the main characteristics of patients (or donors) and their cells, together with relevant data regarding products and materials coming into contact with them, are available at all times. The date and time of each manipulation and identity of all operators and witnesses must be documented throughout the treatment. These records should be kept for the period of time specified by national legislation. All IVF data must be retained for 7 years and any records pertaining to donor gametes must be retained for a minimum of 25 years.

Obviously each specimen of gametes or embryos must be identified by a label. But the "label" is only a tool; the reliability of its use depends on the system within which it is used. It is quite likely that specimens from two different people with the same name coexist in the laboratory. A second person is required to verify the ID check and "witness" the operator performing the process. But "double-witnessing" is also only a tool, not a solution.

There are several electronic witnessing systems created for IVF clinics, with the aim of preventing errors in identification of patients, their gametes, their matching for fertilization process, embryos, and embryo transfer, as well as treatments, such as cryopreservation. These electronic witnessing systems provide a double control system that ensures that all procedures are performed with patient-customized name and barcoded lab-ware and media products [71].

Standard Operational Procedures (SOPs)

SOPs, written in the language commonly understood by the staff of the laboratory, authorized, signed and up-to-date, should be in place for all processes, in order to ensure standardization and uniformity, to optimize outcomes. Standardization in handling of the equipment and ART procedures makes it easier to improve techniques and to test new products. It ensures traceability of all actions performed, renders the processes and procedures more efficient, and improves service quality, which is beneficial for both customers and staff.

SOPs are created to be used in the everyday operation of the laboratory and have a simple description of the method, and include a wide range of management and educational features. The rationale for a particular procedure should always be explained when the procedure is being taught. This is helpful in ensuring that the SOP is respected, and it is also a good way to illustrate how all the processes in the laboratory are interrelated, and how they are each related to physiology. There is no absolute standard for what an SOP must contain or look like. However, the USA National Council for Clinical Laboratory Standards has a set of guidelines on how to prepare SOPs. For medical laboratories, in general, the requirements of the international standards organization (ISO) ISO 15189 standard is the "gold standard" for documenting a laboratory procedure or test. ISO 9000 is a standard for quality management systems, which covers IVF clinics. It is the responsibility of the laboratory director to ensure that the contents of each SOP are complete, current, and have been properly and comprehensively reviewed.

Proper training of the staff is vital and must be provided within an encompassing framework of education. The competency of the staff in different techniques and procedures should be evaluated annually and saved in their personal file.

Quality Management

Quality management is the integration of quality activities, which include QC, quality assurance (QA), and quality improvement of the organization, personnel, equipment and materials, facilities, documentation, and records. This includes defining responsibilities and ensuring that all personnel are qualified and competent, written instructions for each process (SOPs) are in place, proper and periodic equipment maintenance, service, and calibration are performed, specifications conform with requirements, and that risk assessment analysis for all laboratory activities are conducted [57]. There is requirement that a material safety data sheet for each product is available to anyone who comes into contact with it. All relevant data concerning laboratory work must be recorded in a database that allows statistical analysis. Corrections, either written or electronic, should be traceable. Data should include: morphological characteristics of gametes and embryos, detailed information of the procedures, including timing and staff involved, all information needed to comply with the requirements of national and international data registries [57], and participation in Internal Quality Control (IQC) and External Quality Assurance (EQA) programs. A scheme that only reports results in comparison with results from other IVF participating laboratories, with no suggestion as to what the "right answer" was, has limited value. Reference values, even if determined as "consensus" values by averaging the results from a select subgroup of internationally recognized, high-caliber laboratories that participate in the scheme, are essential for quality improvement (EQA).

There are many tools available to support quality and risk management in the IVF laboratory. Inspection is the careful examination of work organization and processes in the IVF laboratory. An audit is a formal examination and verification of an organization's systems or records and supporting documents by a properly qualified professional. An audit system, both internal and external, must be in place. An independent, competent auditor should verify compliance of all procedures with SOPs and requirements. QA provides adequate confidence that a product or service is satisfy in its required quality characteristics and signifies the standards and processes in laboratory practice. Continuous improvement through observation, assessment of procedures, and corrective action after testing and monitoring laboratory equipment (QC) have led to improved culture conditions and increased IVF success, moving clinical embryology from being simply observational and subjective to becoming an objective clinical science [10]. In addition, based on the knowledge of the basic biology and other related scientific disciplines, the embryologist must effectively employ tools and techniques for systems analysis, problem solving, technology development, and quality improvement. Without adequate knowledge of such tools and techniques, the speed of change, and hence, daily quality management implementation, would be slowed.

Daily or periodic examination of all instruments is recommended. Among these instruments are incubators, warming blocks, tube holders, air velocity and pressure gauges, centrifuges, laminar flow hoods, refrigerators, freezers, cryogenic Dewar containers, particle counters, pH sensors, temperature sensors, oxygen sensors, safety systems, monitoring equipment, and VOC sensors.

The laboratory environment must be clean. At all times, there is a release of particles that contaminate all items stored within the benches. Improved laboratory construction methods using clean-room technology are slowly becoming commonplace, with many solutions for maintaining a clean air environment [72]. After a day's work, the surface area must be cleaned, with approved cleaning detergents and following the prescribed cleaning routines.

The following morning and before any handling of gametes or embryos, a routine control of the functionality of the equipment, either via a wireless system or via manual documentation, should be performed.

Equipment must undergo a thorough cleaning. All parts are pre-washed with water for injection, to remove potential contaminants, followed by disinfection by approved ART products, e.g., Oosafe. Avoid 70% ethanol, since it only reduces and fixes, but does not eliminate the contaminants. Hydrogen peroxide should be used with caution, because its might damage the metal parts of the equipment over time. The daily cleaning routines are preferably performed at the end of the day (usually in three steps [water, Oosafe, and water]), so as to avoid cleaning in the morning, with the release of potential toxins from the detergents. Any spillage in between patients should be immediately cleaned with a dry tissue or tissue wetted with water for injection only. A more thorough cleaning is only necessary when no oocytes or embryos are to be evaluated or manipulated.

To avoid contaminations, all culture media handling is performed with powder-free, sterile gloves without chemical additives, accelerants, or emulsifiers.

The dress code must be followed in all aspects and the staff must understand why jewelry, mobile phones, long nails, nail polish, and scented products (cologne, perfume, deodorant, hairspray, body wash or powder, after shave, etc.) cannot be used.

Photocopiers and printers should not be used within the ART suite, as they emit unwanted chemicals, such as solvents and particulate-containing toner dust [73].

It is important to make sure that there are sufficient electrical outlets so all electric equipment is inserted directly into the outlets without any extension cords. All outlets should be fitted so they reside within the wall, which prevents the collection of dust that potentially, over time, could contribute to contaminations within the laboratory.

All services and repairs for each piece of equipment should be registered. Each piece of equipment should be assigned a specific chronological identity and bar code, which is used to register all parameters (QC), services, yearly recertifications, reasons for malfunctioning, and repairs. The heated surface temperature and the heated light source should be calibrated within the most frequently used culture dish, at a specific fan speed, with a surface temperature probe. The surface for the work with oocytes and embryos, and light source temperature should be around 36.5°C, which also causes less damage to the most sensitive status of the oocyte – the meiotic spindle.

Laboratory Safety

The IVF laboratory must have adequate functionalities to minimize any potential damage to reproductive cells, and to ensure good laboratory practice. Attention should be given to operator comfort, to provide a safe working environment that minimizes the risk of distraction and fatigue and thereby making a mistake. Distractions should be minimized, to foster the high degree of attention needed during laboratory work.

Risk reduction and minimization are used in risk management to describe the application of appropriate techniques to reduce the likelihood of an adverse event and its consequences. In the IVF laboratory, risk minimization is strictly practiced in the cryotanks and incubators; usage of LN_2 and gas levels are monitored on a regular basis and tanks are connected to low-level alarms in case of tank/incubator failure, especially outside normal working hours.

Staffing

Personnel are one of the most important elements of an IVF laboratory. For a team to function well there must be mutual trust, respect, and cooperation [9].

The number of laboratory staff should reflect the number of cycles performed per year. Clinics that perform up to 150 retrievals and/or cryopreservation cycles per year should have a minimum of two qualified clinical embryologists [57; 74]. This initial number will increase with both the number of treatments, and the complexity of the procedures, techniques, and tasks undertaken within the laboratory. Other duties, such as administration, training, education, quality management and communication, also require additional staff. The hierarchical laboratory organization will depend on the staff size and can include responsibilities at different levels, e.g., supervisors, clinical embryologists, laboratory technicians, and administrative personnel.

References

1. Pal L, Kidwai N, Kayani J, Grant WB. Donor egg IVF model to assess ecological implications for ART success. *J. Assist. Reprod. Genet.* 2014; **31**:1453–1460.

2. Johansson L. Establishment of an ART clinic: location, construction and design. In: Varghese A, Sjoblom P, Jayaprakasan K, eds., *A Practical Guide to Setting Up an IVF Lab, Embryo Culture Systems and Running the Unit.* New Delhi: Jaypee Brothers Medical Publishers (P) Ltd; 2013; 24–30.

3. Nijs M, Franssen K, Cox A, et al. Reprotoxicity of intrauterine insemination and in vitro fertilization-embryo transfer disposables and products: a 4-year survey. *Fertil. Steril.* 2009; **92**:527–535.

4. Gardner DK, Lane M. Culture systems for the human embryo. In: Gardner D, Weismann A, Howles CM, Shoham Z, eds., *Textbook of Assisted Reproductive Techniques: Laboratory and Clinical Perspectives.* Boca Raton: CRC Press 2017; 200–224.

5. Ottesen LD, Hindkjaer J, Ingerslev J. Light exposure of the ovum and pre-implantation embryo during ART procedures. *J. Assist. Reprod. Genet.* 2007; **24**:99–103.

6. Hua VK, Cooke S. Volatile organic compounds within the IVF laboratory. FSA Australia 2013.

7. Lierman S, De Sutter P, Dhont M, Van der Elst J. Double-quality control reveals high-level toxicity in gloves used for operator protection in assisted reproductive technology. *Fertil. Steril.* 2007; **88**:1266–1267.

8. Brais N. Air disinfection for ART clinics using ultraviolet germicidal irradiation. In: Esteves SC, Varghese AC, Worrilow KC, eds., *Clean Room Technology in ART Clinics: A Practical Guide.* Boca Raton: CRC Press. 2017; 119–132.

9. Mortimer D, Mortimer ST. *Quality and Risk Management in the IVF Laboratory.* Cambridge: Cambridge University Press. 2005.

10. Palmer GA, Kratka C, Szvetecz S, et al. Comparison of 36 assisted reproduction laboratories monitoring environmental conditions and instrument parameters using the same quality-control application. *RBM Online* 2019; **39**:63–74.

11. Mortimer D, Cohen J, Mortimer ST, et al. Cairo consensus on the IVF laboratory environment and air quality: report of an expert meeting. *RBM Online* 2018; **36**:658–674.

12. Esteves SC, Bento FC. Implementation of air quality control in reproductive laboratories in full compliance with the Brazilian Cells and Germinative Tissue Directive. *RBM Online* 2013; **26**:9–21.

13. Munch EM, Sparks AE, Duran HE, Van Voorhis BJ. Lack of carbon air filtration impacts early embryo development. *J. Assist. Reprod. Genet.* 2015; **32**:1009–1017.

14. Heitmann RJ, Hill MJ, James AN, et al. Live births achieved via IVF are increased by improvements in air quality and laboratory environment. *RBM Online* 2015; **31**:364–371.

15. Khoudja RY, Xu Y, Li T, Zhou C. Better IVF outcomes following improvements in laboratory air quality. *J. Assist. Reprod. Genet.* 2013; **30**:69–76.

16. Boone WR, Johnson JE, Locke A-J, Crane MM, Price TM. Control of air quality in an assisted reproductive technology laboratory. *Fertil. Steril.* 1999; **71**:150–154.

17. Swain JE. Decisions for the IVF laboratory: comparative analysis of embryo culture incubators. *RBM Online* 2014; **28**:535–547.

18. Sciorio R, Smith GD. Embryo culture at a reduced oxygen concentration of 5%: a mini review. *Zygote* 2019; **23**:1–7.

19. Edwards RG, Steptoe PC, Purdy JM. Fertilization and cleavage in vitro of preovulator human oocytes. *Nature* 1970; **227**:1307–1309.

20. Hoff A, Khabani A, Khabani C, Hickok L, Marshall L. Reduced oxygen tension helps increase the quality of blastocyst available on D5. *Fertil. Steril.* 2008; **90**:S350.

21. Meintjes M, Chantilis SJ, Douglas JD, et al. A controlled randomized trial evaluating the effect of lowered incubator oxygen tension on live births in a predominantly blastocyst transfer program. *Hum. Reprod.* 2009; **24**:300–307.

22. Nastry CO, Nóbrega BN, Teixeira DM, et al. Low versus atmospheric oxygen tension for embryo culture in assisted reproduction: a systematic review and meta-analysis. *Fertil. Steril.* 2016; **106**:95–104.

23. Mori C, Kuwayama M, Silber S, Kagawa N, Kato H. Water evaporation and osmolality change of human embryo culture media in humid or in dry culture systems. *Fertil. Steril.* 2010; **94**:S151.

24. Fawzy M, Abdel Rahman MY, Zidan MH, et al. Humid versus dry incubator: a prospective, randomized, controlled trial. *Fertil. Steril.* 2017; **108**:277–283.

25. Del Gallego R, Albert C, Marcos J, et al. Humid vs. dry embryo culture conditions on embryo development: a continuous embryo monitoring assessment. *Fertil. Steril.* 2018; **110**:e362.

26. Holmes R, Swain J. Humidification of a dry benchtop IVF incubator: impact on culture media parameters. *Fertil. Steril.* 2018; **110**:e52.

27. Carpenter G, Hammond E, Peek J, Morbeck D. The impact of dry incubation on osmolality of media in time lapse culture dishes. *Hum. Reprod.* 2018; **33**:i61.

28. Swain J. Different mineral oils used for embryo culture microdrop overlay differentially impact media evaporation. *Fertil. Steril.* 2018; **109**:e53.

29. Swain J. Controversies in ART: considerations and risks for uninterrupted embryo culture. *RBM Online* 2019; **39**:19–26.

30. Calhaz-Jorge C, de Geyter C, Kupka MS, et al. Assisted reproductive technology in Europe, 2012: results generated from European registers by ESHRE. *Hum. Reprod.* 2016; **31**:1638–1652.

31. Edwards RG, Purdy JM, Steptoe PC, Walters DE. The growth of human preimplantation embryos in vitro. *Am. J. Obstet. Gynecol.* 1981; **141**:408–416.

32. Wright G, Wiker S, Elsner C, et al. Observations on the morphology of pronuclei and nucleoli in human zygotes and implications for cryopreservation. *Hum. Reprod.* 1990; **5**:109–115.

33. Alikani M, Calderon G, Tomkin G, et al. Cleavage anomalies in early human embryos and survival after prolonged culture in vitro. *Hum. Reprod.* 2000; **15**:2634–2643.

34. Plachot M, Mandelbaum J. Oocyte maturation, fertilization and embryonic growth in vitro. *Br. Med. Bull.* 1990; **46**:675–694.

35. Gardner DK, Lane M, Stevens J, Schlenker T, Schoolcraft WB. Blastocyst score affects implantation and pregnancy outcome: towards single blastocyst transfer. *Fertil. Steril.* 2000; **73**:1155–1158.

36. Meseguer M, Herrero J, Tejera A, et al. The use of morphokinetics as a predictor of embryo implantation. *Hum. Reprod.* 2011; **26**:2658–2671.

37. Ciray HN, Campbell A, Agerholm IE, et al. Proposed guidelines on the nomenclature and annotation of dynamic human embryo monitoring by a time-lapse user group. *Hum. Reprod.* 2014; **29**:2650–2660.

38. Meseguer M, Rubio I, Cruz M, et al. Embryo incubation and selection in a time-lapse monitoring system improves pregnancy outcome compared with a standard incubator: a retrospective cohort study. *Fertil. Steril.* 2012; **98**:1481–1489.

39. Rubio I, Galan A, Larreategui Z, et al. Clinical validation of embryo culture and selection by morphokinetic analysis: a randomized, controlled trial of the EmbryoScope. *Fertil. Steril.* 2014; **102**:1287–1294.

40. Azzarello A, Hoest T, Mikkelsen AL. The impact of pronuclei morphology and dynamicity on live birth outcome after time-lapse culture. *Hum. Reprod.* 2012; **27**:2649–2657.

41. Wong CC, Loewke KE, Bossert NL, et al. Non-invasive imaging of human embryos before embryonic genome activation predicts development to the blastocyst stage. *Nat. Biotechnol.* 2010; **28**:1115–1121.

42. Desai N, Goldberg JM, Austin C, Falcone T. Are cleavage anomalies, multinucleation, or specific cell cycle kinetics observed with time-lapse imaging predictive of embryo developmental capacity or ploidy? *Fertil. Steril.* 2018; **109**:665–674.

43. Liu Y, Chapple V, Roberts P, Ali J, Matson P. Time-lapse videography of human oocytes following intracytoplasmic sperm injection: events up to the first cleavage division. *Reprod. Biol.* 2014; **14**:249–256.

44. Cruz M, Garrido N, Herrero J, et al. Timing of cell division in human cleavage-stage embryos is linked with blastocyst formation and quality. *RBM Online* 2012; **25**:371–381.

45. Kirkegaard K, Agerholm IE, Ingerslev HJ. Time-lapse monitoring as a tool for clinical embryo assessment. *Hum. Reprod.* 2012; **27**:1277–1285.

46. Conaghan J, Chen AA, Willman SP, et al. Improving embryo selection using a computer-automated time-lapse image analysis test plus day 3 morphology: results from a prospective multicenter trial. *Fertil. Steril.* 2013; **100**:412–419.

47. Davies S, Christopikou D, Tsorva E, et al. Delayed cleavage division and a prolonged transition between 2- and 4-cell stages in embryos identified as aneuploidy at the 8-cell stage by array-CGH. *Hum. Reprod.* 2012; **27**:ii84–ii86.

48. Campbell A, Fishel S, Bowman N, et al. Modelling a risk classification of aneuploidy in human embryos using non-invasive morphokinetics. *RBM Online* 2013; **26**:477–485.

49. Reignier A, Lammers J, Barriere P, Freour T. Can time-lapse parameters predict embryo ploidy? A systematic review. *RBM Online* 2018; **36**:380–387.

50. Wong KM, Repping S, Mastenbroek S. Limitations of embryo selection methods. *Semin. Reprod. Med.* 2014; **32**:127–133.

51. Armstrong S, Arroll N, Cree LM, Jordan V, Farquhar C. Time-lapse systems for embryo

incubation and assessment in assisted reproduction. *Cochrane Database Syst. Rev.* 2015; **2**:CD011320. doi:10.1002/14651858.CD011320.pub2.

52. Racowsky C, Kovacs P, Martins WP. A critical appraisal of time-lapse imaging for embryo selection: where are we and where do we need to go? *J. Assist. Reprod. Genet.* 2015; **32**:1025–1030.

53. Armstrong S, Bhide P, Jordan V, et al. Timelapse systems for embryo incubation and assessment in assisted reproduction. *Cochrane Database Syst. Rev.* 2019; **29**:CD011320. doi:10.1002/14651858.CD011320.pub4.

54. Pribenszky C, Nilselid A-M, Montag M. Time-lapse culture with morphokinetic embryo selection improves pregnancy and live birth chances and reduces early pregnancy loss: a meta-analysis. *RBM Online* 2017; **35**:511–520.

55. Mascarenhas M, Fox SJ, Thompson K, Balen AH. Cumulative live birth rates and perinatal outcomes with the use of time-lapse imaging incubators for embryo culture: a retrospective cohort study of 1882 ART cycles. *BJOG* 2018; **126**:280–286.

56. Ferrick L, Lee YSL, Gardner DK. Reducing time to pregnancy and facilitating the birth of healthy children through functional analysis of embryo physiology. *Biol. Reprod.* 2019; **101**:1124–1139. doi:10.1093/biolre/ioz005.

57. European Society of Human Reproduction and Embryology. *Revised guidelines for good practice in IVF laboratories (2015)*. Grimbergen: ESHRE. 2015.

58. Mehta JG, Varghese AC. Gases for embryo culture and volatile organic compounds in incubators. In: Esteves SC, Varghese AC, Worrilow KC, eds., *Clean Room Technology in ART Clinics: A Practical Guide*. Boca Raton: CRC Press. 2017; 99–118.

59. Hunter SK, Scott JR, Hull D, Urry RL. The gamete and embryo compatibility of various synthetic polymers. *Fertil. Steril.* 1988; **50**:110–116.

60. Blake DA, Forsberg AS, Hillensjö T, Wikland M. The practicalities of sequential blastocyst culture. In: *ART, Science and Fiction*, the second international Alpha Congress, Copenhagen (Denmark). 1999; Abstract O28.

61. Kupferschmied HU, Kihm U, Bachman P, Muller KH, Ackerman M. Transmission of IBR/IPV virus in bovine semen: a case report. *Theriogenology* 1986; **25**:439–443.

62. Bielanski A, Bergeron H, Lau PC, Devenish J. Microbial contamination of embryos and semen during long term banking in liquid nitrogen. *Cryobiology* 2003; **46**:146–152.

63. Gilligan AV. Establishing the IVF laboratory: a systems view. In: Carrell DT, Peterson CM, eds., *Reproductive Endocrinology and Infertility: Integrating Modern Clinical and Laboratory Practice*. New York: Springer. 2010; 569–578.

64. Ottosen LDM, Hindkjaer J, Ingerslev J. Light exposure of the ovum and preimplantation embryo during ART procedures. *J. Assist. Reprod. Genet.* 2007; **24**:99–103.

65. Ng KYB, Mingels R, Morgan H, Macklon N, Cheong Y. In vivo oxygen, temperature and pH dynamics in the female reproductive tract and their importance in human conception: a systematic review. *Hum. Reprod. Update* 2018; **24**:15–34.

66. Swain JE, Cabrera L, Xu X, Smith GD. Microdrop preparation factors influence culture-media osmolality, which can impair mouse embryo preimplantation development. *RBM Online* 2012; **24**:142–147.

67. Baum M, Orvieto R, Kon S, et al. Comparison of effects of thawing entire donor sperm vial vs. partial thawing (shaving) on sperm quality. *J. Assist. Reprod. Genet.* 2018; **35**:645–648.

68. Royere D, Hamamah S, Nicolle JC, Lansac J. Chromatin alterations induced by freeze-thawing influence the fertilizing ability of human sperm. *Int. J. Androl.* 1991; **14**:328–332.

69. Sakkas D, Urner F, Bianchi PG, et al. Sperm chromatin anomalies can influence decondensation after intracytoplasmic sperm injection. *Hum. Reprod.* 1996; **11**:837–843.

70. Vutyavanich T, Lattiwongsakorn W, Piromlertamorn W, Samchimchom S. Repeated vitrification/warming of human sperm gives better results than repeated slow programmable freezing. *Asian J. Androl.* 2012; **14**:850–854.

71. Forte M, Faustini F, Maggiulli R, et al. Electronic witness system in IVF—patients perspective. *J. Assist. Reprod. Genet.* 2016; **33**:1215–1222.

72. Varghese AC, Palmer GA. Clean room technology for low resource IVF units. In: Esteves SC, Varghese AC, Worrilow KC, eds., *Clean Room Technology in ART Clinics: A Practical Guide*. Boca Raton: CRC Press. 2017; 347–354.

73. Barrese E, Gioffrè A, Scarpelli M, et al. Indoor pollution in work office: VOCs, formaldehyde and ozone by printer. *Occup. Dis. Environ. Med.* 2014; **2**:49–55.

74. ESHRE Special Interest Group of Embryology and Alpha Scientists in Reproductive Medicine. The Vienna consensus: report of an expert meeting on the development of ART laboratory performance indicators. *RBM Online* 2017; **35**:494–510.

Index

239